Pharmaco-Genomics Handbook

Larisa M. Humma, PharmD, BCPS
Vicki L. Ellingrod, PharmD, BCPP
Jill M. Kolesar, PharmD, FCCP, BCPS

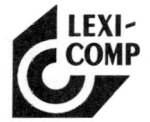

LEXI-COMP

LEXI-COMP'S

Pharmaco-Genomics Handbook

Larisa M. Humma, PharmD, BCPS
Assistant Professor, Section of Cardiology
University of Illinois at Chicago
Chicago, IL

Vicki L. Ellingrod, PharmD, BCPP
Assistant Professor
University of Iowa
Iowa City, IA

Jill M. Kolesar, PharmD, FCCP, BCPS
Associate Professor of Pharmacy
University of Wisconsin
Madison, WI

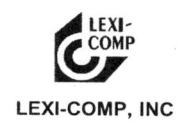

LEXI-COMP, INC

NOTICE

This handbook is intended to serve as a useful reference and not as a complete resource. The explosion of information in many directions, in multiple scientific disciplines, with advances in techniques, and continuing evolution of knowledge requires constant scholarship. The authors, editors, reviewers, contributors, and publishers cannot be responsible for the continued currency of the information or for any errors or omissions in this manual or for any consequences arising therefrom. Because of the dynamic nature of medicine as a discipline, readers are advised that decisions regarding diagnosis and treatment must be based on the independent judgment of the clinician. The editors are not responsible for any inaccuracy of quotation or for any false or misleading implication that may arise due to the text.

The editors, authors, and contributors have written this book in their private capacities. No official support or endorsement by any federal or state agency or pharmaceutical company is intended or inferred.

The publishers have made every effort to trace the copyright holders for borrowed material. If they have inadvertently overlooked any, they will be pleased to make the necessary arrangements at the first opportunity.

If you have any suggestions or questions regarding any information presented in this handbook, please contact our drug information pharmacist at (330) 650-6506.

Copyright © 2003 by Lexi-Comp, Inc. All rights reserved.

Printed in the United States of America. No part of this publication may be reproduced, stored in a retrieval system, or transmitted, in any form or by any means, electronic, mechanical, photocopying, recording, or otherwise, without the prior written permission of the publisher.

This manual was produced using the FormuLex™ Program — a complete publishing service of Lexi-Comp, Inc.

ACKNOWLEDGMENTS

Lexi-Comp's Pharmacogenomics Handbook exists in its present form as the result of the concerted efforts of the following individuals: Robert D. Kerscher, publisher and president of Lexi-Comp, Inc; Lynn D. Coppinger, managing editor; David C. Marcus, director of information systems; Libby Young, product manager; Leslie J. Ruggles, pharmacology database manager; and Tracey J. Reinecke, cover design.

In addition, the authors wish to thank their families, friends, and colleagues who supported them in their efforts to complete this handbook.

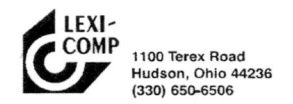

LEXI-COMP
1100 Terex Road
Hudson, Ohio 44236
(330) 650-6506

ISBN 1-59195-060-0

TABLE OF CONTENTS

About the Authors ... 2

Contributing Authors ... 4

Preface ... 5

Description of Sections and Fields in This Handbook ... 6

FDA Name Differentiation Project -
    The Use of Tall-Man Letters ... 8

Definitions / Glossary ... 10

Introduction to Pharmacogenomics ... 12

Introduction to Genetics ... 15

Cytochrome P450 Nomenclature ... 22

Cytochrome P450 Enzymes: Substrates, Inhibitors, and
    Inducers ... 23

ALPHABETICAL LISTING OF DRUGS ... 43

ALPHABETICAL LISTING OF POTENTIAL POLYMORPHISMS ... 159

**INDEX OF POLYMORPHISMS AND DRUGS
    POTENTIALLY AFFECTED** ... 225

ALPHABETICAL INDEX ... 247

INTRODUCTION

ABOUT THE AUTHORS

Larisa M. Humma, PharmD, BCPS

Dr. Humma received her Bachelor of Science in Pharmacy and Doctor of Pharmacy degrees from the University of Georgia, College of Pharmacy. She then completed a one-year pharmacy practice residency with an emphasis in cardiology at the VA Medical Center in Memphis. Dr. Humma subsequently completed a two-year fellowship in cardiovascular pharmacogenomics at the University of Florida, where she was awarded the 1999-2000 American Foundation for Pharmaceutical Education Clinical Pharmacy Post-PharmD Fellowship in the Biomedical Research Sciences. Dr. Humma is presently an Assistant Professor of Pharmacy Practice at the University of Illinois at Chicago and a clinical pharmacist at the University of Illinois Medical Center. Dr. Humma is a Board-Certified Pharmacotherapy Specialist (BCPS) and taught the cardiology and critical care sections of the American College of Clinical Pharmacy-Sponsored Pharmacotherapy Preparatory Course from 2001-2003.

In her current position, Dr. Humma teaches in the cardiovascular section and is actively involved in clinical and basic science research focusing on ethnic and genetic contributions to cardiovascular drug therapy response. She also participates in the student experiential program, serves on several departmental and college committees, serves as a Senator for the College of Pharmacy, and remains actively involved in the care of patients on the cardiology service. Dr. Humma has authored several original research and review articles and has given a number of presentations on the subject of pharmacogenomics at both the state and national levels. She also authored the Pharmacogenetics chapter in the 5th edition of the textbook *Pharmacotherapy: A Pathophysiologic Approach*, DiPiro JT, et al, eds. Dr. Humma is currently a reviewer for the *Annals of Pharmacotherapy* and the 5th edition of the *Pharmacotherapy Self-Assessment Program (PSAP)*.

Dr. Humma is an active member of the American College of Clinical Pharmacy (ACCP), where she serves on the program committee, the Heart Failure Society of America (HFSA), and American Association of Colleges of Pharmacy (AACP).

Vicki L. Ellingrod, PharmD, BCPP

Vicki L. Ellingrod received her bachelor's degree and Doctor of Pharmacy degree from the University of Minnesota. She completed a two-year fellowship in psychopharmacology and pharmacogenetics at the University of Iowa. After completion of her fellowship, Dr. Ellingrod became an Assistant Professor at the University of Iowa and is currently the Director of the Pharmacogenetics Laboratory at the University of Iowa College of Pharmacy. Her research interests include the genetics behind the metabolism of psychiatric medications, as well as the pharmacogenetics of the adverse drug reactions seen with antipsychotics. Currently, her research is primarily funded by the National Institutes of Mental Health through a career development award entitled "The Genetics of Antipsychotic Metabolism." In addition to her research in schizophrenia, Dr. Ellingrod is also actively involved in studies involving antipsychotic use in dementia, as well as serving as a co-investigator on several other projects involving pharmacogenetics and drug metabolism. Dr. Ellingrod has authored numerous journal articles and lectures locally, as well as nationally, on pharmacogenomics in psychiatry.

In her capacity as director of the Pharmacogenetics Laboratory, Dr. Ellingrod is also involved in patient care and is board certified in psychiatric pharmacy. She serves as a reviewer for many psychiatric publications including the *American Journal of Psychiatry*, the *American Journal of Geriatric Psychiatry*, *PharmacoGenomics*, and *Journal of the American Geriatrics Society*. She is actively involved in many pharmacy organizations including the American College of Clinical Pharmacy and the College of Psychiatric and Neurologic Pharmacists. Recently, Dr. Ellingrod was awarded the "Young Investigator Award" by the American College of Clinical Pharmacy for her work in pharmacogenomics.

Jill M. Kolesar, PharmD, FCCP, BCPS

Jill M. Kolesar, Pharm D, FCCP, BCPS, received a Doctor of Pharmacy and completed a specialty practice residency in oncology/hematology and a two-year fellowship in molecular oncology pharmacotherapy at the University of Texas Health Science Center in San Antonio, Texas. She is currently an Associate Professor of Pharmacy at the University of Wisconsin School of Pharmacy and the Director of the Analytical Laboratory and Pharmacogenetics Facility at the University of Wisconsin Comprehensive Cancer Center.

Dr. Kolesar practices in the Hematology and Oncology Clinics at the William S. Middleton VA Hospital in Madison, Wisconsin, managing the pharmacotherapy of ambulatory patients. Her research in pharmacogenomics includes the use of molecular markers to predict response and monitor efficacy of cancer chemotherapy, population genotyping for cancer susceptibility, and the regulation of gene expression of the two electron reductases. She has authored more than 100 abstracts, research articles, and book chapters, and as a principal investigator, she has received more than $350,000 in research funding from the NCI, ACS, and other sources. In addition, she holds two U.S. patents for novel assay methodologies for gene expression and mutation analysis. She has received several research awards from local, national, and international pharmacy organizations and a Merit Award from the American Society of Clinical Oncology (ASCO). Most recently, she received the "Innovations in Teaching Award" from the American Association of Colleges of Pharmacy.

INTRODUCTION

CONTRIBUTING AUTHORS

Mark F. Bonfiglio, BS, PharmD, RPh

Dr. Bonfiglio received his BA in Biology and BS in Pharmacy from the University of Toledo. He earned his Doctor of Pharmacy degree from Ohio State University and subsequently completed a residency in Critical Care Pharmacy at the Ohio State University Hospitals. For the next 8 years, he served on the faculty of the Ohio Northern University College of Pharmacy, maintaining clinical practices in Critical Care and Internal Medicine. Currently, Dr. Bonfiglio is the Director of the Medical Science Division at Lexi-Comp, Inc. He is also an instructor in the Department of Biological Sciences, Kent State University, as well as the College of Nursing, Malone College. Professional memberships include the American Association for the Advancement of Science (AAAS), American College of Clinical Pharmacy (ACCP), American Pharmacists Association (APhA), American Society of Health System Pharmacists (ASHP), and Society for Critical Care Medicine (SCCM).

Matthew A. Fuller, PharmD, BCPS, BCPP, FASHP

Dr. Fuller received his BS in Pharmacy from Ohio Northern University and then earned a Doctor of Pharmacy degree from the University of Cincinnati. A residency in hospital pharmacy was completed at Bethesda Hospital in Zanesville, Ohio. After completion of his training, Dr. Fuller accepted a position at the Veterans Affairs Medical Center in Cleveland, Ohio. Dr. Fuller has over 15 years of experience in psychiatric psychopharmacology in a variety of clinical settings including acute care and ambulatory care. Dr. Fuller is currently a Clinical Pharmacy Specialist in Psychiatry at the Veterans Affairs Medical Center in Cleveland, Ohio. He is also an Associate Clinical Professor of Psychiatry and Clinical Instructor of Psychology at Case Western Reserve University in Cleveland, Ohio and Adjunct Associate Professor of Clinical Pharmacy at the University of Toledo in Toledo, Ohio. He is also the Director of the ASHP accredited Psychopharmacy Residency Program. He has received several awards including the Upjohn Excellence in Research Award and the OSHP Hospital Pharmacist of the Year Award in 1994. In 1996, he received the CSHP Evelyn Gray Scott Award (Pharmacist of the Year). In 2001, he received the OSHP Pharmacy Practice Research Award. Dr. Fuller is Board Certified by the Board of Pharmaceutical Specialties in both Pharmacotherapy and Psychopharmacy. Dr. Fuller is a member of numerous professional organizations, including the American Society of Health-System Pharmacists (ASHP), Ohio Society of Health-System Pharmacists (OSHP), American College of Clinical Pharmacy (ACCP), Ohio College of Clinical Pharmacy, and the Cleveland Society of Health-System Pharmacists (CSHP). He is a member of the National Alliance for the Mentally Ill (NAMI) and also serves as a reviewer for pharmacy and psychiatric journals.

PREFACE

The potential for successful drug therapy outcomes may be enhanced by tailoring dosage to the unique requirements of the individual. For many years, the application of pharmacokinetic principles, coupled with information concerning major organ function, has facilitated the design of dosing regimens to achieve desired serum drug concentrations. However, many of the pharmacokinetic and pharmacodynamic factors responsible for drug response are not addressed by these efforts. The potential to adjust drug selection and/or regimen design to address individual variation in the rate of and/or capacity for drug metabolism, sensitivity to untoward effects, or response at a given serum concentration has been limited.

Recognition of patient factors, such as acetylator status and glucose-6-phosphate dehydrogenase deficiency, provided early evidence of genetic traits which could explain adverse reactions which would otherwise be characterized as "idiosyncratic." Advancing molecular biology techniques, as well as the recent completion of the Human Genome Project, have provided a wealth of information concerning genetic variability. Many of these variations are being examined as predisposing factors for disease, as well as their influence on drug response.

A number of significant advances in our understanding of genetic influences on drug therapy has been made in recent years. As differences in the genes which encode cellular processes are explored, it is hoped that the ability to tailor dosing regimens to individual characteristics will be dramatically expanded.

This book presents information concerning key genetic variations that appear to influence drug disposition and/or sensitivity. Because of the rapidly-changing nature of this field, no static effort to encapsulate the literature will ever be sufficient. However, we believe it is reasonable to provide a snapshot of current knowledge, and attempt to equip the reader with a fundamental understanding of genomic issues. In the process, we hope to establish a paradigm for the incorporation of new information as it unfolds. We look forward to participating in the collection and dissemination of information as we enter the genomic age.

INTRODUCTION

DESCRIPTION OF SECTIONS AND FIELDS IN THIS HANDBOOK

Lexi-Comp's Pharmacogenomics Handbook is divided into five sections.

Section I is a compilation of introductory text pertinent to the use of this book.

Section II is the drug information section of the handbook, and provides a comprehensive listing of selected and pertinent drug monographs.

Information is presented in a consistent format and provides the following:

Generic Name	U.S. adopted name
Pronunciation	Phonetic pronunciation
Polymorphisms of Interest	Listing and cross-reference to the polymorphism affected by the drug
U.S. Brand Names	Trade names found in the United States
Canadian Brand Names	Trade names found in Canada (if different from the U.S.)
Synonyms	Other names or accepted abbreviations for the generic drug
Pharmacologic Class	Unique systematic classification of medications

Section III is the alphabetical listing of potential polymorphisms, and provides a comprehensive listing of polymorphism monographs.

Information is presented in a consistent format and provides the following:

Name	
Synonyms	Other names or accepted abbreviations
Chromosome Location	Nomenclature which identifies the location on the human chromosome
Clinically-Important Polymorphisms	Known gene variance with clinical implications
Discussion	Description of the normal gene function and studies related to effect on individual drugs
May Alter Pharmacokinetics of	Lists drugs for which kinetics may be affected
May Alter Pharmacodynamics of	Lists drugs for which dynamics may be affected

INTRODUCTION

May Affect Disease Predisposition of	Comments on the influence of gene polymorphism on disease risk.
Laboratory Evaluation	Comments on laboratory testing when known.
Clinical Recommendations	Summary of significance in current clinical practice.
Counseling Points	Information for individuals who carry a polymorphism.
References	

Section IV is an alphabetical index of Polymorphisms and Drugs Potentially Affected.

Section V is an alphabetical listing of all polymorphism names, drug names, synonyms, U.S. brand names, and Canadian brand names found in this handbook.

INTRODUCTION

FDA NAME DIFFERENTIATION PROJECT – THE USE OF TALL-MAN LETTERS

Confusion between similar drug names is an important cause of medication errors. For years, The Institute For Safe Medication Practices (ISMP), has urged generic manufacturers to use a combination of large and small letters as well as bolding (ie, chlorpro**MAZINE** and chlorpro**PAMIDE**) to help distinguish drugs with look-alike names, especially when they share similar strengths. Recently, the FDA's Division of Generic Drugs began to issue recommendation letters to manufacturers suggesting this novel way to label their products to help reduce this drug name confusion. Although this project has had marginal success, the method has successfully eliminated problems with products such as diphenhydr**AMINE** and dimenhy**DRINATE**. Hospitals should also follow suit by making similar changes in their own labels, preprinted order forms, computer screens and printouts, and drug storage location labels.

Lexi-Comp uses the "Tall-Man" letters for the drugs suggested by the FDA.

The following is a list of product names and recommended FDA revisions.

Drug Product	Recommended Revision
acetazolamide	aceta**ZOLAMIDE**
acetohexamide	aceto**HEXAMIDE**
bupropion	bu**PROP**ion
buspirone	bus**PIR**one
chlorpromazine	chlorpro**MAZINE**
chlorpropamide	chlorpro**PAMIDE**
clomiphene	clomi**PHENE**
clomipramine	clomi**PRAMINE**
cycloserine	cyclo**SERINE**
cyclosporine	cyclo**SPORINE**
daunorubicin	**DAUNO**rubicin
dimenhydrinate	dimenhy**DRINATE**
diphenhydramine	diphenhydr**AMINE**
dobutamine	**DOBUT**amine
dopamine	**DOP**amine
doxorubicin	**DOXO**rubicin
glipizide	glipi**ZIDE**
glyburide	gly**BURIDE**
hydralazine	hydr**ALAZINE**

INTRODUCTION

hydroxyzine	hydr**OXY**zine
medroxyprogesterone	medroxy**PROGESTER**one
methylprednisolone	methyl**PREDNIS**olone
methyltestosterone	methyl**TESTOSTER**one
nicardipine	ni**CAR**dipine
nifedipine	**NIFE**dipine
prednisolone	predniso**LONE**
prednisone	predni**SONE**
sulfadiazine	sulfa**DIAZINE**
sulfisoxazole	sulfi**SOXAZOLE**
tolazamide	**TOLAZ**amide
tolbutamide	**TOLBUT**amide
vinblastine	vin**BLAS**tine
vincristine	vin**CRIS**tine

Institute for Safe Medication Practices. "New Tall-Man Lettering Will Reduce Mix-Ups Due to Generic Drug Name Confusion," *ISMP Medication Safety Alert*, September 19, 2001. Available at: http://www.ismp.org.

Institute for Safe Medication Practices. "Prescription Mapping, Can Improve Efficiency While Minimizing Errors With Look-Alike Products," *ISMP Medication Safety Alert*, October 6, 1999. Available at: http://www.ismp.org.

U.S. Pharmacopeia, "USP Quality Review: Use Caution-Avoid Confusion," March 2001, No. 76. Available at: http://www.usp.org.

INTRODUCTION

DEFINITIONS / GLOSSARY

Allele: Single copy of a gene (in most cases, everybody has 2 alleles for a given gene). Genes may be polyallelic. For example, the genes for blood type (A, B, and O) are triallelic.

Deletion: Loss of a section of DNA from a gene.

DNA sequencing: Molecular biology technique used to determine the identity and exact pattern of nucleotides in a segment of DNA.

Electrophoresis: Involves the process of separating molecules based on their size and electrical charge, based on passing an electrical current through a gel or similar material with a known pore size.

Gene cloning: Restriction endonucleases are capable of cutting DNA at specific sequences, which may be joined with another fragment of DNA which has been cleaved by a similar process. In this way, DNA fragments can be introduced into systems which allow transcription and analysis of the gene product. The fundamental underpinning of DNA-recombinant technology and the production of insulin, growth factors, and erythropoietin.

Gene frequencies: Frequency of a specific allele in a population.

Genotype: Description of the inherited genes (eg, XY).

Heterozygous: The two copies (alleles) of a gene are different.

Haplotypes: Expression of a set of alleles, signifies one-half of the genetic information for the gene.

Homozygous: Both copies (alleles) of a gene are identical.

Insertion: Addition of a segment of DNA into a gene.

Linkage disequilibrium: Closely-spaced alleles tend to be inherited together. However, when alleles at two distinct loci occur together more frequently than expected based on the known allele frequencies and recombination fraction, the alleles are said to be in linkage disequilibrium. Evidence for linkage disequilibrium is often used to map genes.

Loci: Discrete location or portion of a chromosome where a gene is located.

Microarray: The basic principle of microarray analysis relies on base pairing, or hybridization between strands of nucleotides (between A-T and G-C for DNA and A-U and G-C for RNA). DNA which is complementary to the gene of interest is created and placed in microscopic quantities on solid surfaces. DNA is eluted over the surface, leading to binding of complementary strands. Presence of bound DNA is detected electronically (by fluorescence following laser excitation). Microarrays are often referred to as genome "chips," and are remarkable for the ability to screen large quantities of DNA (high-throughput). Microarrays require specialized robotics and imaging equipment. An experiment with a single DNA chip can provide researchers information on thousands of genes simultaneously. DNA-microarray technology may be used to identify DNA sequences (identify mutation), and to determine the level of expression of specific genes. Gene expression signatures for molecular diagnosis of leukemias is not currently employed in routine clinical practice.

INTRODUCTION

Mutation or mutant: Copy of a gene which differs from the "wild type;" often assigned a numerical designation (*2, *3, etc). The "mutant" allele may be a misnomer as the allele generally occurs commonly in the human population, and in some instances, occurs more commonly than the "wild-type" allele.

Open reading frame (ORF): A stretch of DNA that has the potential to encode a protein. To qualify, it must begin with a start codon and terminate with one of the three "stop" codons. An ORF is not usually considered equivalent to a gene until a phenotype has been associated with a mutation in the ORF or a specific gene product has been identified.

Phenotype: Expression of the genotype/genome, appearance or metabolism (eg, male).

Polymerase chain reaction: A method of creating multiple copies of specific fragments of DNA. PCR rapidly amplifies a single DNA molecule into many billions of molecules. In a typical application, small samples of DNA, such as those found in a strand of hair at a crime scene, can produce sufficient copies to carry out forensic tests.

Restriction fragment: The result of enzymatic digestion by an enzyme capable of cleaving DNA based on the recognition of a specific nucleic acid sequence. Digestion produces a reproducible group of DNA fragments. A number of restriction enzymes are available, with unique recognition sequences, resulting in a distinct pattern of fragments. The fragments are detected by electrophoresis/Southern blotting of a gene of interest.

Restriction fragment length polymorphism (RFLP): Variation in DNA sequence which introduces a new site for the activity of a restriction enzyme (or removes a site); this variation results in a change in the banding pattern seen on electrophoresis and subsequent Southern blotting. For a given gene, different restriction enzymes may be tested to identify an enzyme which results in a different pattern between two individuals (an RFLP).

"Signatures:" Groupings of genes of interest. Identifies the notion that many genes may group together to create phenotypes which dictate response. This may be the most clinically-relevant term.

SNP: "Snips" - changes in a gene involving the substitution of one nucleotide base for another. Often designated as the normal base, location of exchange, and secondary base (C825T).

"Wild-type:" Refers to an allele or genotype that was either the first described or that occurs in the majority of the population (often designated as *1). It is important to note that in some cases, the "wild-type" occurs at a lower frequency than the "mutant." Also, given that the frequency of genetic polymorphisms often varies among racial groups, the most commonly occurring allele/genotype in one racial group may be the least commonly occurring allele/genotype in another group.

INTRODUCTION TO PHARMACOGENOMICS

Genetic Variation: Polymorphisms

Each gene is encoded in a sequence of nucleic acid bases (see "Introduction to Genetics"). Common variations in the genome are termed polymorphisms. Polymorphisms are mutations which occur in >1% of the population. It is important to note that polymorphisms may occur in any segment of the gene, including exon regions, which encode the final protein, noncoding intron sequences, and gene promoter regions, which regulate gene transcription. The variability may result in a change in the final protein, altered mRNA processing, or a difference in the regulation of gene expression. Some of the more common types of polymorphisms include single nucleotide changes (SNP or "snips"), insertions, deletions, or tandem repeats.

Single nucleotide polymorphisms occur when one nucleotide is replaced by another. Over 1.4 million SNPs have been identified in the human genome, and it has been estimated that as many as 3 million SNPs may be present. This yields a frequency of as many as 1 SNP per every 1000 base pairs. A SNP may result in a change in the amino acid sequence of the final protein product. However, given the redundancy in the human genetic code (one codon may code for more than one amino acid, as discussed in the "Introduction to Genetics") some SNPs may not result in an amino acid change. Single nucleotide polymorphisms that result in amino acid changes are termed nonsynonymous. Those that do not result in an amino acid change are called synonymous. For example, in the sequence CCA and CCG, adenine has been replaced by guanine; however, both triads encode the amino acid proline, and no overall change in the encoded protein would result from this substitution.

Specific mutations are frequently assigned "shorthand" designations. Single nucleotide pairs, for example, are often identified by the two bases which are exchanged, along with a designation of the position on the gene where the substitution occurs. An example of this is C825T, where thymidine is substituted for cytosine at nucleotide position 825. This may also be designated as C825→T. Nonsynonymous SNPs are usually designated by the usual amino acid, codon (amino acid) position, and substituted amino acid (eg, Arg389Gly or Arg389→Gly indicates that glycine replaces arginine at codon 389), and may be represented by the amino acid symbol (eg, Arg389Gly may be abbreviated as R389G); see table of abbreviations below.

A	Ala	G	Gly	M	Met	S	Ser
C	Cys	H	His	N	Asn	T	Thr
D	Asp	I	Ile	P	Pro	V	Val
E	Glu	K	Lys	Q	Gln	W	Trp
F	Phe	L	Leu	R	Arg	Y	Tyr

Insertions and deletions refer to changes of greater than one base pair, in which a section of DNA is either added or deleted. These may be designated by the I or D alleles. For insertions and deletions, the typical nomenclature specifies the I (insertion) allele or the D (deletion) allele. The total genotype may be expressed as I/I or D/D for homozygotes (those who carry two I or D alleles) or I/D for heterozygotes (those who carry one I allele and one D allele) of the gene of interest. Tandem repeats are segments of DNA in which the same nucleotide sequence is repeated multiple times.

In some cases, insertion of a segment of DNA which is not divisible by three will lead to a frameshift mutation, since the codon:anticodon pattern will be disturbed for all DNA which lies downstream from the insertion. Some polymorphisms alter the stability of mRNA, which may result in the synthesis of a reduced number of proteins. In addition, differences may result in changes in post-translational modifications of the final protein product, yielding a protein with altered functionality. Finally, polymorphisms may lead to the creation of stop codons, which would terminate translation prior to formation of the final gene product.

In addition to the nomenclature mentioned above for SNPs and insertion/deletions, mutations may be expressed in a manner which relates to their discovery and/or naming. In these cases, the first form of the gene (usually, but not always, the most common, or "wild-type"), is designated as the *1 genotype (CYP3A4*1). Subsequent mutations may be designated numerically (CYP3A4*2, CYP3A4*3, etc).

Pharmacokinetic and Pharmacodynamic Consequences

Since proteins may participate as enzymes, transporters, receptors, or structural elements of the cell, the final expression of the polymorphism may take a variety of forms. Specific effects on pharmacologic activities may result from altered metabolism of a drug (pharmacokinetic differences), or changes in sensitivity to a drug's action at any given concentration (pharmacodynamic differences).

An example of pharmacokinetic consequences is the relationship between mercaptopurine and the enzyme thiopurine methyltransferase (TPMT). This enzyme has a number of polymorphisms, which lead to the expression of three basic phenotypes. Approximately 89% to 94% of the population demonstrate "high activity" of this enzyme, while 6% to 11% display "intermediate activity." Importantly, a segment of the population, approximately 0.3%, displays very low activity. In a single study of 147 patients receiving mercaptopurine for the treatment of ALL, homozygotes for the low metabolic activity demonstrated severe hematologic toxicity despite a 50% reduction in dose. Formerly, this type of observation would be idiotypic, without sufficient explanation. With the advent of pharmacogenomic analysis, it is possible to identify patients at risk of this reaction prior to administration of mercaptopurine, as well as other drugs metabolized by this enzyme.

INTRODUCTION TO PHARMACOGENOMICS
(Continued)

Other polymorphisms which may result in pronounced pharmacokinetic variability include polymorphisms of cytochrome P450 enzymes (CYP isoenzyme variants), drug transporters (such as P-glycoprotein), and various activating enzymes, such as DPD (required to activate fluorouracil).

Several pharmacodynamic consequences of drug polymorphisms are also well documented. For example, specific alleles of the β_2-adrenergic receptor may alter receptor sensitivity and response to β_2-receptor agonists.

Web Sites

http://snp500cancer.nci.nih.gob/snp.cfm

http://www.genomica.net/RICERCA/HAPMAP/HAPMAP_consorzio.htm

http://snp.cshl.org

INTRODUCTION TO GENETICS

Structure of DNA

The central dogma of molecular genetics states that genes encoded in DNA are transcribed to RNA and translated into protein products. Therefore, all potential products of the genome are encoded on DNA, located in the nucleus of a cell. Despite its complex functions, the molecular structure of DNA is based on only four nucleic acid molecules, or nucleotides. In humans, these four nucleotide bases are adenine, cytosine, guanine, and thymidine. Each base binds preferentially to one complementary nucleotide, leading to two fundamental associations: Guanine with cytosine (G-C pairs) and adenine with thymidine (A-T pairs). These associations are illustrated in Figure 1.

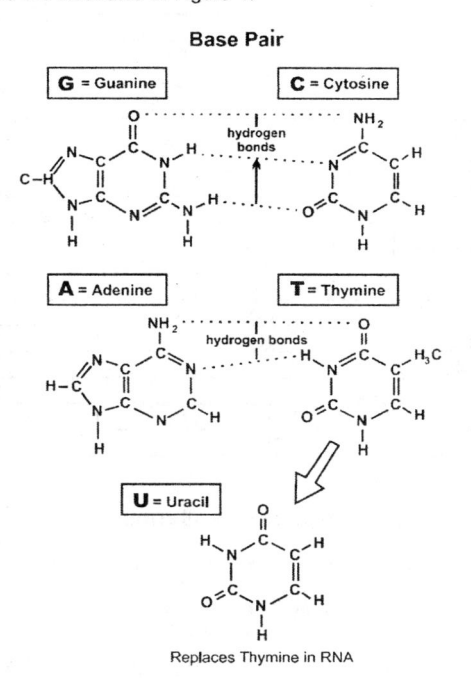

Base Pair

Figure 1. Base pairs of nucleic acids. Adenine pairs with thymidine by hydrogen bonding in DNA. Thymidine is replaced by uracil in the RNA transcript.

INTRODUCTION TO GENETICS *(Continued)*

DNA is arranged in a double helix. The helix is formed by two strands of nucleotide bases, linked to each other by bonds between complementary pairs of nucleotides. A strand of nucleotides, associated with its complementary strand, forms a structure which may be likened to a twisted ladder, with the "rungs" of the ladder corresponding to the linkage between bases of opposite strands. One side of the DNA encodes the sequence for a protein (sense strand) while the opposite mirror-image strand does not encode protein (anti-sense strand). The length of a DNA segment is often described by the number of base pairs in the segment (ie, 1600 bp for a segment consisting of 1600 sequential nucleotide bases).

Genetic Code Showing How Nucleotide Combinations Determine the Amino Acid Encoded

1st Position	2nd Position				3rd Position
	U	C	A	G	
U	Phe	Ser	Tyr	Cys	U
	Phe	Ser	Tyr	Cys	C
	Leu	Ser	STOP	STOP	A
	Leu	Ser	STOP	Trp	G
C	Leu	Pro	His	Arg	U
	Leu	Pro	His	Arg	C
	Leu	Pro	Gln	Arg	A
	Leu	Pro	Gln	Arg	G
A	Ile	Thr	Asn	Ser	U
	Ile	Thr	Asn	Ser	C
	Ile	Thr	Lys	Arg	A
	Met	Thr	Lys	Arg	G
G	Val	Ala	Asp	Gly	U
	Val	Ala	Asp	Gly	C
	Val	Ala	Glu	Gly	A
	Val	Ala	Glu	Gly	G

Inheritance: Dominant / Recessive Genes

The human genome contains 46 chromosomes (23 pairs). The Human Genome Project is an international research effort to determine the DNA sequence of the entire human genome. The complete genome has been sequenced with remarkable implications for health and disease.

The inheritance of genetic information depends on the segregation of chromosomes as individual gametes are formed. This results in one-half of the genetic information needed by the individual's progeny. A haplotype refers to the pattern of single nucleotide polymorphisms on a chromosome in a block. Since the ultimate human genome results from the contribution

INTRODUCTION TO GENETICS

of two copies of each chromosome (with the exception of the X and Y chromosomes), each individual inherits two copies of each gene.

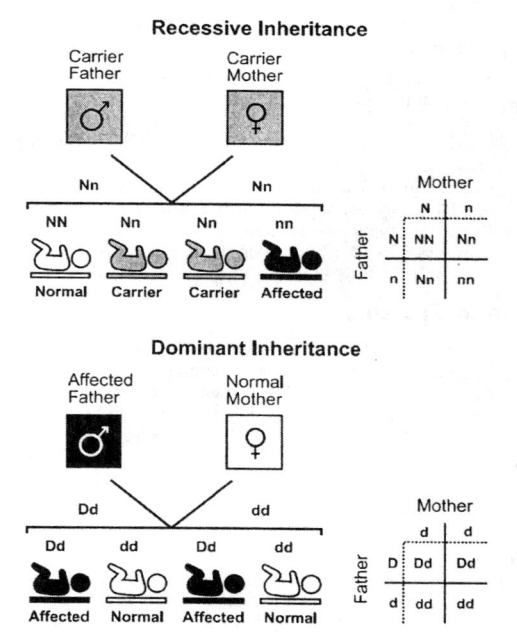

Figure 2. Examples of dominant and recessive single-gene inheritance. A gene which is inherited as a recessive trait requires both alleles to encode this trait (small letter "n" in the first example) before the trait will be expressed. In dominant inheritance, any combination in which the dominant allele ("D" in the second example) is included will result in expression of the trait.

In some cases, one gene is described as being expressed in preference over another. This concept of "dominant" and "recessive" genes is a useful illustration of simple inheritance patterns, and correlates with many physical traits such as eye and hair pigmentation. Dominant and recessive genes are often further identified as being autosomal or sex-linked (residing on the X or Y chromosome). Basic education in genetics frequently focuses on this simple pattern of inheritance, which is illustrated in Figure 2.

However, in many cases, simple dominant and recessive concepts do not adequately characterize gene expression. In some cases, genes exhibit codominance, in which both alleles are expressed. Many genes are polyallelic (for example, blood type is determined by A, B, and O gene

INTRODUCTION TO GENETICS *(Continued)*

products). In addition, many cellular processes are the result of multiple gene products, and it is difficult to predict an individual phenotype based on a change in only one of the involved genes.

Additional factors that moderate the phenotype include variable expression and incomplete penetrance. Variable expression of either allele results in intermediate expression of the individual genes. In some cases, this expression may be complex, and may relate to developmental stage or other cellular conditions. The term "penetrance" describes the degree to which a specific gene is expressed in the phenotype of the individual. As an extension of the concept of penetrance, if an individual carries the gene for a specific disease, and the disease usually develops in these patients, the gene is said to exhibit a high phenotypic penetrance.

Genes and Proteins

Genetic material contains the code for sequences of amino acids. The amino acid sequence determines the production of functional proteins. To translate from code to protein, two distinct steps must occur. First, the code must be transferred from the nucleic acids within the nucleus to the "machinery" of protein synthesis within the cytoplasm, the ribosome. Second, the code must be interpreted to allow assembly of the appropriate amino acids from the nucleic acid template. These two processes are known as transcription and translation. Figure 3 illustrates the steps of transcription and translation.

All cellular processes are determined by the activity of specific proteins. The individual's genotype is a representation of the inherited set of genes that provides the "code" for these proteins. Each individual inherits a pair of alleles, or forms of the gene, one from each parent. An allele is defined as the amino acid sequence at a given chromosomal locus. The phenotype of an individual refers to the actual physical or metabolic traits that result from expression of the inherited genes. Since a variety of processes regulate expression of a particular gene, the relationship between genotype and phenotype may be complex. For example, the genetic regulation of blood pressure involves a large number of physiologic processes, and other physiologic regulatory processes may compensate for a polymorphism in any single gene.

Transcription

During transcription, DNA segments are used to prepare complementary strands of RNA, that are later used as a template for protein synthesis (messenger RNA or mRNA). As encoded on DNA, individual genes have characteristics that regulate their transcription. For example, the segment of the DNA that encodes the information to "switch" the gene from active transcription to suppression is known as the promoter region.

Transcription is accomplished by specific proteins within the nucleus. The key transcriptional protein is RNA polymerase, that "reads" the DNA code

INTRODUCTION TO GENETICS

and translates it into corresponding mRNA sequences. RNA polymerase requires several other proteins, called transcription factors, to initiate this process. These proteins assemble in the promoter region of the gene, and recognize a specific DNA sequence called the TATA box. With remarkable consistency, this sequence is located 25 nucleotides away from the site where transcription will be initiated.

When transcription terminates, the mRNA contains segments that encode the final protein (exons) as well as segments that do not encode protein (introns). Prior to being translocated to the cytoplasm, introns are spliced out of the mRNA to yield a strand that will correspond to the amino acid sequence the ribosome will assemble. It is important to note that the splicing process may introduce additional complexity into the gene expression process. Alternative splicing, in which one or more exons are shared among multiple transcripts, may lead to the production of different proteins from the same DNA sequence. Sometimes, the two products are very similar in terms of activities but, in other cases, the activities of the two proteins have no clear association.

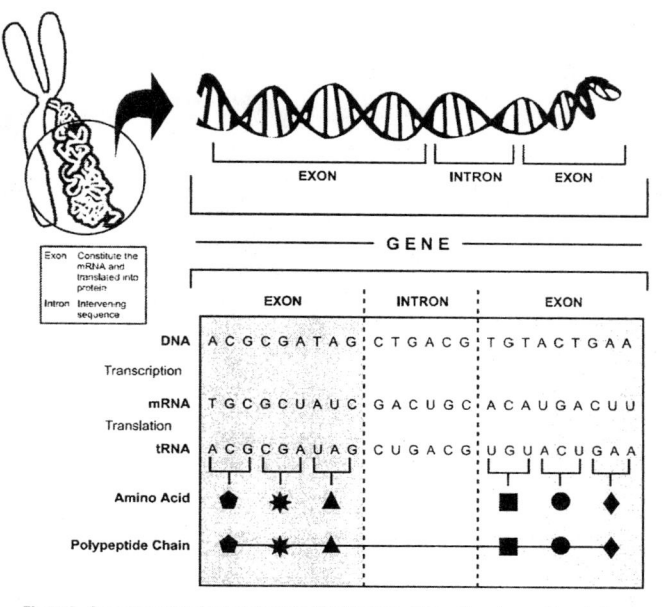

Figure 3. Gene expression: Transcription from DNA to mRNA within nucleus, transport to cytoplasmic ribosome for translation by tRNA + amino acids. Exon translation occurs within the ribosome.

INTRODUCTION TO GENETICS (Continued)

Translation

In the translation process, the nucleic acid code is used to guide the assembly of amino acids to yield protein products. The translation process occurs on ribosomes, within the cytoplasm of the cell. Transfer RNA (tRNA) shuttles a specific amino acid to the ribosome. Sequences on the tRNA portion of an amino-acid-containing complex correspond to the complementary base pairs of the mRNA.

Translation is initiated at the start codon, AUG. Translation requires the recognition of discrete sequences of three nucleic acids (codons) that determine a "vocabulary" of amino acids. The corresponding tRNA is called the anticodon. Since there are 4 nucleic acids, the requirement that these be arranged in triplets, the potential number of codons is 64 (4 x 4 x 4). However, only 20 amino acids are used in human protein synthesis, so a single amino acid may be encoded by more than one codon (therefore, the code is referred to as "degenerate"). Some codons do not correspond to an amino acid, and terminate protein synthesis ("stop" codons). The string of amino acids is manufactured by joining amino acids from their carboxy-terminus to the amino terminal. Figure 4 illustrates the relationship between RNA sequence and amino acid codons.

RNA
Ribonucleic acid

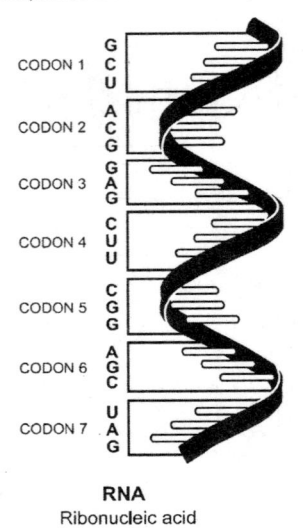

Figure 4. Organization of nucleic acid triplets into codons.

If an alteration occurs in the DNA, the triad of nucleic acids is disturbed. In some cases, there is no change because of the redundancy of the genetic code. In some cases, this leads to the coding of one amino acid rather than another during protein synthesis. This may result in altered activity of the synthesized protein. In other cases, the substitution results in a triad that cannot be recognized (as stop codon), and synthesis of the protein terminates (non-sense mutation). Mutations are genetic variations which occur in <1% of the population. A polymorphism refers to a genetic variation present in ≥1% of a population. Variation may also occur within the regions of DNA that regulate the production or processing of mRNA.

Post-Translational Modification

Following synthesis of the initial polypeptide chain, a number of modifications may be required before the amino acid sequence becomes a functional protein. For example, insulin is only active following the removal of C-peptide (this is often used as a marker of endogenous synthesis). The two-dimensional polypeptide folds into a three-dimensional structure, as determined by hydrophobic/hydrophilic characteristics, as well as the formation of stabilizing bonds within the internal structure. In many cases, enzymes within the cell assist in modification by cleaving segments of the amino acid chain, assisting in the formation of bonds (for example, disulfide bonds between cysteine groups), and the addition of polysaccharide groups to the initial chain.

Learning More

This brief introduction is intended to review basic principles of genetics and inheritance. Interested readers are encouraged to access additional resources, including the National Human Genome Research Institute (www.genome.gov) and Access Excellence, a project of the National Health Museum (www.nationalhealthmuseum.org).

CYTOCHROME P450 NOMENCLATURE

Cytochrome P450 refers to an important group of enzymes responsible for a variety of Phase I reactions including epoxidation, N-dealkylation, O-dealkylation, S-oxidation, and hydroxylation. The designation "P450" refers to the original identification of these enzymes as a pigment (P) with a characteristic absorption of light at a wavelength of 450 nm.

A large portion of cytochrome P450 enzymes exist in the liver and small intestine. They are also found in the skin, kidneys, lungs, and brain. CYP enzymes are localized in the microsomal portion of the cytoplasm, which includes the endoplasmic reticulum. CYP enzymes are responsible for the metabolism of xenobiotics, but are also involved in the formation of steroidal compounds, cholesterol, and arachadonic acid metabolites.

After its original identification, it became clear that "Cytochrome P450" actually consisted of a large number of enzymes with individual substrate specificity and separate genetic coding. These are referred to as isoforms, or variants. Isoforms are classified according to the similarities within their amino-acid sequences.

CYP isoforms are divided into families which contain substantial homology in their genetic sequence (at least 40% homology). At least 18 families have been identified in humans, and a total of over 70 families have been identified across various animal species. Families are assigned a numerical designation, such as CYP3. Isoenzyme families are further divided into subfamilies, which have at least 60% sequence homology. Subfamilies are designated by a letter after the specific CYP numerical designation. Finally, an individual gene is designated by an additional Arabic numeral. The following example illustrates the increasing specificity of these designations.

Family: CYP3

Subfamily: CYP3A

Genetic designation: CYP3A4

Individual isoforms may also have allelic variants, which are designated by an additional * symbol (CYP3A*2). The ability to classify CYP isoenzymes has been an important advance in terms of the ability to predict drug interactions between inhibitors, inducers, and substrates of this enzyme system. Additional investigation and potential profiling may allow more sophisticated analysis of drug metabolism, yielding greater accuracy in the prediction of interactions, and the tailoring of a dosing regimen to the specific capabilities of individual patients.

CYTOCHROME P450 ENZYMES: SUBSTRATES, INHIBITORS, AND INDUCERS

Introduction

Most drugs are eliminated from the body, at least in part, by being chemically altered to less lipid-soluble products (ie, metabolized), and thus more likely to be excreted via the kidneys or the bile. Phase I metabolism includes drug hydrolysis, oxidation, and reduction, and results in drugs that are more polar in their chemical structure, while Phase II metabolism involves the attachment of an additional molecule onto the drug (or partially metabolized drug) in order to create an inactive and/or more water soluble compound. Phase II processes include (primarily) glucuronidation, sulfation, glutathione conjugation, acetylation, and methylation.

Virtually any of the Phase I and II enzymes can be inhibited by some xenobiotic or drug. Some of the Phase I and II enzymes can be induced. Inhibition of the activity of metabolic enzymes will result in increased concentrations of the substrate (drug), whereas induction of the activity of metabolic enzymes will result in decreased concentrations of the substrate. For example, the well-documented enzyme-inducing effects of phenobarbital may include a combination of Phase I and II enzymes. Phase II glucuronidation may be increased via induced UDP-glucuronosyltransferase (UGT) activity, whereas Phase I oxidation may be increased via induced cytochrome P450 (CYP) activity. However, for most drugs, the primary route of metabolism (and the primary focus of drug-drug interaction) is Phase I oxidation, and specifically, metabolism.

CYP enzymes may be responsible for the metabolism (at least partial metabolism) of approximately 75% of all drugs, with the CYP3A subfamily responsible for nearly half of this activity. Found throughout plant, animal, and bacterial species, CYP enzymes represent a superfamily of xenobiotic metabolizing proteins. There have been several hundred CYP enzymes identified in nature, each of which has been assigned to a family (1, 2, 3, etc), subfamily (A, B, C, etc) and given a specific enzyme number (1, 2, 3, etc) according to the similarity in amino acid sequence that it shares with other enzymes. Of these many enzymes, only a few are found in humans, and even fewer appear to be involved in the metabolism of xenobiotics (eg, drugs). The key human enzyme subfamilies include CYP1A, CYP2A, CYP2B, CYP2C, CYP2D, CYP2E, and CYP3A.

CYP enzymes are found in the endoplasmic reticulum of cells in a variety of human tissues (eg, skin, kidneys, brain, lungs), but their predominant sites of concentration and activity are the liver and intestine. Though the abundance of CYP enzymes throughout the body is relatively equally distributed among the various subfamilies, the relative contribution to drug metabolism is (in decreasing order of magnitude) CYP3A4 (nearly 50%), CYP2D6 (nearly 25%), CYP2C8/9 (nearly 15%), then CYP1A2,

CYTOCHROME P450 ENZYMES: SUBSTRATES, INHIBITORS, AND INDUCERS *(Continued)*

CYP2C19, CYP2A6, and CYP2E1. Owing to their potential for numerous drug-drug interactions, those drugs that are identified in preclinical studies as substrates of CYP3A enzymes are often given a lower priority for continued research and development in favor of drugs that appear to be less affected by (or less likely to affect) this enzyme subfamily.

Each enzyme subfamily possesses unique selectivity toward potential substrates. For example, CYP1A2 preferentially binds medium-sized, planar, lipophilic molecules, while CYP2D6 preferentially binds molecules that possess a basic nitrogen atom. Some CYP subfamilies exhibit polymorphism (ie, multiple allelic variants that manifest differing catalytic properties). The best described polymorphisms involve CYP2C9, CYP2C19, and CYP2D6. Individuals possessing "wild type" gene alleles exhibit normal functioning CYP capacity. Others, however, possess allelic variants that leave the person with a subnormal level of catalytic potential (so called "poor metabolizers"). Poor metabolizers would be more likely to experience toxicity from drugs metabolized by the affected enzymes (or less effects if the enzyme is responsible for converting a prodrug to it's active form as in the case of codeine). The percentage of people classified as poor metabolizers varies by enzyme and population group. As an example, approximately 7% of Caucasians and only about 1% of Orientals appear to be CYP2D6 poor metabolizers.

CYP enzymes can be both inhibited and induced by other drugs, leading to increased or decreased serum concentrations (along with the associated effects), respectively. Induction occurs when a drug causes an increase in the amount of smooth endoplasmic reticulum, secondary to increasing the amount of the affected CYP enzymes in the tissues. This "revving up" of the CYP enzyme system may take several days to reach peak activity, and likewise, may take several days, even months, to return to normal following discontinuation of the inducing agent.

CYP inhibition occurs via several potential mechanisms. Most commonly, a CYP inhibitor competitively (and reversibly) binds to the active site on the enzyme, thus preventing the substrate from binding to the same site, and preventing the substrate from being metabolized. The affinity of an inhibitor for an enzyme may be expressed by an inhibition constant (Ki) or IC50 (defined as the concentration of the inhibitor required to cause 50% inhibition under a given set of conditions). In addition to reversible competition for an enzyme site, drugs may inhibit enzyme activity by binding to sites on the enzyme other than that to which the substrate would bind, and thereby cause a change in the functionality or physical structure of the enzyme. A drug may also bind to the enzyme in an irreversible (ie, "suicide") fashion. In such a case, it is not the concentration of drug at the enzyme site that is important (constantly binding and releasing), but the number of molecules available for binding (once bound, always bound).

Although an inhibitor or inducer may be known to affect a variety of CYP subfamilies, it may only inhibit one or two in a clinically important fashion.

Likewise, although a substrate is known to be at least partially metabolized by a variety of CYP enzymes, only one or two enzymes may contribute significantly enough to its overall metabolism to warrant concern when used with potential inducers or inhibitors. Therefore, when attempting to predict the level of risk of using two drugs that may affect each other via altered CYP function, it is important to identify the relative effectiveness of the inhibiting/inducing drug on the CYP subfamilies that significantly contribute to the metabolism of the substrate. The contribution of a specific CYP pathway to substrate metabolism should be considered not only in light of other known CYP pathways, but also other nonoxidative pathways for substrate metabolism (eg, glucuronidation) and transporter proteins (eg, P-glycoprotein) that may affect the presentation of a substrate to a metabolic pathway.

How to Use the Tables

The following CYP SUBSTRATES, INHIBITORS, and INDUCERS tables provide a comprehensive perspective on drugs that are affected by, or affect, cytochrome P450 (CYP) enzymes.

The CYP Substrates table contains a list of drugs reported to be metabolized, at least in part, by one or more CYP enzymes. An enzyme that appears to play a clinically significant role in a drug's metabolism is marked with a solid dot "•", and an enzyme whose role does not appear to be clinically significant is marked with an open dot "o". The designation of clinically significant is the result of a two-phase review. The first phase considered the clinical relevance of a substrate's concentration being increased twofold, or decreased by one-half. If either of these changes (which might occur in the presence of an effective enzyme inhibitor or inducer) was considered to present a clinically significant concern, the drug was subjected to a second phase. The second phase considered the contribution of each CYP enzyme to the overall metabolism of the drug. The enzyme pathway was considered clinically relevant if it was responsible for at least 30% of the metabolism of the drug.

The CYP Inhibitors table contains a list of drugs that are reported to inhibit one or more CYP enzymes. Enzymes that appear to be effectively inhibited by a drug are marked with a solid dot "•", and enzymes that do not appear to be effectively inhibited are marked with an open dot "o". The designation of "effectively inhibited" is the compiled result of the authors' review of published clinical reports, available Ki data, and assessments published by other experts in the field.

The CYP Inducers table contains a list of drugs that are reported to induce one or more CYP enzymes. Enzymes that appear to be effectively induced by a drug are marked with a solid dot "•", and enzymes that do not appear to be effectively induced are marked with an open dot "o". The designation of "effectively induced" is the compiled result of the authors' review of published clinical reports and assessments published by other experts in the field.

In all cases, only those enzymes marked with either a solid or open dot should be considered relevant to the drug identified at the beginning of the

CYTOCHROME P450 ENZYMES: SUBSTRATES, INHIBITORS, AND INDUCERS *(Continued)*

row. In general, clinically significant interactions are more likely to occur between substrates and either inhibitors or inducers of the same enzyme(s), all of which have been marked with a solid dot "•". However, these assessments possess a degree of subjectivity on behalf of the authors, at times based on limited indications regarding the significance of CYP effects of particular agents. The authors have attempted to balance a conservative, clinically-sensitive presentation of the data with a desire to avoid the numbing effect of a "beware of everything" approach. Even so, other potential interactions (ie, those involving enzymes marked with an open dot "o") may warrant consideration in some cases. It is important to note that information related to CYP metabolism of drugs is expanding at a rapid pace, and thus, the contents of this table should only be considered to represent a "snapshot" of the information available at the time of publication.

Selected Readings

Drug-Drug Interactions, Rodrigues AD, ed, New York, NY: Marcel Dekker, Inc, 2002.

Metabolic Drug Interactions, Levy R, Thummel K, Trager W, et al, eds, Philadephia, PA: Lippincott Williams & Wilkins, 2000.

Michalets EL, "Update: Clinically Significant Cytochrome P-450 Drug Interactions," *Pharmacotherapy*, 1998, 18(1):84-112.

Thummel KE and Wilkinson GR, "*In vitro* and *in vivo* Drug Interactions Involving Human CYP3A," *Annu Rev Pharmacol Toxicol*, 1998, 38:389-430.

Zhang Y and Benet LZ, "The Gut as a Barrier to Drug Absorption: Combined Role of Cytochrome P450 3A and P-Glycoprotein," *Clin Pharmacokinet*, 2001, 40(3):159-68.

Selected Websites

http://www.gentest.com

http://www.imm.ki.se/CYPalleles

http://medicine.iupui.edu/flockhart

http://www.mhc.com/Cytochromes

CYTOCHROME INFORMATION

CYP Substrates

Drug	1A2	2A6	2B6	2C8/9	2C19	2D6	2E1	3A4
Acetaminophen	o	o		o		o	o	o
Albendazole	o							o
Albuterol								•
Alfentanil								•
Almotriptan						o		o
Alosetron	o			•				o
Alprazolam								•
Aminophylline	•						o	o
Amiodarone	o			•	o	o		o
Amitriptyline	o		o	o	o	•		o
Amlodipine								•
Amoxapine						•		
Amphetamine						o		
Amprenavir				o				•
Aprepitant	o				o			•
Argatroban								o
Aripiprazole						•		•
Aspirin				o				
Atomoxetine					o	•		
Atorvastatin								•
Azelastine	o			o	o			o
Azithromycin								o
Benzphetamine			o					•
Benztropine						o		
Betaxolol	•					•		
Bexarotene								o
Bezafibrate								o
Bisoprolol						o		•
Bosentan				•				•
Brinzolamide								o
Bromazepam								•
Bromocriptine								•
Budesonide								o
Bupivacaine	o				o	o		o
Buprenorphine								•
BuPROPion	o	o	•	o		o	o	o
BusPIRone						o		•
Busulfan								•
Caffeine	•			o		o	o	o
Candesartan				o				
Capsaicin							o	
Captopril						•		
Carbamazepine				o				•
Carisoprodol					•			
Carteolol						o		
Carvedilol	o			•		•	o	o
Celecoxib				o				o

CYTOCHROME INFORMATION
CYTOCHROME P450 ENZYMES: SUBSTRATES, INHIBITORS, AND INDUCERS *(Continued)*

CYP Substrates *(continued)*

Drug	1A2	2A6	2B6	2C8/9	2C19	2D6	2E1	3A4
Cerivastatin								•
Cetirizine								o
Cevimeline						o		o
Chlordiazepoxide								•
Chloroquine						•		•
Chlorpheniramine						o		•
ChlorproMAZINE	o					•		o
ChlorproPAMIDE					o			
Chlorzoxazone	o	o				o	•	o
Cilostazol	o				o	o		o
Cisapride	o	o	o	o	o			•
Citalopram					•	o		•
Clarithromycin								•
Clobazam								•
Clofibrate								o
ClomiPRAMINE	•				•	•		o
Clonazepam								•
Clopidogrel	o							o
Clorazepate								•
Clozapine	•	o		o	o	o		o
Cocaine								•
Codeine						•		o
Colchicine								•
Cyclobenzaprine	•					o		o
Cyclophosphamide		o	•	o	•			o
CycloSPORINE								•
Dacarbazine	•						•	
Dantrolene								•
Dapsone				o	o		o	•
Delavirdine						o		•
Desipramine	o					•		
Desogestrel					•			
Dexamethasone								o
Dexmedetomidine		•						
Dextroamphetamine						•		
Dextromethorphan		o		o	o	•	o	o
Diazepam	o		o	o	•			•
Diclofenac	o		o	o	o	o		o
Dicumarol					•			
Digitoxin								•
Digoxin								o
Dihydrocodeine compound						•		
Dihydroergotamine								•
Diltiazem				o		o		•

28

CYP Substrates *(continued)*

Drug	1A2	2A6	2B6	2C8/9	2C19	2D6	2E1	3A4
Dirithromycin								o
Disopyramide								•
Disulfiram	o	o	o			o	o	o
Docetaxel								•
Dofetilide								o
Dolasetron				o				o
Domperidone								o
Donepezil						o		o
Dorzolamide				o				o
Doxepin	•					•		•
DOXOrubicin						•		•
Doxycycline								•
Drospirenone								o
Dutasteride								o
Efavirenz			•					•
Electriptan								•
Enalapril								•
Enflurane							•	
Eplerenone								•
Ergoloid mesylates								•
Ergonovine								•
Ergotamine								•
Erythromycin				o				•
Escitalopram						•		•
Esomeprazole					•			o
Estazolam								o
Estradiol	•	o	o	o	o	o	o	•
Estrogens, conjugated A/synthetic	•	o	o	o	o	o	o	•
Estrogens, conjugated equine	•	o	o	o	o	o	o	•
Estrogens, conjugated esterified	•		o	o			o	•
Estrone	•		o	o			o	•
Estropipate	•		o	o			o	•
Ethinyl estradiol								•
Ethosuximide								•
Etonogestrel								o
Etoposide	o						o	•
Exemestane								o
Felbamate							o	•
Felodipine								•
Fenofibrate								o
Fentanyl								•
Fexofenadine								o
Finasteride								o
Flecainide	o					•		

CYTOCHROME INFORMATION

CYTOCHROME P450 ENZYMES: SUBSTRATES, INHIBITORS, AND INDUCERS (Continued)

CYP Substrates (continued)

Drug	1A2	2A6	2B6	2C8/9	2C19	2D6	2E1	3A4
Fluoxetine	o		o	•	o	•	o	o
Fluphenazine						•		
Flurazepam								•
Flurbiprofen				o				
Flutamide	•							•
Fluticasone								o
Fluvastatin				o		o		o
Fluvoxamine	•					•		
Formoterol		o		o	o	o		
Fosphenytoin (as phenytoin)				•	•			o
Frovatriptan	o							
Fulvestrant								•
Galantamine						o		o
Gefitinib								•
Gemfibrozil								o
Glimepiride				•				
GlipiZIDE				•				
Granisetron								o
Guanabenz	•							
Halazepam								o
Halofantrine				o		o		•
Haloperidol	o					•		•
Halothane		o	o	o		o	•	o
Hydrocodone						•		
Hydrocortisone								o
Ibuprofen				o	o			
Ifosfamide		•	o	•	•			•
Imatinib	o			o	o	o		•
Imipramine	o		o		•	•		o
Imiquimod	o							o
Indinavir						o		•
Indomethacin				o	o			
Irbesartan				o				
Irinotecan			•					•
Isoflurane							•	
Isoniazid							•	
Isosorbide								•
Isosorbide dinitrate								•
Isosorbide mononitrate								•
Isradipine								•
Itraconazole								•
Ivermectin								o
Ketamine			•	•				•

CYP Substrates *(continued)*

Drug	1A2	2A6	2B6	2C8/9	2C19	2D6	2E1	3A4
Ketoconazole								•
Labetalol						•		
Lansoprazole				o	•			•
Letrozole		o						•
Levobupivacaine	o							o
Levomethadyl acetate hydrochloride			o					•
Levonorgestrel								•
Lidocaine	o	o	o	o		•		•
Lomustine						•		
Lopinavir								o
Loratadine						o		o
Losartan				•				•
Lovastatin								•
Maprotiline						•		
MedroxyPROGESTERone								•
Mefenamic acid				o				
Mefloquine								•
Meloxicam				o				o
Mephenytoin			o	•	•			
Mephobarbital			o	o	•			
Mestranol				•				•
Methadone				o	o	o		•
Methamphetamine						•		
Methoxsalen		o						
Methsuximide					•			
Methylergonovine								•
Methylphenidate						•		
MethylPREDNISolone								o
Methysergide								•
Metoclopramide	o					o		
Metoprolol					o	•		
Mexiletine	•					•		
Miconazole								•
Midazolam			o					•
Mifepristone								o
Mirtazapine	•			o		•		•
Moclobemide					•	•		
Modafinil								•
Mometasone furoate								o
Montelukast				•				•
Moricizine								•
Morphine sulfate						o		
Naproxen	o			o				
Nateglinide				•				•
Nefazodone						•		•
Nelfinavir				o	•	o		•

CYTOCHROME INFORMATION

CYTOCHROME P450 ENZYMES: SUBSTRATES, INHIBITORS, AND INDUCERS *(Continued)*

CYP Substrates *(continued)*

Drug	1A2	2A6	2B6	2C8/9	2C19	2D6	2E1	3A4
Nevirapine			o			o		•
NiCARdipine	o			o		o	o	•
Nicotine	o	o	o	o	o	o	o	o
NIFEdipine						o		•
Nilutamide					•			
Nimodipine								•
Nisoldipine								•
Nitrendipine								•
Norelgestromin								o
Norethindrone								•
Norgestrel								•
Nortriptyline	o				o	•		o
Olanzapine	o					o		
Omeprazole		o		o	•	o		o
Ondansetron	o			o		o	o	•
Orphenadrine	o		o			o		o
Oxybutynin								o
Oxycodone						•		
Paclitaxel				•				•
Pantoprazole					•			o
Paroxetine						•		
Pentamidine					•			
Pergolide								•
Perphenazine	o			o	o	•		o
Phencyclidine								•
Phenobarbital				o	•		o	
Phenytoin				•	•			o
Pimecrolimus								o
Pimozide	•							•
Pindolol						•		
Pioglitazone				•				•
Pipecuronium				o				
Piroxicam				o				
Pravastatin								o
Prazepam								o
PrednisoLONE								o
PredniSONE								o
Primaquine								•
Procainamide						•		
Progesterone	o	o		o	•	o		•
Proguanil	o				o			o
Promethazine			•			•		
Propafenone	o					•		o
Propofol	o	o	•	•	o	o	o	o

CYP Substrates *(continued)*

Drug	1A2	2A6	2B6	2C8/9	2C19	2D6	2E1	3A4
Propranolol	•				•	•		o
Quazepam								o
Quetiapine						o		•
Quinidine				o			o	•
Quinine	o				o			o
Rabeprazole					•			•
Ranitidine	o				o	o		
Repaglinide				o				•
Rifabutin	•							•
Rifampin		•		•				•
Riluzole	•							
Risperidone						•		o
Ritonavir	o		o			•		•
Rofecoxib				o				
Ropinirole	•							o
Ropivacaine	o		o			o		o
Rosiglitazone				•				
Rosuvastatin				o				o
Saquinavir						o		•
Selegiline	o	o	•	•		o		o
Sertraline			•	•	•	o		•
Sevoflurane		o	o				•	o
Sibutramine								•
Sildenafil				o				•
Simvastatin								•
Sirolimus								•
Spiramycin								•
Sufentanil								•
SulfaDIAZINE				•			o	o
Sulfamethoxazole				•				o
Sulfinpyrazone				•				o
SulfiSOXAZOLE				•				
Suprofen				o				
Tacrine	•							
Tacrolimus								•
Tamoxifen		o	o	•		•	o	•
Tamsulosin						•		•
Temazepam			o	o	o			o
Teniposide								•
Terbinafine								•
Testosterone			o	o	o			o
Tetracycline								•
Theophylline	•			o		o	•	•
Thiabendazole	o							
Thioridazine					o	•		
Thiothixene	•							
Tiagabine								•

CYTOCHROME P450 ENZYMES: SUBSTRATES, INHIBITORS, AND INDUCERS (Continued)

CYP Substrates (continued)

Drug	1A2	2A6	2B6	2C8/9	2C19	2D6	2E1	3A4
Ticlopidine								•
Timolol						•		
TOLBUTamide				•	o			
Tolcapone (metabolites)		o						o
Tolterodine				o	o	•		•
Toremifene	o							•
Torsemide				•				
Tramadol						•		o
Trazodone						o		•
Tretinoin		o	o	o				
Triazolam								•
Trifluoperazine	•							
Trimethadione				o	o		•	o
Trimethoprim				•				•
Trimipramine					•	•		•
Troleandomycin								•
Valdecoxib				o				o
Valproic acid		o	o	o	o		o	
Venlafaxine				o	o	•		•
Verapamil	o		o	o			o	•
VinBLAStine						o		•
VinCRIStine								•
Vinorelbine						o		•
Voriconazole				•	•			o
Warfarin	o			•	o			o
Yohimbine						o		
Zafirlukast				•				
Zaleplon								o
Zidovudine		o		o	o			o
Zileuton	o			o				o
Ziprasidone	o							o
Zolmitriptan	o							
Zolpidem	o			o	o	o		•
Zonisamide					o			•
Zopiclone				•				•
Zuclopenthixol						•		

CYTOCHROME INFORMATION

CYP Inhibitors

Drug	1A2	2A6	2B6	2C8/9	2C19	2D6	2E1	3A4
Acebutolol						o		
AcetaZOLAMIDE								o
Albendazole	o							
Alosetron	o						o	
Amiodarone	o	o	o	•	o	•		•
Amitriptyline	o			o	o	o	o	
Amlodipine			o	o		o		o
Amphetamine						o		
Amprenavir					o			•
Anastrozole	o			o				o
Aprepitant								o
Atorvastatin								o
Azelastine			o	o	o	•		o
Azithromycin								o
Bepridil						o		
Betamethasone								o
Betaxolol						o		
Biperiden						o		
Bromazepam							o	
Bromocriptine								•
BuPROPion						•		
Caffeine	•							
Candesartan				o				
Celecoxib						o		
Cerivastatin								o
Chloramphenicol				o				o
Chloroquine						o		
Chlorpheniramine						•		
ChlorproMAZINE						o	o	
Chlorzoxazone							o	o
Cholecalciferol				o	o	o		
Cimetidine	•			o	o	•	o	•
Ciprofloxacin	•							•
Cisapride						o		
Citalopram	o		o		o	o		
Clarithromycin	o							•
Clemastine						•		o
Clofazimine								o
Clofibrate		o						
ClomiPRAMINE						•		
Clopidogrel				o				
Clotrimazole		o		o			o	o
Clozapine				o		o		o
Cocaine						•		o
Codeine						o		
Cyclophosphamide								o
CycloSPORINE				o				o

35

CYTOCHROME INFORMATION

CYTOCHROME P450 ENZYMES: SUBSTRATES, INHIBITORS, AND INDUCERS *(Continued)*

CYP Inhibitors *(continued)*

Drug	1A2	2A6	2B6	2C8/9	2C19	2D6	2E1	3A4
Danazol								o
Delavirdine	o			o	o	o		o
Desipramine						o	o	
Dexmedetomidine	o			o		•		o
Dextromethorphan						o		
Diazepam					o			o
Diclofenac				o			o	
Dihydroergotamine								o
Diltiazem				o		o		•
Dimethyl sulfoxide				o	o			
DiphenhydrAMINE						o		
Disulfiram	o	o	o	o		o	•	o
Docetaxel								o
Dolasetron						o		
DOXOrubicin						o		o
Doxycycline								o
Drospirenone	o			o	o			o
Econazole							o	
Efavirenz				o	o			o
Enoxacin	•							•
Entacapone	o	o		o	o	o	o	o
Eprosartan				o				
Ergotamine								o
Erythromycin	o							•
Escitalopram						o		
Estradiol	o							
Estrogens, conjugated A/synthetic	o							
Estrogens, conjugated equine	o							
Ethinyl estradiol	o		o		o			o
Ethotoin					o			
Etoposide				o				o
Felbamate					o			
Felodipine				o		o		o
Fentanyl								o
Fexofenadine						o		
Flecainide						o		
Fluconazole	o			•	•			•
Fluoxetine	o		•	o	o	•		o
Fluphenazine	o					o	o	
Flurazepam							o	
Flurbiprofen				o				
Flutamide	o							

CYP Inhibitors *(continued)*

Drug	1A2	2A6	2B6	2C8/9	2C19	2D6	2E1	3A4
Fluvastatin	o			•		o		o
Fluvoxamine	•		•	o	•	o		•
Fomepizole		•						
Gefitinib					o	o		
Grapefruit juice								•
Halofantrine						o		
Haloperidol						•		
HydrALAZINE								o
HydrOXYzine						o		
ibuprofen				o				
Ifosfamide								o
Imatinib				o		o		•
Imipramine	o				o	o	o	
Indinavir				o	o	o		•
Indomethacin				o	o			
interferon alfa-2a	o							
Interferon alfa-2b	o							
Interferon gamma-1b	o						o	
Irbesartan				o				o
Isoflurane			o					
Isoniazid	o			o	o	o	o	o
Itraconazole								•
Ketoconazole	o	o	o	o	o	o		•
Ketoprofen				o				
Labetalol						o		
Lansoprazole				o	•	o		o
Leflunomide				o				
Letrozole		o			o			
Levofloxacin	•							
Lidocaine	o					o		
Lomefloxacin	•							
Lomustine						o		o
Losartan	o			o	o			o
Lovastatin				o		o		
Mefenamic acid				o				
Mefloquine								o
Meloxicam				o				
Mephobarbital					o			
Mestranol	o		o		o			o
Methadone						•		o
Methimazole	o	o	o	o	o	o	o	o
Methoxsalen	•	•		o	o	o	o	o
Methsuximide					o			
Methylphenidate						o		
MethylPREDNISolone								o
Metoclopramide						o		
Metoprolol						o		

CYTOCHROME INFORMATION

CYTOCHROME P450 ENZYMES: SUBSTRATES, INHIBITORS, AND INDUCERS *(Continued)*

CYP Inhibitors *(continued)*

Drug	1A2	2A6	2B6	2C8/9	2C19	2D6	2E1	3A4
Metronidazole				o				o
Metyrapone		o						
Mexiletine	o							
Miconazole		o		o			o	o
Midazolam					o			o
Mifepristone						o		o
Mirtazapine	o							o
Mitoxantrone								o
Moclobemide	o				o	o		
Modafinil				o	o			
Montelukast				o				
Nalidixic acid	•							
Nateglinide				o				
Nefazodone	o		o			o		•
Nelfinavir	o		o	o	o	o		•
Nevirapine	o					o		o
NiCARdipine				o	o			o
Nicotine		o						
NIFEdipine	o			o		o		o
Nilutamide					o			
Nisoldipine	o							o
Nitrendipine								o
Norfloxacin	•							o
Nortriptyline						o	o	
Ofloxacin	o							
Olanzapine	o			o	o	o		o
Omeprazole				o	•	o		•
Ondansetron	o			o		o		
Orphenadrine	o	o	o	o	o	o	o	•
Oxcarbazepine					o			
Oxprenolol						o		
Oxybutynin						o		o
Paroxetine	o		•	o	o	•		o
Peginterferon alfa-2a	o							
Peginterferon alfa-2b	o							
Pentamidine						o		
Pentoxifylline	o							
Pergolide						•		o
Perphenazine	o					•		
Phencyclidine								o
Pilocarpine		o					o	o
Pimozide						•		o
Pindolol						o		
Pioglitazone				o	o			

CYP Inhibitors *(continued)*

Drug	1A2	2A6	2B6	2C8/9	2C19	2D6	2E1	3A4
Pipecuronium				o				
Pravastatin				o		o		o
Praziquantel						o		
PrednisoLONE								o
Primaquine						o		o
Probenecid					o			
Progesterone				o	o			
Promethazine						o		
Propafenone	o					o		
Propofol	o			o		o	o	o
Propoxyphene				o		o		o
Propranolol	o					o		
Pyrimethamine						o		
Quinidine				o		•		o
Quinine				o		•		o
Quinupristin								o
Rabeprazole					o			o
Ranitidine	o					o		
Risperidone						o		o
Ritonavir				o	o	•	o	•
Rofecoxib	•							
Ropinirole	o					•		
Rosiglitazone				o				
Saquinavir				o	o	o		•
Selegiline	o	o		o	o	o	o	o
Sertraline	o		•	o	•	o		o
Sildenafil	o			o	o	o	o	o
Simvastatin				o		o		
Sirolimus								o
Sparfloxacin	•							
SulfaDIAZINE				o				
Sulfamethoxazole				o				
Sulfinpyrazone				o				
SulfiSOXAZOLE				o				
Tacrine	o							
Tacrolimus								o
Tamoxifen			o	o				o
Telmisartan					o			
Teniposide				o				o
Tenofovir	o							
Terbinafine						o		
Testosterone								o
Tetracycline								o
Theophylline	o							
Thioridazine	o					•	o	
Thiotepa			o					
Thiothixene						o		

CYTOCHROME P450 ENZYMES: SUBSTRATES, INHIBITORS, AND INDUCERS *(Continued)*

CYP Inhibitors *(continued)*

Drug	1A2	2A6	2B6	2C8/9	2C19	2D6	2E1	3A4
Ticlopidine	•			•	•	o		
Timolol						o		
Tocainide	o							
TOLBUTamide				o				
Tolcapone				o				
Topiramate					o			
Torsemide					o			
Tranylcypromine	o	•		o	o	o	o	o
Trazodone						o		
Tretinoin				o				
Triazolam				o				
Trimethoprim				o				
Tripelennamine						o		
Triprolidine						o		
Troleandomycin								•
Valdecoxib				o	o			
Valproic acid				o	o	o		o
Valsartan				o				
Venlafaxine			o			o		o
Verapamil	o			o		o		•
VinBLAStine						o		o
VinCRIStine								o
Vinorelbine						o		o
Voriconazole				o	o			•
Warfarin				o	o			
Yohimbine						o		
Zafirlukast	o			o	o	o		o
Zileuton	o							
Ziprasidone						o		o

CYTOCHROME INFORMATION

CYP Inducers

Drug	1A2	2A6	2B6	2C8/9	2C19	2D6	2E1	3A4
Aminoglutethimide	•				•			•
Amobarbital		•						
Aprepitant				o				o
Azatadine								o
Bexarotene								o
Bosentan				o				o
Calcitriol								o
Carbamazepine	•		•	•	•			•
Clofibrate			o				o	o
Colchicine				o			o	o
Cyclophosphamide			o	o				
Dexamethasone		o	o	o				o
Dicloxacillin								o
Efavirenz (in liver only)			o					o
Estradiol								o
Estrogens, conjugated A/synthetic								o
Estrogens, conjugated equine								o
Felbamate								o
Fosphenytoin (as phenytoin)			•	•	•			•
Griseofulvin	o			o				o
Hydrocortisone								o
Ifosfamide				o				
Insulin preparations	o							
Isoniazid (after D/C)							o	
Lansoprazole	o							
MedroxyPROGESTERone								o
Mephobarbital		o						
Metyrapone								o
Modafinil	o		o					o
Moricizine	o							o
Nafcillin								•
Nevirapine			•					•
Norethindrone					o			
Omeprazole	o							
Oxcarbazepine								•
Paclitaxel								o
Pantoprazole	o							o
Pentobarbital		•						•
Phenobarbital	•	•	•	•				•
Phenytoin			•	•	•			•
Pioglitazone								o
PredniSONE					o			o
Primaquine	o							
Primidone	•			•	•			•

CYTOCHROME P450 ENZYMES: SUBSTRATES, INHIBITORS, AND INDUCERS *(Continued)*

CYP Inducers *(continued)*

Drug	1A2	2A6	2B6	2C8/9	2C19	2D6	2E1	3A4
Rifabutin								•
Rifampin	•	•	•	•	•			•
Rifapentine				•				•
Ritonavir (long-term)	o			o				o
Rofecoxib								o
Secobarbital		•		•				
Sulfinpyrazone								o
Terbinafine								o
Topiramate								o
Tretinoin							o	
Troglitazone								o
Valproic acid		o						

ALPHABETICAL LISTING OF DRUGS

Abacavir (a BAK a veer)
Gene(s) of Interest Human Leukocyte Antigen *on page 206*
U.S. Brand Names Ziagen®
Pharmacologic Class Antiretroviral Agent, Reverse Transcriptase Inhibitor (Nucleoside)

Abciximab (ab SIK si mab)
Gene(s) of Interest
Glycoprotein IIIa Receptor *on page 196*
U.S. Brand Names ReoPro®
Synonyms C7E3; 7E3
Pharmacologic Class Antiplatelet Agent, Glycoprotein IIb/IIIa Inhibitor

- **Abilify™** *see* Aripiprazole *on page 51*
- **Accolate®** *see* Zafirlukast *on page 156*
- **AccuNeb™** *see* Albuterol *on page 46*
- **Accupril®** *see* Quinapril *on page 133*
- **ACE** *see* Captopril *on page 60*

Acebutolol (a se BYOO toe lole)
Gene(s) of Interest
Angiotensin-Converting Enzyme *on page 163*
Beta-1 Adrenergic Receptor *on page 171*
Gs Protein Alpha-Subunit *on page 198*
U.S. Brand Names Sectral®
Canadian Brand Names Apo®-Acebutolol; Gen-Acebutolol; Monitan®; Novo-Acebutolol; Nu-Acebutolol; Rhotral
Pharmacologic Class Antiarrhythmic Agent, Class II; Beta Blocker With Intrinsic Sympathomimetic Activity

- **Aceon®** *see* Perindopril Erbumine *on page 126*

Acetaminophen and Codeine
(a seet a MIN oh fen & KOE deen)
Gene(s) of Interest
COMT *on page 180*
CYP2D6 *on page 186*
U.S. Brand Names Capital® and Codeine; Phenaphen® With Codeine; Tylenol® With Codeine
Canadian Brand Names Emtec-30; Lenoltec; Triatec-8; Triatec-8 Strong; Triatec-30
Synonyms Codeine and Acetaminophen
Pharmacologic Class Analgesic, Narcotic

- **Acetaminophen and Hydrocodone** *see* Hydrocodone and Acetaminophen *on page 94*
- **Acetaminophen and Oxycodone** *see* Oxycodone and Acetaminophen *on page 123*

Acetaminophen and Phenyltoloxamine
(a seet a MIN oh fen & fen il to LOKS a meen)
Gene(s) of Interest
COMT *on page 180*
U.S. Brand Names
Genesec® [OTC]; Percogesic® [OTC]; Phenylgesic® [OTC]
Synonyms
Phenyltoloxamine and Acetaminophen
Pharmacologic Class
Analgesic, Non-narcotic

◆ **Acetaminophen and Propoxyphene** *see* Propoxyphene and Acetaminophen *on page 132*

Acetaminophen and Tramadol
(a seet a MIN oh fen & TRA ma dole)
Gene(s) of Interest
COMT *on page 180*
CYP2D6 *on page 186*

U.S. Brand Names
Ultracet™

Synonyms
APAP and Tramadol; Tramadol Hydrochloride and Acetaminophen

Pharmacologic Class
Analgesic, Non-narcotic; Analgesic, Miscellaneous

◆ **Acetaminophen, Caffeine, Codeine, and Butalbital** *see* Butalbital, Acetaminophen, Caffeine, and Codeine *on page 58*

Acetophenazine
(a set oh FEN a zeen) *Not available in the U.S.*
Gene(s) of Interest
Alpha-1 Adrenergic Receptor *on page 161*
D2 Receptor *on page 190*
Pharmacologic Class
Antipsychotic Agent, Phenothiazine, Piperazine

◆ **Acetoxymethylprogesterone** *see* MedroxyPROGESTERone *on page 107*
◆ **Acetylsalicylic Acid** *see* Aspirin *on page 51*
◆ **Achromycin** *see* Tetracycline *on page 146*
◆ **Aciclovir** *see* Acyclovir *on page 45*
◆ **Aciphex®** *see* Rabeprazole *on page 134*
◆ **Actiq®** *see* Fentanyl *on page 86*
◆ **Actonel®** *see* Risedronate *on page 137*
◆ **Actos®** *see* Pioglitazone *on page 128*
◆ **Acular®** *see* Ketorolac *on page 101*
◆ **Acular® PF** *see* Ketorolac *on page 101*
◆ **ACV** *see* Acyclovir *on page 45*
◆ **Acycloguanosine** *see* Acyclovir *on page 45*

Acyclovir
(ay SYE kloe veer)
Gene(s) of Interest
None known
U.S. Brand Names
Zovirax®
(Continued)

Acyclovir *(Continued)*
Canadian Brand Names Alti-Acyclovir; Apo®-Acyclovir; Gen-Acyclovir; Nu-Acyclovir; ratio-Acyclovir
Synonyms Aciclovir; ACV; Acycloguanosine
Pharmacologic Class Antiviral Agent

- **Adalat® CC** *see* NIFEdipine *on page 118*
- **Adderall®** *see* Dextroamphetamine and Amphetamine *on page 72*
- **Adderall XR™** *see* Dextroamphetamine and Amphetamine *on page 72*
- **Adoxa™** *see* Doxycycline *on page 76*
- **ADR** *see* DOXOrubicin *on page 76*
- **Adria** *see* DOXOrubicin *on page 76*
- **Adriamycin PFS®** *see* DOXOrubicin *on page 76*
- **Adriamycin RDF®** *see* DOXOrubicin *on page 76*
- **Adrucil®** *see* Fluorouracil *on page 87*
- **Advair™ Diskus®** *see* Fluticasone and Salmeterol *on page 89*
- **Advil® [OTC]** *see* Ibuprofen *on page 96*
- **Advil® Children's [OTC]** *see* Ibuprofen *on page 96*
- **Advil® Infants' Concentrated Drops [OTC]** *see* Ibuprofen *on page 96*
- **Advil® Junior [OTC]** *see* Ibuprofen *on page 96*
- **Advil® Migraine [OTC]** *see* Ibuprofen *on page 96*
- **Aggrastat®** *see* Tirofiban *on page 149*
- **Aggrenox™** *see* Aspirin and Dipyridamole *on page 52*
- **A-hydroCort®** *see* Hydrocortisone *on page 95*
- **Akne-Mycin®** *see* Erythromycin *on page 79*
- **AK-Sulf®** *see* Sulfacetamide *on page 142*
- **Alavert™ [OTC]** *see* Loratadine *on page 105*

Albuterol (al BYOO ter ole)
Gene(s) of Interest
Beta-2 Adrenergic Receptor *on page 171*
U.S. Brand Names AccuNeb™; Proventil®; Proventil® HFA; Proventil® Repetabs®; Ventolin®; Ventolin® HFA; Volmax®; VoSpire ER™
Canadian Brand Names Airomir; Alti-Salbutamol; Apo®-Salvent; Gen-Salbutamol; PMS-Salbutamol; ratio-Inspra-Sal; ratio-Salbutamol; Rhoxal-salbutamol; Salbu-2; Salbu-4; Ventolin® Diskus; Ventrodisk
Synonyms Salbutamol
Pharmacologic Class Beta$_2$ Agonist

- **Albuterol and Ipratropium** *see* Ipratropium and Albuterol *on page 98*
- **Aldactone®** *see* Spironolactone *on page 142*

Alendronate (a LEN droe nate)
Gene(s) of Interest None known
U.S. Brand Names Fosamax®
Pharmacologic Class Bisphosphonate Derivative

- **Alesse®** *see* Ethinyl Estradiol and Levonorgestrel *on page 83*
- **Aleve® [OTC]** *see* Naproxen *on page 117*
- **Alfenta®** *see* Alfentanil *on page 47*

Alfentanil (al FEN ta nil)
Gene(s) of Interest
COMT *on page 180*
CYP3A4 *on page 189*
U.S. Brand Names Alfenta®
Pharmacologic Class Analgesic, Narcotic

- **Allegra®** *see* Fexofenadine *on page 87*
- **Aller-Chlor® [OTC]** *see* Chlorpheniramine *on page 63*

Allopurinol (al oh PURE i nole)
Gene(s) of Interest None known
U.S. Brand Names Aloprim™; Zyloprim®
Canadian Brand Names Apo®-Allopurinol
Synonyms Allopurinol Sodium Injection
Pharmacologic Class Xanthine Oxidase Inhibitor

- **Allopurinol Sodium Injection** *see* Allopurinol *on page 47*
- **Aloprim™** *see* Allopurinol *on page 47*
- **Alora®** *see* Estradiol *on page 80*

Alprazolam (al PRAY zoe lam)
Gene(s) of Interest
CYP3A4 *on page 189*
U.S. Brand Names Alprazolam Intensol®; Xanax®; Xanax XR®
Canadian Brand Names Alti-Alprazolam; Apo®-Alpraz; Gen-Alprazolam; Novo-Alprazol; Nu-Alprax; Xanax TS™
Pharmacologic Class Benzodiazepine

- **Alprazolam Intensol®** *see* Alprazolam *on page 47*
- **Altace®** *see* Ramipril *on page 135*
- **Altocor™** *see* Lovastatin *on page 106*
- **Alupent®** *see* Metaproterenol *on page 109*
- **Amaryl®** *see* Glimepiride *on page 92*
- **Ambien®** *see* Zolpidem *on page 157*
- **A-Methapred®** *see* MethylPREDNISolone *on page 111*

Amiloride (a MIL oh ride)
Gene(s) of Interest
Epithelial Sodium Channel Beta-Subunit *on page 194*
U.S. Brand Names Midamor®
Pharmacologic Class Diuretic, Potassium Sparing

- **2-Amino-6-Mercaptopurine** *see* Thioguanine *on page 147*
- **2-Amino-6-Trifluoromethoxy-Benzothiazole** *see* Riluzole *on page 136*

Aminophylline (am in OFF i lin)
Gene(s) of Interest
CYP1A2 *on page 181*
Canadian Brand Names Phyllocontin®; Phyllocontin®-350
Synonyms Theophylline Ethylenediamine
Pharmacologic Class Theophylline Derivative

Amiodarone (a MEE oh da rone)
Gene(s) of Interest
Cardiac Potassium Ion Channel *on page 177*
Cardiac Sodium Channel *on page 178*
CYP2C9 *on page 183*
CYP2D6 *on page 186*
P-Glycoprotein *on page 213*
U.S. Brand Names Cordarone®; Pacerone®
Canadian Brand Names Alti-Amiodarone; Gen-Amiodarone; Novo-Amiodarone; Rhoxal-amiodarone
Pharmacologic Class Antiarrhythmic Agent, Class III

Amitriptyline (a mee TRIP ti leen)
Gene(s) of Interest
Alpha-1 Adrenergic Receptor *on page 161*
Cardiac Potassium Ion Channel *on page 177*
Cardiac Sodium Channel *on page 178*
G-Protein Beta-3 Subunit *on page 197*
Gs Protein Alpha-Subunit *on page 198*
P-Glycoprotein *on page 213*
TNF-Alpha *on page 222*
U.S. Brand Names Elavil®; Vanatrip®
Canadian Brand Names Apo®-Amitriptyline; Levate®; PMS-Amitriptyline
Pharmacologic Class Antidepressant, Tricyclic (Tertiary Amine)

Amitriptyline and Chlordiazepoxide
(a mee TRIP ti leen & klor dye az e POKS ide)
Gene(s) of Interest
Alpha-1 Adrenergic Receptor *on page 161*
Cardiac Potassium Ion Channel *on page 177*
Cardiac Sodium Channel *on page 178*
CYP3A4 *on page 189*
G-Protein Beta-3 Subunit *on page 197*
Gs Protein Alpha-Subunit *on page 198*
P-Glycoprotein *on page 213*
TNF-Alpha *on page 222*
U.S. Brand Names Limbitrol®; Limbitrol® DS
Synonyms Chlordiazepoxide and Amitriptyline
Pharmacologic Class Antidepressant, Tricyclic (Tertiary Amine); Benzodiazepine

Amitriptyline and Perphenazine
(a mee TRIP ti leen & per FEN a zeen)
Gene(s) of Interest
Alpha-1 Adrenergic Receptor *on page 161*
Cardiac Potassium Ion Channel *on page 177*
Cardiac Sodium Channel *on page 178*
CYP2D6 *on page 186*
D2 Receptor *on page 190*
G-Protein Beta-3 Subunit *on page 197*
Gs Protein Alpha-Subunit *on page 198*
P-Glycoprotein *on page 213*
TNF-Alpha *on page 222*
U.S. Brand Names Etrafon®; Triavil®
Synonyms Perphenazine and Amitriptyline
Pharmacologic Class Antidepressant, Tricyclic (Tertiary Amine); Antipsychotic Agent, Phenothiazine, Piperazine

Amlodipine (am LOE di peen)
Gene(s) of Interest
CYP3A4 *on page 189*
U.S. Brand Names Norvasc®
Pharmacologic Class Calcium Channel Blocker

Amlodipine and Benazepril
(am LOE di peen & ben AY ze pril)
Gene(s) of Interest
Aldosterone Synthase *on page 160*
Angiotensin-Converting Enzyme *on page 163*
Angiotensin II Type 1 Receptor *on page 166*
Angiotensinogen *on page 167*
Bradykinin B2 Receptor *on page 175*
CYP3A4 *on page 189*
U.S. Brand Names Lotrel®
Synonyms Benazepril and Amlodipine
Pharmacologic Class Antihypertensive Agent Combination

Amoxapine (a MOKS a peen)
Gene(s) of Interest
Alpha-1 Adrenergic Receptor *on page 161*
G-Protein Beta-3 Subunit *on page 197*
Gs Protein Alpha-Subunit *on page 198*
Synonyms Asendin [DSC]
Pharmacologic Class Antidepressant, Tricyclic (Secondary Amine)

Amoxicillin (a moks i SIL in)
Gene(s) of Interest None known
U.S. Brand Names Amoxil®; Moxilin®; Trimox®
(Continued)

AMOXICILLIN AND CLAVULANATE POTASSIUM

Amoxicillin *(Continued)*
Canadian Brand Names Apo®-Amoxi; Gen-Amoxicillin; Lin-Amox; Novamoxin®; Nu-Amoxi
Synonyms Amoxycillin; *p*-Hydroxyampicillin
Pharmacologic Class Antibiotic, Penicillin

Amoxicillin and Clavulanate Potassium
(a moks i SIL in & klav yoo LAN ate poe TASS ee um)
Gene(s) of Interest None known
U.S. Brand Names Augmentin®; Augmentin ES-600®; Augmentin XR™
Canadian Brand Names Alti-Amoxi-Clav®; Apo®-Amoxi-Clav; Clavulin®; ratio-AmoxiClav
Synonyms Amoxicillin and Clavulanic Acid
Pharmacologic Class Antibiotic, Penicillin

- **Amoxicillin and Clavulanic Acid** *see* Amoxicillin and Clavulanate Potassium *on page 50*
- **Amoxil®** *see* Amoxicillin *on page 49*
- **Amoxycillin** *see* Amoxicillin *on page 49*
- **Amphetamine and Dextroamphetamine** *see* Dextroamphetamine and Amphetamine *on page 72*
- **Anafranil®** *see* ClomiPRAMINE *on page 66*
- **Anaprox®** *see* Naproxen *on page 117*
- **Anaprox® DS** *see* Naproxen *on page 117*
- **Androderm®** *see* Testosterone *on page 146*
- **AndroGel®** *see* Testosterone *on page 146*
- **Anestacon®** *see* Lidocaine *on page 103*
- **Anexsia®** *see* Hydrocodone and Acetaminophen *on page 94*
- **Ansaid®** *see* Flurbiprofen *on page 89*
- **Ansamycin** *see* Rifabutin *on page 136*
- **Antabuse®** *see* Disulfiram *on page 75*
- **Antihist-1® [OTC]** *see* Clemastine *on page 65*
- **Antivert®** *see* Meclizine *on page 107*
- **Anturane** *see* Sulfinpyrazone *on page 143*
- **Anucort-HC®** *see* Hydrocortisone *on page 95*
- **Anusol-HC®** *see* Hydrocortisone *on page 95*
- **Anusol® HC-1 [OTC]** *see* Hydrocortisone *on page 95*
- **APAP and Tramadol** *see* Acetaminophen and Tramadol *on page 45*

Aprepitant (ap RE pi tant)
Gene(s) of Interest
CYP3A4 *on page 189*
U.S. Brand Names Emend®
Synonyms L 754030; MK869
Pharmacologic Class Antiemetic

- **Apresoline [DSC]** *see* HydrALAZINE *on page 94*

ASPIRIN

- **Apri®** *see* Ethinyl Estradiol and Desogestrel *on page 82*
- **Aquanil™ HC [OTC]** *see* Hydrocortisone *on page 95*
- **Aquatensen®** *see* Methyclothiazide *on page 110*
- **Aquazide® H** *see* Hydrochlorothiazide *on page 94*
- **Aralen® Phosphate** *see* Chloroquine *on page 62*
- **Aricept®** *see* Donepezil *on page 75*

Aripiprazole (ay ri PIP ray zole)
Gene(s) of Interest
Alpha-1 Adrenergic Receptor *on page 161*
CYP3A4 *on page 189*
D2 Receptor *on page 190*
D3 Receptor *on page 191*
5HT1A Receptor *on page 200*
5HT2A Receptor *on page 201*
5HT2C Receptor *on page 202*
U.S. Brand Names Abilify™
Synonyms BMS 337039; OPC14597
Pharmacologic Class Antipsychotic Agent, Quinolinone

- **Aristocort®** *see* Triamcinolone *on page 151*
- **Aristocort® A** *see* Triamcinolone *on page 151*
- **Aristocort® Forte** *see* Triamcinolone *on page 151*
- **Aristospan®** *see* Triamcinolone *on page 151*

Arsenic Trioxide (AR se nik tri OKS id)
Gene(s) of Interest
Cardiac Potassium Ion Channel *on page 177*
Cardiac Sodium Channel *on page 178*
U.S. Brand Names Trisenox™
Synonyms NSC-706363
Pharmacologic Class Antineoplastic Agent, Miscellaneous

- **Arthrotec®** *see* Diclofenac and Misoprostol *on page 72*
- **ASA** *see* Aspirin *on page 51*
- **Ascriptin® [OTC]** *see* Aspirin *on page 51*
- **Ascriptin® Arthritis Pain [OTC]** *see* Aspirin *on page 51*
- **Ascriptin® Enteric [OTC]** *see* Aspirin *on page 51*
- **Ascriptin® Extra Strength [OTC]** *see* Aspirin *on page 51*
- **Asendin [DSC]** *see* Amoxapine *on page 49*
- **Aspercin [OTC]** *see* Aspirin *on page 51*
- **Aspercin Extra [OTC]** *see* Aspirin *on page 51*
- **Aspergum® [OTC]** *see* Aspirin *on page 51*

Aspirin (AS pir in)
Gene(s) of Interest
Glycoprotein IIIa Receptor *on page 196*
Leukotriene C4 Synthase *on page 206*
U.S. Brand Names Ascriptin® [OTC]; Ascriptin® Arthritis Pain [OTC]; Ascriptin® Enteric [OTC]; Ascriptin® Extra Strength [OTC]; Aspercin
(Continued)

ASPIRIN AND CODEINE

Aspirin *(Continued)*
[OTC]; Aspercin Extra [OTC]; Aspergum® [OTC]; Bayer® Aspirin [OTC]; Bayer® Aspirin Extra Strength [OTC]; Bayer® Aspirin Regimen Adult Low Strength [OTC]; Bayer® Aspirin Regimen Adult Low Strength with Calcium [OTC]; Bayer® Aspirin Regimen Children's [OTC]; Bayer® Aspirin Regimen Regular Strength [OTC]; Bayer® Plus Extra Strength [OTC]; Bufferin® [OTC]; Bufferin® Arthritis Strength [OTC]; Bufferin® Extra Strength [OTC]; Easprin®; Ecotrin® [OTC]; Ecotrin® Low Adult Strength [OTC]; Ecotrin® Maximum Strength [OTC]; Halfprin® [OTC]; St. Joseph® Pain Reliever [OTC]; Sureprin 81™ [OTC]; ZORprin®

Canadian Brand Names Asaphen; Asaphen E.C.; Entrophen®; Novasen

Synonyms Acetylsalicylic Acid; ASA

Pharmacologic Class Salicylate

Aspirin and Codeine (AS pir in & KOE deen)
Gene(s) of Interest
COMT *on page 180*
CYP2D6 *on page 186*
Glycoprotein IIIa Receptor *on page 196*
Leukotriene C4 Synthase *on page 206*

Canadian Brand Names Coryphen® Codeine

Synonyms Codeine and Aspirin

Pharmacologic Class Analgesic, Narcotic

Aspirin and Dipyridamole (AS pir in & dye peer ID a mole)
Gene(s) of Interest
Glycoprotein IIIa Receptor *on page 196*
Leukotriene C4 Synthase *on page 206*
P-Glycoprotein *on page 213*

U.S. Brand Names Aggrenox™

Synonyms Aspirin and Extended-Release Dipyridamole; Dipyridamole and Aspirin

Pharmacologic Class Antiplatelet Agent

- **Aspirin and Extended-Release Dipyridamole** *see* Aspirin and Dipyridamole *on page 52*
- **Aspirin and Hydrocodone** *see* Hydrocodone and Aspirin *on page 94*
- **Aspirin and Oxycodone** *see* Oxycodone and Aspirin *on page 123*
- **Aspirin and Propoxyphene** *see* Propoxyphene and Aspirin *on page 132*
- **Aspirin, Caffeine, and Dihydrocodeine** *see* Dihydrocodeine, Aspirin, and Caffeine *on page 73*
- **Aspirin, Caffeine, Codeine, and Butalbital** *see* Butalbital, Aspirin, Caffeine, and Codeine *on page 59*
- **Astelin®** *see* Azelastine *on page 54*
- **Astramorph/PF™** *see* Morphine Sulfate *on page 115*
- **Atacand®** *see* Candesartan *on page 59*

• **Atarax®** *see* HydrOXYzine *on page 96*

Atenolol (a TEN oh lole)
Gene(s) of Interest
Angiotensin-Converting Enzyme *on page 163*
Beta-1 Adrenergic Receptor *on page 171*
Gs Protein Alpha-Subunit *on page 198*
U.S. Brand Names Tenormin®
Canadian Brand Names Apo®-Atenol; Gen-Atenolol; Novo-Atenol; Nu-Atenol; PMS-Atenolol; Rhoxal-atenolol; Tenolin
Pharmacologic Class Beta Blocker, Beta$_1$ Selective

• **Ativan®** *see* Lorazepam *on page 105*

Atomoxetine (AT oh mox e teen)
Gene(s) of Interest
CYP2D6 *on page 186*
U.S. Brand Names Strattera™
Synonyms LY139603; Tomoxetine
Pharmacologic Class Norepinephrine Reuptake Inhibitor, Selective

Atorvastatin (a TORE va sta tin)
Gene(s) of Interest
Angiotensin-Converting Enzyme *on page 163*
Apolipoprotein E *on page 168*
Beta-Fibrinogen *on page 174*
Cholesteryl Ester Transfer Protein *on page 179*
CYP3A4 *on page 189*
Glycoprotein IIIa Receptor *on page 196*
Low-Density Lipoprotein Receptor *on page 209*
P-Glycoprotein *on page 213*
Stromelysin-1 *on page 219*
U.S. Brand Names Lipitor®
Pharmacologic Class Antilipemic Agent, HMG-CoA Reductase Inhibitor

• **Atromid-S®** *see* Clofibrate *on page 66*
• **A/T/S®** *see* Erythromycin *on page 79*
• **Augmentin®** *see* Amoxicillin and Clavulanate Potassium *on page 50*
• **Augmentin ES-600®** *see* Amoxicillin and Clavulanate Potassium *on page 50*
• **Augmentin XR™** *see* Amoxicillin and Clavulanate Potassium *on page 50*
• **Avandia®** *see* Rosiglitazone *on page 138*
• **Avapro®** *see* Irbesartan *on page 99*
• **Avelox®** *see* Moxifloxacin *on page 115*
• **Avelox® I.V.** *see* Moxifloxacin *on page 115*
• **Aventyl® HCl** *see* Nortriptyline *on page 120*
• **Aviane™** *see* Ethinyl Estradiol and Levonorgestrel *on page 83*
• **Avinza™** *see* Morphine Sulfate *on page 115*

AZATHIOPRINE

- **Avlosulfon [DSC]** *see* Dapsone *on page 70*
- **Aygestin®** *see* Norethindrone *on page 119*

Azathioprine (ay za THYE oh preen)
Gene(s) of Interest
Thiopurine Methyltransferase *on page 220*
U.S. Brand Names Imuran®
Canadian Brand Names Alti-Azathioprine; Apo®-Azathioprine; Gen-Azathioprine
Pharmacologic Class Immunosuppressant Agent

Azelastine (a ZEL as teen)
Gene(s) of Interest
CYP2D6 *on page 186*
P-Glycoprotein *on page 213*
U.S. Brand Names Astelin®; Optivar™
Pharmacologic Class Antihistamine

Azithromycin (az ith roe MYE sin)
Gene(s) of Interest None known
U.S. Brand Names Zithromax®
Synonyms Zithromax® TRI-PAK™; Zithromax® Z-PAK®
Pharmacologic Class Antibiotic, Macrolide

- **Azmacort®** *see* Triamcinolone *on page 151*
- **Azulfidine®** *see* Sulfasalazine *on page 143*
- **Azulfidine® EN-tabs®** *see* Sulfasalazine *on page 143*
- **Bactrim™** *see* Sulfamethoxazole and Trimethoprim *on page 143*
- **Bactrim™ DS** *see* Sulfamethoxazole and Trimethoprim *on page 143*
- **Bactroban®** *see* Mupirocin *on page 116*
- **Bactroban® Nasal** *see* Mupirocin *on page 116*
- **BAL** *see* Dimercaprol *on page 74*
- **BAL in Oil®** *see* Dimercaprol *on page 74*
- **Bancap HC®** *see* Hydrocodone and Acetaminophen *on page 94*
- **Band-Aid® Hurt-Free™ Antiseptic Wash [OTC]** *see* Lidocaine *on page 103*
- **Bayer® Aspirin [OTC]** *see* Aspirin *on page 51*
- **Bayer® Aspirin Extra Strength [OTC]** *see* Aspirin *on page 51*
- **Bayer® Aspirin Regimen Adult Low Strength [OTC]** *see* Aspirin *on page 51*
- **Bayer® Aspirin Regimen Adult Low Strength with Calcium [OTC]** *see* Aspirin *on page 51*
- **Bayer® Aspirin Regimen Children's [OTC]** *see* Aspirin *on page 51*
- **Bayer® Aspirin Regimen Regular Strength [OTC]** *see* Aspirin *on page 51*
- **Bayer® Plus Extra Strength [OTC]** *see* Aspirin *on page 51*

Belladonna and Opium (bel a DON a & OH pee um)
Gene(s) of Interest
COMT *on page 180*
U.S. Brand Names B&O Supprettes®
Synonyms Opium and Belladonna
Pharmacologic Class Analgesic Combination (Narcotic); Antispasmodic Agent, Urinary

Benazepril (ben AY ze pril)
Gene(s) of Interest
Aldosterone Synthase *on page 160*
Angiotensin-Converting Enzyme *on page 163*
Angiotensin II Type 1 Receptor *on page 166*
Angiotensinogen *on page 167*
Bradykinin B2 Receptor *on page 175*
U.S. Brand Names Lotensin®
Pharmacologic Class Angiotensin-Converting Enzyme (ACE) Inhibitor

♦ **Benazepril and Amlodipine** *see* Amlodipine and Benazepril *on page 49*

Bendroflumethiazide (ben droe floo meth EYE a zide)
Gene(s) of Interest
Alpha-Adducin *on page 162*
G-Protein Beta-3 Subunit *on page 197*
U.S. Brand Names Naturetin®
Pharmacologic Class Diuretic, Thiazide

♦ **Benemid [DSC]** *see* Probenecid *on page 130*
♦ **Benicar™** *see* Olmesartan *on page 122*

Benzonatate (ben ZOE na tate)
Gene(s) of Interest None known
U.S. Brand Names Tessalon®
Pharmacologic Class Antitussive

Benzphetamine (benz FET a meen)
Gene(s) of Interest
CYP3A4 *on page 189*
U.S. Brand Names Didrex®
Pharmacologic Class Anorexiant

Bepridil (BE pri dil)
Gene(s) of Interest
Cardiac Potassium Ion Channel *on page 177*
Cardiac Sodium Channel *on page 178*
U.S. Brand Names Vascor®
Pharmacologic Class Calcium Channel Blocker

♦ **Betapace®** *see* Sotalol *on page 141*
♦ **Betapace AF®** *see* Sotalol *on page 141*

Betaxolol (be TAKS oh lol)
Gene(s) of Interest
Beta-1 Adrenergic Receptor *on page 171*
CYP1A2 *on page 181*
CYP2D6 *on page 186*
Gs Protein Alpha-Subunit *on page 198*
U.S. Brand Names Betoptic® S; Kerlone®
Pharmacologic Class Beta Blocker, Beta₁ Selective

- **Betimol®** *see* Timolol *on page 148*
- **Betoptic® S** *see* Betaxolol *on page 56*
- **Bextra®** *see* Valdecoxib *on page 153*

Bezafibrate (be za FYE brate)
Gene(s) of Interest
Angiotensin-Converting Enzyme *on page 163*
Cholesteryl Ester Transfer Protein *on page 179*
Canadian Brand Names Bezalip®; PMS-Bezafibrate
Pharmacologic Class Antilipemic Agent, Fibric Acid

- **Biaxin®** *see* Clarithromycin *on page 65*
- **Biaxin® XL** *see* Clarithromycin *on page 65*
- **Biocef** *see* Cephalexin *on page 62*
- **Bishydroxycoumarin** *see* Dicumarol *on page 72*

Bisoprolol (bis OH proe lol)
Gene(s) of Interest
Angiotensin-Converting Enzyme *on page 163*
Beta-1 Adrenergic Receptor *on page 171*
CYP3A4 *on page 189*
Gs Protein Alpha-Subunit *on page 198*
U.S. Brand Names Zebeta®
Canadian Brand Names Monocor®
Pharmacologic Class Beta Blocker, Beta₁ Selective

Bitolterol (bye TOLE ter ole)
Gene(s) of Interest
Beta-2 Adrenergic Receptor *on page 171*
Canadian Brand Names Tornalate®
Synonyms Tornalate [DSC]
Pharmacologic Class Beta₂ Agonist

- **Bleph®-10** *see* Sulfacetamide *on page 142*
- **Blocadren®** *see* Timolol *on page 148*
- **BMS 337039** *see* Aripiprazole *on page 51*
- **Bonine® [OTC]** *see* Meclizine *on page 107*

Bosentan (boe SEN tan)
Gene(s) of Interest
CYP2C9 *on page 183*

CYP3A4 *on page 189*
U.S. Brand Names Tracleer™
Pharmacologic Class Endothelin Antagonist

- **B&O Supprettes®** *see Belladonna and Opium on page 55*
- **Brethine®** *see Terbutaline on page 146*

Bretylium (bre TIL ee um)
Gene(s) of Interest
Cardiac Potassium Ion Channel *on page 177*
Cardiac Sodium Channel *on page 178*
Pharmacologic Class Antiarrhythmic Agent, Class III

- **Brevibloc®** *see Esmolol on page 80*
- **Brevicon®** *see Ethinyl Estradiol and Norethindrone on page 84*
- **British Anti-Lewisite** *see Dimercaprol on page 74*

Bromazepam (broe MA ze pam)
Gene(s) of Interest
CYP3A4 *on page 189*
Canadian Brand Names Apo®-Bromazepam; Gen-Bromazepam; Lectopam®; Novo-Bromazepam; Nu-Bromazepam
Pharmacologic Class Benzodiazepine

Bromocriptine (broe moe KRIP teen)
Gene(s) of Interest
CYP3A4 *on page 189*
U.S. Brand Names Parlodel®
Canadian Brand Names Apo® Bromocriptine; PMS-Bromocriptine
Pharmacologic Class Anti-Parkinson's Agent, Dopamine Agonist; Ergot Derivative

Budesonide (byoo DES oh nide)
Gene(s) of Interest None known
U.S. Brand Names Entocort™ EC; Pulmicort Respules®; Pulmicort Turbuhaler®; Rhinocort® [DSC]; Rhinocort® Aqua™
Canadian Brand Names Gen-Budesonide AQ; Pulmicort®; Rhinocort® Turbuhaler®
Pharmacologic Class Corticosteroid, Inhalant (Oral); Corticosteroid, Nasal; Corticosteroid, Systemic

- **Bufferin® [OTC]** *see Aspirin on page 51*
- **Bufferin® Arthritis Strength [OTC]** *see Aspirin on page 51*
- **Bufferin® Extra Strength [OTC]** *see Aspirin on page 51*
- **Buprenex®** *see Buprenorphine on page 57*

Buprenorphine (byoo pre NOR feen)
Gene(s) of Interest
COMT *on page 180*
CYP3A4 *on page 189*
U.S. Brand Names Buprenex®; Subutex®
Pharmacologic Class Analgesic, Narcotic

Buprenorphine and Naloxone
(byoo pre NOR feen & nal OKS one)

Gene(s) of Interest
COMT *on page 180*
CYP3A4 *on page 189*

U.S. Brand Names Suboxone®

Synonyms Buprenorphine Hydrochloride and Naloxone Hydrochloride Dihydrate; Naloxone and Buprenorphine; Naloxone Hydrochloride Dihydrate and Buprenorphine Hydrochloride

Pharmacologic Class Analgesic, Narcotic

- **Buprenorphine Hydrochloride and Naloxone Hydrochloride Dihydrate** *see* Buprenorphine and Naloxone *on page 58*

BuPROPion (byoo PROE pee on)
Gene(s) of Interest
CYP2D6 *on page 186*

U.S. Brand Names Wellbutrin®; Wellbutrin SR®; Zyban®

Pharmacologic Class Antidepressant, Dopamine-Reuptake Inhibitor; Smoking Cessation Aid

- **Burnamycin [OTC]** *see* Lidocaine *on page 103*
- **Burn Jel [OTC]** *see* Lidocaine *on page 103*
- **Burn-O-Jel [OTC]** *see* Lidocaine *on page 103*
- **BuSpar®** *see* BusPIRone *on page 58*

BusPIRone (byoo SPYE rone)
Gene(s) of Interest
CYP3A4 *on page 189*

U.S. Brand Names BuSpar®

Canadian Brand Names Apo®-Buspirone; Buspirex; Gen-Buspirone; Lin-Buspirone; Novo-Buspirone; Nu-Buspirone; PMS-Buspirone

Pharmacologic Class Antianxiety Agent, Miscellaneous

Busulfan (byoo SUL fan)
Gene(s) of Interest
CYP3A4 *on page 189*

U.S. Brand Names Busulfex®; Myleran®

Pharmacologic Class Antineoplastic Agent, Alkylating Agent

- **Busulfex®** *see* Busulfan *on page 58*

Butalbital, Acetaminophen, Caffeine, and Codeine
(byoo TAL bi tal, a seet a MIN oh fen, KAF een, & KOE deen)

Gene(s) of Interest
COMT *on page 180*
CYP2D6 *on page 186*

U.S. Brand Names Fioricet® with Codeine

Synonyms Acetaminophen, Caffeine, Codeine, and Butalbital; Caffeine, Acetaminophen, Butalbital, and Codeine; Codeine, Acetaminophen, Butalbital, and Caffeine

Pharmacologic Class Analgesic Combination (Narcotic); Barbiturate

Butalbital, Aspirin, Caffeine, and Codeine
(byoo TAL bi tal, AS pir in, KAF een, & KOE deen)

Gene(s) of Interest
COMT *on page 180*
CYP2D6 *on page 186*

U.S. Brand Names Fiorinal® With Codeine

Canadian Brand Names Fiorinal®-C 1/2; Fiorinal®-C 1/4; Tecnal C 1/2; Tecnal C 1/4

Synonyms Aspirin, Caffeine, Codeine, and Butalbital; Butalbital Compound and Codeine; Caffeine, Codeine, Butalbital Compound, and Aspirin; Codeine and Butalbital Compound; Codeine, Butalbital, Aspirin, and Caffeine

Pharmacologic Class Analgesic Combination (Narcotic); Barbiturate

♦ **Butalbital Compound and Codeine** *see* Butalbital, Aspirin, Caffeine, and Codeine *on page 59*

Butorphanol (byoo TOR fa nole)
Gene(s) of Interest
COMT *on page 180*

U.S. Brand Names Stadol®; Stadol® NS

Canadian Brand Names Apo®-Butorphanol

Pharmacologic Class Analgesic, Narcotic

♦ **C7E3** *see* Abciximab *on page 44*
♦ **Cafergot®** *see* Ergotamine *on page 79*
♦ **Caffeine, Acetaminophen, Butalbital, and Codeine** *see* Butalbital, Acetaminophen, Caffeine, and Codeine *on page 58*
♦ **Caffeine, Aspirin, and Dihydrocodeine** *see* Dihydrocodeine, Aspirin, and Caffeine *on page 73*
♦ **Caffeine, Codeine, Butalbital Compound, and Aspirin** *see* Butalbital, Aspirin, Caffeine, and Codeine *on page 59*
♦ **Calan®** *see* Verapamil *on page 154*
♦ **Calan® SR** *see* Verapamil *on page 154*
♦ **CaldeCORT® [OTC]** *see* Hydrocortisone *on page 95*
♦ **Camila™** *see* Norethindrone *on page 119*
♦ **Camphorated Tincture of Opium** *see* Paregoric *on page 124*
♦ **Camptosar®** *see* Irinotecan *on page 99*
♦ **Camptothecin-11** *see* Irinotecan *on page 99*

Candesartan (kan de SAR tan)
Gene(s) of Interest
Aldosterone Synthase *on page 160*
Angiotensin-Converting Enzyme *on page 163*
Angiotensin II Type I Receptor *on page 166*
Angiotensinogen *on page 167*
(Continued)

Candesartan *(Continued)*
U.S. Brand Names Atacand®
Pharmacologic Class Angiotensin II Receptor Blocker

Capecitabine (ka pe SITE a been)
Gene(s) of Interest
Dihydropyrimidine Dehydrogenase *on page 193*
U.S. Brand Names Xeloda®
Pharmacologic Class Antineoplastic Agent, Antimetabolite

- **Capital® and Codeine** *see* Acetaminophen and Codeine *on page 44*
- **Capoten®** *see* Captopril *on page 60*

Captopril (KAP toe pril)
Gene(s) of Interest
Aldosterone Synthase *on page 160*
Angiotensin-Converting Enzyme *on page 163*
Angiotensin II Type I Receptor *on page 166*
Angiotensinogen *on page 167*
Bradykinin B2 Receptor *on page 175*
U.S. Brand Names Capoten®
Canadian Brand Names Alti-Captopril; Apo®-Capto; Gen-Captopril; Novo-Captopril; Nu-Capto®; PMS-Captopril®
Synonyms ACE
Pharmacologic Class Angiotensin-Converting Enzyme (ACE) Inhibitor

- **Carac™** *see* Fluorouracil *on page 87*

Carbamazepine (kar ba MAZ e peen)
Gene(s) of Interest
CYP3A4 *on page 189*
U.S. Brand Names Carbatrol®; Epitol®; Tegretol®; Tegretol®-XR
Canadian Brand Names Apo®-Carbamazepine; Apo®-Carbamazepine CR; Gen-Carbamazepine CR; Novo-Carbamaz; Nu-Carbamazepine®; PMS-Carbamazepine; Taro-Carbamazepine Chewable
Synonyms CBZ
Pharmacologic Class Anticonvulsant, Miscellaneous

- **Carbatrol®** *see* Carbamazepine *on page 60*
- **Cardene®** *see* NiCARdipine *on page 118*
- **Cardene® I.V.** *see* NiCARdipine *on page 118*
- **Cardene® SR** *see* NiCARdipine *on page 118*
- **Cardizem®** *see* Diltiazem *on page 74*
- **Cardizem® CD** *see* Diltiazem *on page 74*
- **Cardizem® LA** *see* Diltiazem *on page 74*
- **Cardizem® SR** *see* Diltiazem *on page 74*
- **Cardura®** *see* Doxazosin *on page 76*
- **Carisoprodate** *see* Carisoprodol *on page 61*

Carisoprodol (kar eye soe PROE dole)
Gene(s) of Interest
CYP2C19 on page 185
U.S. Brand Names Soma®
Synonyms Carisoprodate; Isobamate
Pharmacologic Class Skeletal Muscle Relaxant

- **Carmol® Scalp** see Sulfacetamide on page 142
- **Cartia XT™** see Diltiazem on page 74

Carvedilol (KAR ve dil ole)
Gene(s) of Interest
Angiotensin-Converting Enzyme on page 163
Beta-1 Adrenergic Receptor on page 171
CYP2C9 on page 183
CYP2D6 on page 186
Gs Protein Alpha-Subunit on page 198
P-Glycoprotein on page 213
U.S. Brand Names Coreg®
Pharmacologic Class Beta Blocker With Alpha-Blocking Activity

- **Cataflam®** see Diclofenac on page 72
- **Catapres®** see Clonidine on page 66
- **Catapres-TTS®-1** see Clonidine on page 66
- **Catapres-TTS®-2** see Clonidine on page 66
- **Catapres-TTS®-3** see Clonidine on page 66
- **CBZ** see Carbamazepine on page 60

Cefdinir (SEF di ner)
Gene(s) of Interest None known
U.S. Brand Names Omnicef®
Synonyms CFDN
Pharmacologic Class Antibiotic, Cephalosporin (Third Generation)

Cefprozil (sef PROE zil)
Gene(s) of Interest None known
U.S. Brand Names Cefzil®
Pharmacologic Class Antibiotic, Cephalosporin (Second Generation)

- **Cefzil®** see Cefprozil on page 61
- **Celebrex®** see Celecoxib on page 61

Celecoxib (se le KOKS ib)
Gene(s) of Interest
Leukotriene C4 Synthase on page 206
U.S. Brand Names Celebrex®
Pharmacologic Class Nonsteroidal Anti-inflammatory Drug (NSAID), COX-2 Selective

- **Celexa™** see Citalopram on page 64
- **Celontin®** see Methsuximide on page 110

- **Cenestin®** *see* Estrogens (Conjugated A/Synthetic) *on page 81*

Cephalexin (sef a LEKS in)
Gene(s) of Interest None known
U.S. Brand Names Biocef; Keflex®; Keftab®
Canadian Brand Names Apo®-Cephalex; Novo-Lexin®; Nu-Cephalex®
Pharmacologic Class Antibiotic, Cephalosporin (First Generation)

- **Cerebyx®** *see* Fosphenytoin *on page 90*
- **C.E.S.** *see* Estrogens (Conjugated/Equine) *on page 81*
- **Cetacort®** *see* Hydrocortisone *on page 95*
- **Ceta-Plus®** *see* Hydrocodone and Acetaminophen *on page 94*

Cetirizine (se TI ra zeen)
Gene(s) of Interest None known
U.S. Brand Names Zyrtec®
Canadian Brand Names Apo®-Cetirizine; Reactine™
Synonyms P-071; UCB-P071
Pharmacologic Class Antihistamine

- **CFDN** *see* Cefdinir *on page 61*
- **CGP 57148B** *see* Imatinib *on page 97*
- **Chlo-Amine® [OTC]** *see* Chlorpheniramine *on page 63*

Chloramphenicol (klor am FEN i kole)
Gene(s) of Interest
  Glucose-6-Phosphate Dehydrogenase *on page 195*
U.S. Brand Names Chloromycetin®; Chloroptic®; Ocu-Chlor®
Canadian Brand Names Diochloram®; Pentamycetin®
Pharmacologic Class Antibiotic, Ophthalmic; Antibiotic, Otic; Antibiotic, Miscellaneous

Chlordiazepoxide (klor dye az e POKS ide)
Gene(s) of Interest
  CYP3A4 *on page 189*
U.S. Brand Names Librium®
Canadian Brand Names Apo®-Chlordiazepoxide
Synonyms Methaminodiazepoxide Hydrochloride
Pharmacologic Class Benzodiazepine

- **Chlordiazepoxide and Amitriptyline** *see* Amitriptyline and Chlordiazepoxide *on page 48*
- **Chlormeprazine** *see* Prochlorperazine *on page 130*
- **Chloromycetin®** *see* Chloramphenicol *on page 62*
- **Chloroptic®** *see* Chloramphenicol *on page 62*

Chloroquine (KLOR oh kwin)
Gene(s) of Interest
  Glucose-6-Phosphate Dehydrogenase *on page 195*

U.S. Brand Names Aralen® Phosphate
Pharmacologic Class Aminoquinoline (Antimalarial)

Chlorothiazide (klor oh THYE a zide)
Gene(s) of Interest
  Alpha-Adducin *on page 162*
  G-Protein Beta-3 Subunit *on page 197*
U.S. Brand Names Diuril®
Pharmacologic Class Diuretic, Thiazide

Chlorpheniramine (klor fen IR a meen)
Gene(s) of Interest
  CYP2D6 *on page 186*
  CYP3A4 *on page 189*
U.S. Brand Names Aller-Chlor® [OTC]; Chlo-Amine® [OTC]; Chlor-Trimeton® [OTC]
Canadian Brand Names Chlor-Tripolon®
Synonyms CTM
Pharmacologic Class Antihistamine

ChlorproMAZINE (klor PROE ma zeen)
Gene(s) of Interest
  Alpha-1 Adrenergic Receptor *on page 161*
  Cardiac Potassium Ion Channel *on page 177*
  Cardiac Sodium Channel *on page 178*
  D2 Receptor *on page 190*
  P-Glycoprotein *on page 213*
U.S. Brand Names Thorazine®
Canadian Brand Names Apo®-Chlorpromazine; Largactil®; Novo-Chlorpromazine
Synonyms CPZ
Pharmacologic Class Antipsychotic Agent, Phenothiazine, Aliphatic

Chlorprothixene (klor proe THIKS een)
Gene(s) of Interest
  Alpha-1 Adrenergic Receptor *on page 161*
  Cardiac Potassium Ion Channel *on page 177*
  Cardiac Sodium Channel *on page 178*
  D2 Receptor *on page 190*
Pharmacologic Class Antipsychotic Agent, Thioxanthene Derivative

Chlorthalidone (klor THAL i done)
Gene(s) of Interest
  Alpha-Adducin *on page 162*
  G-Protein Beta-3 Subunit *on page 197*
U.S. Brand Names Thalitone®
Canadian Brand Names Apo®-Chlorthalidone
Synonyms Hygroton [DSC]
Pharmacologic Class Diuretic, Thiazide

♦ **Chlor-Trimeton® [OTC]** *see* Chlorpheniramine *on page 63*

Cilazapril (sye LAY za pril)
Gene(s) of Interest
Aldosterone Synthase *on page 160*
Angiotensin-Converting Enzyme *on page 163*
Angiotensin II Type I Receptor *on page 166*
Angiotensinogen *on page 167*
Bradykinin B2 Receptor *on page 175*
Canadian Brand Names Inhibace®
Pharmacologic Class Angiotensin-Converting Enzyme (ACE) Inhibitor

Cilostazol (sil OH sta zol)
Gene(s) of Interest
Glycoprotein IIIa Receptor *on page 196*
U.S. Brand Names Pletal®
Synonyms OPC13013
Pharmacologic Class Antiplatelet Agent; Phosphodiesterase Enzyme Inhibitor

♦ **Ciloxan®** *see* Ciprofloxacin *on page 64*

Cimetidine (sye MET i deen)
Gene(s) of Interest
CYP2D6 *on page 186*
P-Glycoprotein *on page 213*
U.S. Brand Names Tagamet®; Tagamet® HB 200 [OTC]
Canadian Brand Names Apo®-Cimetidine; Gen-Cimetidine; Novo-Cimetidine; Nu-Cimet®; PMS-Cimetidine; Tagamet® HB
Pharmacologic Class Histamine H_2 Antagonist

♦ **Cipro®** *see* Ciprofloxacin *on page 64*

Ciprofloxacin (sip roe FLOKS a sin)
Gene(s) of Interest None known
U.S. Brand Names Ciloxan®; Cipro®; Cipro® XR
Pharmacologic Class Antibiotic, Ophthalmic; Antibiotic, Quinolone

♦ **Cipro® XR** *see* Ciprofloxacin *on page 64*

Cisapride (SIS a pride)
Gene(s) of Interest
Cardiac Potassium Ion Channel *on page 177*
Cardiac Sodium Channel *on page 178*
CYP3A4 *on page 189*
U.S. Brand Names Propulsid®
Pharmacologic Class Gastrointestinal Agent, Prokinetic

Citalopram (sye TAL oh pram)
Gene(s) of Interest
CYP2C19 *on page 185*
CYP3A4 *on page 189*
G-Protein Beta-3 Subunit *on page 197*

Gs Protein Alpha-Subunit *on page 198*
5HT Transporter *on page 204*
U.S. Brand Names Celexa™
Synonyms Nitalapram
Pharmacologic Class Antidepressant, Selective Serotonin Reuptake Inhibitor

- **CI-719** *see Gemfibrozil on page 91*
- **Cla** *see Clarithromycin on page 65*
- **Clarinex®** *see Desloratadine on page 71*

Clarithromycin (kla RITH roe mye sin)
Gene(s) of Interest
Cardiac Potassium Ion Channel *on page 177*
Cardiac Sodium Channel *on page 178*
CYP3A4 *on page 189*
P-Glycoprotein *on page 213*
U.S. Brand Names Biaxin®; Biaxin® XL
Synonyms Cla
Pharmacologic Class Antibiotic, Macrolide

- **Claritin® [OTC]** *see Loratadine on page 105*

Clemastine (KLEM as teen)
Gene(s) of Interest
CYP2D6 *on page 186*
U.S. Brand Names Antihist-1® [OTC]; Tavist®; Tavist®-1 [OTC]
Pharmacologic Class Antihistamine

- **Cleocin®** *see Clindamycin on page 65*
- **Cleocin HCl®** *see Clindamycin on page 65*
- **Cleocin Pediatric®** *see Clindamycin on page 65*
- **Cleocin Phosphate®** *see Clindamycin on page 65*
- **Cleocin T®** *see Clindamycin on page 65*
- **Climara®** *see Estradiol on page 80*
- **Clindagel™** *see Clindamycin on page 65*

Clindamycin (klin da MYE sin)
Gene(s) of Interest None known
U.S. Brand Names Cleocin®; Cleocin HCl®; Cleocin Pediatric®; Cleocin Phosphate®; Cleocin T®; Clindagel™; Clindets®
Canadian Brand Names Alti-Clindamycin; Dalacin® C; Dalacin® T; Dalacin® Vaginal
Pharmacologic Class Antibiotic, Miscellaneous

- **Clindets®** *see Clindamycin on page 65*
- **Clinoril®** *see Sulindac on page 144*

Clobazam (KLOE ba zam)
Gene(s) of Interest
CYP3A4 *on page 189*
(Continued)

Clobazam *(Continued)*
Canadian Brand Names Alti-Clobazam; Frisium®; Novo-Clobazam; PMS-Clobazam
Pharmacologic Class Benzodiazepine

Clofibrate (kloe FYE brate)
Gene(s) of Interest
Angiotensin-Converting Enzyme *on page 163*
Cholesteryl Ester Transfer Protein *on page 179*
U.S. Brand Names Atromid-S®
Pharmacologic Class Antilipemic Agent, Fibric Acid

ClomiPRAMINE (kloe MI pra meen)
Gene(s) of Interest
Alpha-1 Adrenergic Receptor *on page 161*
CYP1A2 *on page 181*
CYP2C19 *on page 185*
CYP2D6 *on page 186*
G-Protein Beta-3 Subunit *on page 197*
Gs Protein Alpha-Subunit *on page 198*
U.S. Brand Names Anafranil®
Canadian Brand Names Apo®-Clomipramine; Gen-Clomipramine; Novo-Clopramine
Pharmacologic Class Antidepressant, Tricyclic (Tertiary Amine)

Clonazepam (kloe NA ze pam)
Gene(s) of Interest
CYP3A4 *on page 189*
U.S. Brand Names Klonopin™
Canadian Brand Names Alti-Clonazepam; Apo®-Clonazepam; Clonapam; Gen-Clonazepam; Novo-Clonazepam; Nu-Clonazepam; PMS-Clonazepam; Rho-Clonazepam; Rivotril®
Pharmacologic Class Benzodiazepine

Clonidine (KLON i deen)
Gene(s) of Interest None known
U.S. Brand Names Catapres®; Catapres-TTS®-1; Catapres-TTS®-2; Catapres-TTS®-3; Duraclon™
Canadian Brand Names Apo®-Clonidine; Carapres®; Dixarit®; Novo-Clonidine®; Nu-Clonidine®
Pharmacologic Class Alpha$_2$-Adrenergic Agonist

Clopidogrel (kloh PID oh grel)
Gene(s) of Interest
Glycoprotein IIIa Receptor *on page 196*
U.S. Brand Names Plavix®
Pharmacologic Class Antiplatelet Agent

Clorazepate (klor AZ e pate)
Gene(s) of Interest
 CYP3A4 *on page 189*
U.S. Brand Names Tranxene®
Canadian Brand Names Apo®-Clorazepate; Novo-Clopate®
Pharmacologic Class Benzodiazepine

Clozapine (KLOE za peen)
Gene(s) of Interest
 Alpha-1 Adrenergic Receptor *on page 161*
 Beta-3 Adrenergic Receptor *on page 174*
 CYP1A2 *on page 181*
 D2 Receptor *on page 190*
 D3 Receptor *on page 191*
 D4 Receptor *on page 192*
 G-Protein Beta-3 Subunit *on page 197*
 Gs Protein Alpha-Subunit *on page 198*
 Histamine 1 and 2 Receptors *on page 199*
 HLA-A1 *on page 200*
 5HT1A Receptor *on page 200*
 5HT2A Receptor *on page 201*
 5HT2C Receptor *on page 202*
 5HT6 Receptor *on page 203*
 5HT Transporter *on page 204*
 TNF-Alpha *on page 222*
U.S. Brand Names Clozaril®
Canadian Brand Names Rhoxal-clozapine
Pharmacologic Class Antipsychotic Agent, Dibenzodiazepine

♦ **Clozaril®** *see* Clozapine *on page 67*

Cocaine (koe KANE)
Gene(s) of Interest
 CYP2D6 *on page 186*
 CYP3A4 *on page 189*
Pharmacologic Class Local Anesthetic

Codeine (KOE deen)
Gene(s) of Interest
 COMT *on page 180*
 CYP2D6 *on page 186*
Synonyms Methylmorphine
Pharmacologic Class Analgesic, Narcotic; Antitussive

♦ **Codeine, Acetaminophen, Butalbital, and Caffeine** *see* Butalbital, Acetaminophen, Caffeine, and Codeine *on page 58*
♦ **Codeine and Acetaminophen** *see* Acetaminophen and Codeine *on page 44*
♦ **Codeine and Aspirin** *see* Aspirin and Codeine *on page 52*
♦ **Codeine and Butalbital Compound** *see* Butalbital, Aspirin, Caffeine, and Codeine *on page 59*

COLCHICINE

- **Codeine and Promethazine** see Promethazine and Codeine on page 131
- **Codeine, Butalbital, Aspirin, and Caffeine** see Butalbital, Aspirin, Caffeine, and Codeine on page 59
- **Co-Gesic®** see Hydrocodone and Acetaminophen on page 94
- **Cognex®** see Tacrine on page 144

Colchicine (KOL chi seen)
Gene(s) of Interest
CYP3A4 on page 189
Canadian Brand Names ratio-Colchicine
Pharmacologic Class Colchicine

- **Colocort™** see Hydrocortisone on page 95
- **Combivent®** see Ipratropium and Albuterol on page 98
- **Compazine®** see Prochlorperazine on page 130
- **Compound F** see Hydrocortisone on page 95
- **Compro™** see Prochlorperazine on page 130
- **Concerta®** see Methylphenidate on page 111
- **Cordarone®** see Amiodarone on page 48
- **Coreg®** see Carvedilol on page 61
- **Corgard®** see Nadolol on page 116
- **CortaGel® Maximum Strength [OTC]** see Hydrocortisone on page 95
- **Cortaid® Intensive Therapy [OTC]** see Hydrocortisone on page 95
- **Cortaid® Maximum Strength [OTC]** see Hydrocortisone on page 95
- **Cortaid® Sensitive Skin With Aloe [OTC]** see Hydrocortisone on page 95
- **Cortef®** see Hydrocortisone on page 95
- **Corticool® [OTC]** see Hydrocortisone on page 95
- **Cortifoam®** see Hydrocortisone on page 95
- **Cortisol** see Hydrocortisone on page 95
- **Cortizone®-5 [OTC]** see Hydrocortisone on page 95
- **Cortizone®-10 Maximum Strength [OTC]** see Hydrocortisone on page 95
- **Cortizone®-10 Plus Maximum Strength [OTC]** see Hydrocortisone on page 95
- **Cortizone® 10 Quick Shot [OTC]** see Hydrocortisone on page 95
- **Cortizone® for Kids [OTC]** see Hydrocortisone on page 95
- **Corvert®** see Ibutilide on page 97
- **Co-Trimoxazole** see Sulfamethoxazole and Trimethoprim on page 143
- **Coumadin®** see Warfarin on page 155
- **Covera-HS®** see Verapamil on page 154
- **Cozaar®** see Losartan on page 105
- **CPM** see Cyclophosphamide on page 69

- **CPT-11** see Irinotecan on page 99
- **CPZ** see ChlorproMAZINE on page 63
- **Crinone®** see Progesterone on page 131
- **Cryselle™** see Ethinyl Estradiol and Norgestrel on page 84
- **Crystodigin** see Digitoxin on page 73
- **CSA** see CycloSPORINE on page 69
- **CTM** see Chlorpheniramine on page 63
- **CTX** see Cyclophosphamide on page 69
- **Cutivate®** see Fluticasone on page 89
- **CyA** see CycloSPORINE on page 69
- **Cyclessa®** see Ethinyl Estradiol and Desogestrel on page 82

Cyclobenzaprine (sye kloe BEN za preen)
Gene(s) of Interest
CYP1A2 on page 181
U.S. Brand Names Flexeril®
Canadian Brand Names Apo®-Cyclobenzaprine; Flexitec; Gen-Cyclobenzaprine; Novo-Cycloprine®; Nu-Cyclobenzaprine
Pharmacologic Class Skeletal Muscle Relaxant

Cyclophosphamide (sye kloe FOS fa mide)
Gene(s) of Interest
CYP2C19 on page 185
U.S. Brand Names Cytoxan®; Neosar®
Canadian Brand Names Procytox®
Synonyms CPM; CTX; CYT; NSC-26271
Pharmacologic Class Antineoplastic Agent, Alkylating Agent

- **Cyclosporin A** see CycloSPORINE on page 69

CycloSPORINE (SYE kloe spor een)
Gene(s) of Interest
CYP3A4 on page 189
P-Glycoprotein on page 213
U.S. Brand Names Gengraf™; Neoral®; Restasis™; Sandimmune®
Canadian Brand Names Rhoxal-cyclosporine; Sandimmune® I.V.
Synonyms CSA; CyA; Cyclosporin A
Pharmacologic Class Immunosuppressant Agent

- **CYT** see Cyclophosphamide on page 69
- **Cytochrome P450 Enzymes: Substrates, Inhibitors, and Inducers** see page 23
- **Cytoxan®** see Cyclophosphamide on page 69

Dacarbazine (da KAR ba zeen)
Gene(s) of Interest
CYP1A2 on page 181
U.S. Brand Names DTIC-Dome®
Canadian Brand Names DTIC®
(Continued)

Dacarbazine *(Continued)*
Synonyms DIC; Dimethyl Triazeno Imidazol Carboxamide; DTIC; Imidazol Carboxamide Dimethyltriazene; Imidazole Carboxamide; WR-139007
Pharmacologic Class Antineoplastic Agent, Alkylating Agent (Triazene)

- **Dalmane®** *see* Flurazepam *on page 88*
- **Damason-P®** *see* Hydrocodone and Aspirin *on page 94*
- **Dantrium®** *see* Dantrolene *on page 70*

Dantrolene (DAN troe leen)
Gene(s) of Interest
CYP3A4 *on page 189*
U.S. Brand Names Dantrium®
Pharmacologic Class Skeletal Muscle Relaxant

Dapsone (DAP sone)
Gene(s) of Interest
CYP3A4 *on page 189*
Glucose-6-Phosphate Dehydrogenase *on page 195*
Synonyms Avlosulfon [DSC]; Diaminodiphenylsulfone
Pharmacologic Class Antibiotic, Miscellaneous

- **Darvocet-N® 50** *see* Propoxyphene and Acetaminophen *on page 132*
- **Darvocet-N® 100** *see* Propoxyphene and Acetaminophen *on page 132*
- **Darvon®** *see* Propoxyphene *on page 132*
- **Darvon® Compound-65 Pulvules®** *see* Propoxyphene and Aspirin *on page 132*
- **Darvon-N®** *see* Propoxyphene *on page 132*
- **Daypro®** *see* Oxaprozin *on page 123*
- **Dehydrobenzperidol** *see* Droperidol *on page 76*
- **Delatestryl®** *see* Testosterone *on page 146*
- **Delestrogen®** *see* Estradiol *on page 80*
- **Deltacortisone** *see* PredniSONE *on page 129*
- **Deltadehydrocortisone** *see* PredniSONE *on page 129*
- **Deltasone®** *see* PredniSONE *on page 129*
- **Demadex®** *see* Torsemide *on page 150*
- **Demerol®** *see* Meperidine *on page 108*
- **Demulen®** *see* Ethinyl Estradiol and Ethynodiol Diacetate *on page 83*
- **Depacon®** *see* Valproic Acid and Derivatives *on page 153*
- **Depakene®** *see* Valproic Acid and Derivatives *on page 153*
- **Depakote® Delayed Release** *see* Valproic Acid and Derivatives *on page 153*
- **Depakote® ER** *see* Valproic Acid and Derivatives *on page 153*
- **Depakote® Sprinkle®** *see* Valproic Acid and Derivatives *on page 153*

DEXRAZOXANE

- **Depo®-Estradiol** *see Estradiol on page 80*
- **Depo-Medrol®** *see MethylPREDNISolone on page 111*
- **Depo-Provera®** *see MedroxyPROGESTERone on page 107*
- **Depo-Provera® Contraceptive** *see MedroxyPROGESTERone on page 107*
- **Depo®-Testosterone** *see Testosterone on page 146*
- **Deprenyl** *see Selegiline on page 139*
- **Dermarest Dricort® [OTC]** *see Hydrocortisone on page 95*
- **Dermtex® HC [OTC]** *see Hydrocortisone on page 95*

Desipramine (des IP ra meen)
Gene(s) of Interest
Alpha-1 Adrenergic Receptor *on page 161*
G-Protein Beta-3 Subunit *on page 197*
Gs Protein Alpha-Subunit *on page 198*
P-Glycoprotein *on page 213*
U.S. Brand Names Norpramin®
Canadian Brand Names Alti-Desipramine; Apo®-Desipramine; Novo-Desipramine; Nu-Desipramine; PMS-Desipramine
Synonyms Desmethylimipramine Hydrochloride
Pharmacologic Class Antidepressant, Tricyclic (Secondary Amine)

Desloratadine (des lor AT a deen)
Gene(s) of Interest None known
U.S. Brand Names Clarinex®
Canadian Brand Names Aerius®
Pharmacologic Class Antihistamine, Nonsedating

- **Desmethylimipramine Hydrochloride** *see Desipramine on page 71*
- **Desogen®** *see Ethinyl Estradiol and Desogestrel on page 82*
- **Desogestrel and Ethinyl Estradiol** *see Ethinyl Estradiol and Desogestrel on page 82*
- **Desyrel®** *see Trazodone on page 151*
- **Detrol®** *see Tolterodine on page 149*
- **Detrol® LA** *see Tolterodine on page 149*

Dexmedetomidine (deks MED e toe mi deen)
Gene(s) of Interest
CYP2D6 *on page 186*
U.S. Brand Names Precedex™
Pharmacologic Class Alpha$_2$-Adrenergic Agonist; Sedative

Dexrazoxane (deks ray ZOKS ane)
Gene(s) of Interest
P-Glycoprotein *on page 213*
U.S. Brand Names Zinecard®
Synonyms ICRF-187
Pharmacologic Class Cardioprotectant

Dextroamphetamine and Amphetamine
(deks troe am FET a meen & am FET a meen)
Gene(s) of Interest None known
U.S. Brand Names Adderall®; Adderall XR™
Synonyms Amphetamine and Dextroamphetamine
Pharmacologic Class Stimulant

- **Dextropropoxyphene** *see* Propoxyphene *on page 132*
- **DHE** *see* Dihydroergotamine *on page 73*
- **D.H.E. 45®** *see* Dihydroergotamine *on page 73*
- **Diaβeta®** *see* GlyBURIDE *on page 92*
- **Diaminodiphenylsulfone** *see* Dapsone *on page 70*
- **Diastat® Rectal Delivery System** *see* Diazepam *on page 72*

Diazepam (dye AZ e pam)
Gene(s) of Interest
CYP2C19 *on page 185*
CYP3A4 *on page 189*
U.S. Brand Names Diastat® Rectal Delivery System; Diazepam Intensol®; Valium®
Canadian Brand Names Apo®-Diazepam; Diastat®; Diazemuls®
Pharmacologic Class Benzodiazepine

- **Diazepam Intensol®** *see* Diazepam *on page 72*
- **DIC** *see* Dacarbazine *on page 69*

Diclofenac (dye KLOE fen ak)
Gene(s) of Interest
Leukotriene C4 Synthase *on page 206*
U.S. Brand Names Cataflam®; Solaraze™; Voltaren®; Voltaren Ophthalmic®; Voltaren®-XR
Canadian Brand Names Apo®-Diclo; Apo®-Diclo Rapide; Apo®-Diclo SR; Diclotec; Novo-Difenac®; Novo-Difenac K; Novo-Difenac-SR®; Nu-Diclo; Nu-Diclo-SR; PMS-Diclofenac; PMS-Diclofenac SR; Riva-Diclofenac; Riva-Diclofenac-K, Voltaren Ophtha®; Voltaren Rapide®
Pharmacologic Class Nonsteroidal Anti-inflammatory Drug (NSAID)

Diclofenac and Misoprostol
(dye KLOE fen ak & mye soe PROST ole)
Gene(s) of Interest
Leukotriene C4 Synthase *on page 206*
U.S. Brand Names Arthrotec®
Synonyms Misoprostol and Diclofenac
Pharmacologic Class Nonsteroidal Anti-inflammatory Drug (NSAID); Prostaglandin

Dicumarol (dye KOO ma role)
Gene(s) of Interest
CYP2C9 *on page 183*
Synonyms Bishydroxycoumarin
Pharmacologic Class Anticoagulant, Coumarin Derivative

- **Didrex®** *see Benzphetamine on page 55*
- **Diflucan®** *see Fluconazole on page 87*

Diflunisal (dye FLOO ni sal)
Gene(s) of Interest
Leukotriene C4 Synthase *on page 206*
U.S. Brand Names Dolobid®
Canadian Brand Names Apo®-Diflunisal; Novo-Diflunisal; Nu-Diflunisal
Pharmacologic Class Nonsteroidal Anti-inflammatory Drug (NSAID)

- **Digitek®** *see Digoxin on page 73*

Digitoxin (di ji TOKS in)
Gene(s) of Interest
CYP3A4 *on page 189*
Synonyms Crystodigin
Pharmacologic Class Antiarrhythmic Agent, Class IV

Digoxin (di JOKS in)
Gene(s) of Interest
P-Glycoprotein *on page 213*
U.S. Brand Names Digitek®; Lanoxicaps®; Lanoxin®
Canadian Brand Names Digoxin CSD; Novo-Digoxin
Pharmacologic Class Antiarrhythmic Agent, Class IV; Cardiac Glycoside

Dihydrocodeine, Aspirin, and Caffeine
(dye hye droe KOE deen, AS pir in, & KAF een)
Gene(s) of Interest
COMT *on page 180*
CYP2D6 *on page 186*
U.S. Brand Names Synalgos®-DC
Synonyms Aspirin, Caffeine, and Dihydrocodeine; Caffeine, Aspirin, and Dihydrocodeine; Dihydrocodeine Compound
Pharmacologic Class Analgesic, Narcotic

- **Dihydrocodeine Compound** *see Dihydrocodeine, Aspirin, and Caffeine on page 73*

Dihydroergotamine (dye hye droe er GOT a meen)
Gene(s) of Interest
CYP3A4 *on page 189*
U.S. Brand Names D.H.E. 45®; Migranal®
Synonyms DHE
Pharmacologic Class Ergot Derivative

- **Dihydroergotoxine** *see Ergoloid Mesylates on page 79*
- **Dihydrogenated Ergot Alkaloids** *see Ergoloid Mesylates on page 79*
- **Dihydrohydroxycodeinone** *see Oxycodone on page 123*
- **Dihydromorphinone** *see Hydromorphone on page 96*

DILTIAZEM

- **Dihydroxydeoxynorvinkaleukoblastine** *see* Vinorelbine *on page 155*
- **Dilacor® XR** *see* Diltiazem *on page 74*
- **Dilantin®** *see* Phenytoin *on page 127*
- **Dilatrate®-SR** *see* Isosorbide Dinitrate *on page 100*
- **Dilaudid®** *see* Hydromorphone *on page 96*
- **Dilaudid-HP®** *see* Hydromorphone *on page 96*
- **Diltia XT®** *see* Diltiazem *on page 74*

Diltiazem (dil TYE a zem)
Gene(s) of Interest
CYP3A4 *on page 189*
P-Glycoprotein *on page 213*
U.S. Brand Names Cardizem®; Cardizem® CD; Cardizem® LA; Cardizem® SR; Cartia XT™; Dilacor® XR; Diltia XT®; Tiazac®
Canadian Brand Names Alti-Diltiazem CD; Apo®-Diltiaz; Apo®-Diltiaz CD; Apo®-Diltiaz SR; Gen-Diltiazem; Gen-Diltiazem SR; Med-Diltiazem; Novo-Diltazem; Novo-Diltiazem-CD; Novo-Diltiazem SR; Nu-Diltiaz; Nu-Diltiaz-CD; ratio-Diltiazem CD; Rhoxal-diltiazem CD; Rhoxal-diltiazem SR; Syn-Diltiazem®
Pharmacologic Class Calcium Channel Blocker

Dimercaprol (dye mer KAP role)
Gene(s) of Interest
Glucose-6-Phosphate Dehydrogenase *on page 195*
U.S. Brand Names BAL in Oil®
Synonyms BAL; British Anti-Lewisite; Dithioglycerol
Pharmacologic Class Antidote

- **Dimethyl Triazeno Imidazol Carboxamide** *see* Dacarbazine *on page 69*
- **Diovan®** *see* Valsartan *on page 153*
- **Diphenylhydantoin** *see* Phenytoin *on page 127*
- **Diprivan®** *see* Propofol *on page 131*
- **Dipropylacetic Acid** *see* Valproic Acid and Derivatives *on page 153*

Dipyridamole (dye peer ID a mole)
Gene(s) of Interest
Glycoprotein IIIa Receptor *on page 196*
P-Glycoprotein *on page 213*
U.S. Brand Names Persantine®
Canadian Brand Names Apo®-Dipyridamole FC; Novo-Dipiradol
Pharmacologic Class Antiplatelet Agent; Vasodilator

- **Dipyridamole and Aspirin** *see* Aspirin and Dipyridamole *on page 52*

Disopyramide (dye soe PEER a mide)
Gene(s) of Interest
Cardiac Potassium Ion Channel *on page 177*

DONEPEZIL

Cardiac Sodium Channel *on page 178*
CYP3A4 *on page 189*
U.S. Brand Names Norpace®; Norpace® CR
Canadian Brand Names Rythmodan®; Rythmodan®-LA
Pharmacologic Class Antiarrhythmic Agent, Class Ia

Disulfiram (dye SUL fi ram)
Gene(s) of Interest
P-Glycoprotein *on page 213*
U.S. Brand Names Antabuse®
Pharmacologic Class Aldehyde Dehydrogenase Inhibitor

- **Dithioglycerol** *see* Dimercaprol *on page 74*
- **Diucardin® [DSC]** *see* Hydroflumethiazide *on page 95*
- **Diuril®** *see* Chlorothiazide *on page 63*
- **Divalproex Sodium** *see* Valproic Acid and Derivatives *on page 153*

Docetaxel (doe se TAKS el)
Gene(s) of Interest
CYP3A4 *on page 189*
U.S. Brand Names Taxotere®
Synonyms NSC-628503; RP-6976
Pharmacologic Class Antineoplastic Agent, Natural Source (Plant) Derivative

Dofetilide (doe FET il ide)
Gene(s) of Interest
Cardiac Potassium Ion Channel *on page 177*
Cardiac Sodium Channel *on page 178*
U.S. Brand Names Tikosyn™
Synonyms UK-68-798
Pharmacologic Class Antiarrhythmic Agent, Class III

- **Dolobid®** *see* Diflunisal *on page 73*
- **Dolophine®** *see* Methadone *on page 110*

Domperidone (dom PE ri done)
Gene(s) of Interest
Cardiac Potassium Ion Channel *on page 177*
Cardiac Sodium Channel *on page 178*
Canadian Brand Names Alti-Domperidone; Apo®-Domperidone; Dom-Domperidone; FTP-Domperidone Maleate; Motilium®; Novo-Domperidone; Nu-Domperidone; Ratio-Domperidone
Pharmacologic Class Dopamine Antagonist, Peripheral

Donepezil (doh NEP e zil)
Gene(s) of Interest
Apolipoprotein E *on page 168*
U.S. Brand Names Aricept®
Synonyms E2020
(Continued)

Donepezil *(Continued)*
Pharmacologic Class Acetylcholinesterase Inhibitor (Central)

♦ **Doryx®** *see* Doxycycline *on page 76*

Doxazosin (doks AY zoe sin)
Gene(s) of Interest None known
U.S. Brand Names Cardura®
Canadian Brand Names Alti-Doxazosin; Apo®-Doxazosin; Cardura-1™; Cardura-2™; Cardura-4™; Gen-Doxazosin; Novo-Doxazosin
Pharmacologic Class Alpha$_1$ Blocker

Doxepin (DOKS e pin)
Gene(s) of Interest
  Alpha-1 Adrenergic Receptor *on page 161*
  CYP1A2 *on page 181*
  CYP3A4 *on page 189*
  G-Protein Beta-3 Subunit *on page 197*
  Gs Protein Alpha-Subunit *on page 198*
  P-Glycoprotein *on page 213*
U.S. Brand Names Prudoxin™; Sinequan®; Zonalon®
Canadian Brand Names Apo®-Doxepin; Novo-Doxepin
Pharmacologic Class Antidepressant, Tricyclic (Tertiary Amine); Topical Skin Product

DOXOrubicin (doks oh ROO bi sin)
Gene(s) of Interest
  CYP3A4 *on page 189*
U.S. Brand Names Adriamycin PFS®; Adriamycin RDF®; Rubex®
Canadian Brand Names Adriamycin®
Synonyms ADR; Adria; Hydroxydaunomycin Hydrochloride; NSC-123127
Pharmacologic Class Antineoplastic Agent, Anthracycline

♦ **Doxy-100®** *see* Doxycycline *on page 76*

Doxycycline (doks i SYE kleen)
Gene(s) of Interest None known
U.S. Brand Names Adoxa™; Doryx®; Doxy-100®; Monodox®; Periostat®; Vibramycin®; Vibra-Tabs®
Canadian Brand Names Apo®-Doxy; Apo®-Doxy Tabs; Doxycin; Doxytec; Novo-Doxylin; Nu-Doxycycline
Pharmacologic Class Antibiotic, Tetracycline Derivative

♦ **DPA** *see* Valproic Acid and Derivatives *on page 153*
♦ **DPH** *see* Phenytoin *on page 127*
♦ **Dramamine® Less Drowsy Formula [OTC]** *see* Meclizine *on page 107*

Droperidol (droe PER i dole)
Gene(s) of Interest
  Alpha-1 Adrenergic Receptor *on page 161*

ELETRIPTAN

    Cardiac Potassium Ion Channel *on page 177*
    Cardiac Sodium Channel *on page 178*
    D2 Receptor *on page 190*
  U.S. Brand Names Inapsine®
  Synonyms Dehydrobenzperidol
  Pharmacologic Class Antiemetic; Antipsychotic Agent, Butyrophenone

- **Drospirenone and Ethinyl Estradiol** *see* Ethinyl Estradiol and Drospirenone *on page 82*
- **DTIC** *see* Dacarbazine *on page 69*
- **DTIC-Dome®** *see* Dacarbazine *on page 69*
- **DTO** *see* Opium Tincture *on page 122*
- **DuoNeb™** *see* Ipratropium and Albuterol *on page 98*
- **DuP 753** *see* Losartan *on page 105*
- **Duraclon™** *see* Clonidine *on page 66*
- **Duragesic®** *see* Fentanyl *on page 86*
- **Duramorph®** *see* Morphine Sulfate *on page 115*
- **Dynacin®** *see* Minocycline *on page 113*
- **DynaCirc®** *see* Isradipine *on page 100*
- **DynaCirc® CR** *see* Isradipine *on page 100*
- **E_2C and MPA** *see* Estradiol and Medroxyprogesterone *on page 81*
- **7E3** *see* Abciximab *on page 44*
- **E2020** *see* Donepezil *on page 75*
- **EarSol® HC** *see* Hydrocortisone *on page 95*
- **Easprin®** *see* Aspirin *on page 51*
- **EC-Naprosyn®** *see* Naproxen *on page 117*
- **Ecotrin® [OTC]** *see* Aspirin *on page 51*
- **Ecotrin® Low Adult Strength [OTC]** *see* Aspirin *on page 51*
- **Ecotrin® Maximum Strength [OTC]** *see* Aspirin *on page 51*
- **E.E.S.®** *see* Erythromycin *on page 79*
- **Effexor®** *see* Venlafaxine *on page 154*
- **Effexor® XR** *see* Venlafaxine *on page 154*
- **Efudex®** *see* Fluorouracil *on page 87*
- **ELA-Max® [OTC]** *see* Lidocaine *on page 103*
- **ELA-Max® 5 [OTC]** *see* Lidocaine *on page 103*
- **Elavil®** *see* Amitriptyline *on page 48*
- **Eldepryl®** *see* Selegiline *on page 139*

Eletriptan (el e TRIP tan)
  Gene(s) of Interest
    CYP3A4 *on page 189*
  U.S. Brand Names Relpax®
  Pharmacologic Class Serotonin 5-HT$_{1B,\ 1D}$ Receptor Agonist

- **Elitek™** *see* Rasburicase *on page 135*
- **Elixophyllin®** *see* Theophylline *on page 147*
- **Elocon®** *see* Mometasone Furoate *on page 114*
- **Emend®** *see* Aprepitant *on page 50*

- **Emgel®** *see Erythromycin on page 79*
- **EMLA®** *see Lidocaine and Prilocaine on page 104*
- **ENA 713** *see Rivastigmine on page 137*

Enalapril (e NAL a pril)
Gene(s) of Interest
Aldosterone Synthase *on page 160*
Angiotensin-Converting Enzyme *on page 163*
Angiotensin II Type I Receptor *on page 166*
Angiotensinogen *on page 167*
Bradykinin B2 Receptor *on page 175*
U.S. Brand Names Vasotec®; Vasotec® I.V.
Synonyms Enalaprilat
Pharmacologic Class Angiotensin-Converting Enzyme (ACE) Inhibitor

- **Enalaprilat** *see Enalapril on page 78*
- **Endocet®** *see Oxycodone and Acetaminophen on page 123*
- **Endodan®** *see Oxycodone and Aspirin on page 123*
- **Enduron®** *see Methyclothiazide on page 110*
- **Enpresse™** *see Ethinyl Estradiol and Levonorgestrel on page 83*
- **Entocort™ EC** *see Budesonide on page 57*
- **Epipodophyllotoxin** *see Etoposide on page 85*
- **Epitol®** *see Carbamazepine on page 60*

Eplerenone (e PLER en one)
Gene(s) of Interest
CYP3A4 *on page 189*
U.S. Brand Names Inspra™
Pharmacologic Class Antihypertensive; Selective Aldosterone Blocker

Eprosartan (ep roe SAR tan)
Gene(s) of Interest
Aldosterone Synthase *on page 160*
Angiotensin-Converting Enzyme *on page 163*
Angiotensin II Type I Receptor *on page 166*
Angiotensinogen *on page 167*
U.S. Brand Names Teveten®
Pharmacologic Class Angiotensin II Receptor Blocker

- **EPT** *see Teniposide on page 146*

Eptifibatide (ep TIF i ba tide)
Gene(s) of Interest
Glycoprotein IIIa Receptor *on page 196*
U.S. Brand Names Integrilin®
Synonyms Intrifiban
Pharmacologic Class Antiplatelet Agent, Glycoprotein IIb/IIIa Inhibitor

Ergoloid Mesylates (ER goe loid MES i lates)
Gene(s) of Interest
CYP3A4 *on page 189*
Canadian Brand Names Hydergine®
Synonyms Dihydroergotoxine; Dihydrogenated Ergot Alkaloids; Hydergine [DSC]
Pharmacologic Class Ergot Derivative

- **Ergomar®** *see Ergotamine on page 79*
- **Ergometrine Maleate** *see Ergonovine on page 79*

Ergonovine (er goe NOE veen)
Gene(s) of Interest
CYP3A4 *on page 189*
Synonyms Ergometrine Maleate
Pharmacologic Class Ergot Derivative

Ergotamine (er GOT a meen)
Gene(s) of Interest
CYP3A4 *on page 189*
U.S. Brand Names Cafergot®; Ergomar®; Wigraine®
Canadian Brand Names Cafergor®
Synonyms Ergotamine Tartrate and Caffeine
Pharmacologic Class Ergot Derivative

- **Ergotamine Tartrate and Caffeine** *see Ergotamine on page 79*
- **Errin™** *see Norethindrone on page 119*
- **Eryc®** *see Erythromycin on page 79*
- **Erycette®** *see Erythromycin on page 79*
- **Eryderm®** *see Erythromycin on page 79*
- **Erygel®** *see Erythromycin on page 79*
- **EryPed®** *see Erythromycin on page 79*
- **Ery-Tab®** *see Erythromycin on page 79*
- **Erythra-Derm™** *see Erythromycin on page 79*
- **Erythrocin®** *see Erythromycin on page 79*

Erythromycin (er ith roe MYE sin)
Gene(s) of Interest
Cardiac Potassium Ion Channel *on page 177*
Cardiac Sodium Channel *on page 178*
CYP3A4 *on page 189*
P-Glycoprotein *on page 213*
U.S. Brand Names Akne-Mycin®; A/T/S®; E.E.S.®; Emgel®; Eryc®; Erycette®; Eryderm®; Erygel®; EryPed®; Ery-Tab®; Erythra-Derm™; Erythrocin®; PCE®; Romycin®; Staticin®; Theramycin Z®; T-Stat®
Canadian Brand Names Apo®-Erythro Base; Apo®-Erythro E-C; Apo®-Erythro-ES; Apo®-Erythro-S; Diomycin®; Erybid™; Eryc®; Erythromid®; Nu-Erythromycin-S; PMS-Erythromycin
Pharmacologic Class Antibiotic, Macrolide; Antibiotic, Ophthalmic; Antibiotic, Topical; Topical Skin Product; Topical Skin Product, Acne

Erythromycin and Sulfisoxazole
(er ith roe MYE sin & sul fi SOKS a zole)
Gene(s) of Interest
CYP2C9 *on page 183*
Cardiac Potassium Ion Channel *on page 177*
Cardiac Sodium Channel *on page 178*
CYP3A4 *on page 189*
Glucose-6-Phosphate Dehydrogenase *on page 195*
N-Acetyltransferase 2 Enzyme *on page 211*
P-Glycoprotein *on page 213*
U.S. Brand Names Eryzole®; Pediazole®
Synonyms Sulfisoxazole and Erythromycin
Pharmacologic Class Antibiotic, Macrolide; Antibiotic, Macrolide Combination; Antibiotic, Sulfonamide Derivative

♦ **Eryzole®** *see* Erythromycin and Sulfisoxazole *on page 80*

Escitalopram (es sye TAL oh pram)
Gene(s) of Interest
CYP2C19 *on page 185*
CYP3A4 *on page 189*
G-Protein Beta-3 Subunit *on page 197*
Gs Protein Alpha-Subunit *on page 198*
5HT Transporter *on page 204*
U.S. Brand Names Lexapro™
Synonyms Lu-26-054; S-Citalopram
Pharmacologic Class Antidepressant, Selective Serotonin Reuptake Inhibitor

♦ **Esclim®** *see* Estradiol *on page 80*

Esmolol (ES moe lol)
Gene(s) of Interest
Beta-1 Adrenergic Receptor *on page 171*
Gs Protein Alpha-Subunit *on page 198*
U.S. Brand Names Brevibloc®
Pharmacologic Class Antiarrhythmic Agent, Class II; Beta Blocker, Beta₁ Selective

Esomeprazole (es oh ME pray zol)
Gene(s) of Interest None known
U.S. Brand Names Nexium®
Pharmacologic Class Proton Pump Inhibitor

♦ **Esterified Estrogens** *see* Estrogens (Esterified) *on page 82*
♦ **Estrace®** *see* Estradiol *on page 80*
♦ **Estraderm®** *see* Estradiol *on page 80*

Estradiol (es tra DYE ole)
Gene(s) of Interest
CYP1A2 *on page 181*

Factor V *on page 194*
Prothrombin *on page 219*

U.S. Brand Names Alora®; Climara®; Delestrogen; Depo®-Estradiol; Esclim®; Estrace®; Estraderm®; Estring®; Femring™; Gynodiol®; Vagifem®; Vivelle®; Vivelle-Dot®

Canadian Brand Names Estradot®; Estrogel®; Oesclim®

Pharmacologic Class Estrogen Derivative

Estradiol and Medroxyprogesterone
(es tra DYE ole & me DROKS ee proe JES te rone)

Gene(s) of Interest
CYP1A2 *on page 181*
BRCA Genes *on page 176*
Factor V *on page 194*
Prothrombin *on page 219*

U.S. Brand Names Lunelle™

Synonyms E_2C and MPA; Medroxyprogesterone Acetate and Estradiol Cypionate; Medroxyprogesterone and Estradiol

Pharmacologic Class Contraceptive

- **Estratab® [DSC]** *see* Estrogens (Esterified) *on page 82*
- **Estring®** *see* Estradiol *on page 80*
- **Estrogenic Substances, Conjugated** *see* Estrogens (Conjugated/Equine) *on page 81*

Estrogens (Conjugated A/Synthetic)
(ES troe jenz, KON joo gate ed, aye, sin THET ik)

Gene(s) of Interest
CYP1A2 *on page 181*
Factor V *on page 194*
Prothrombin *on page 219*

U.S. Brand Names Cenestin®

Pharmacologic Class Estrogen Derivative

Estrogens (Conjugated/Equine)
(ES troe jenz KON joo gate ed, EE kwine)

Gene(s) of Interest
CYP1A2 *on page 181*
Factor V *on page 194*
Prothrombin *on page 219*

U.S. Brand Names Premarin®

Canadian Brand Names Cenestin; C.E.S.®; Congest

Synonyms C.E.S.; Estrogenic Substances, Conjugated

Pharmacologic Class Estrogen Derivative

Estrogens (Conjugated/Equine) and Medroxyprogesterone
(ES troe jenz KON joo gate ed & me DROKS ee proe JES te rone)

Gene(s) of Interest
Factor V *on page 194*
(Continued)

ESTROGENS (ESTERIFIED)

Estrogens (Conjugated/Equine) and Medroxyprogesterone *(Continued)*
Prothrombin *on page 219*
U.S. Brand Names Premphase®; Prempro™
Canadian Brand Names Premplus®
Synonyms Medroxyprogesterone and Estrogens (Conjugated); MPA and Estrogens (Conjugated)
Pharmacologic Class Estrogen Derivative

Estrogens (Esterified) (ES troe jenz, es TER i fied)
Gene(s) of Interest
CYP1A2 *on page 181*
Factor V *on page 194*
Prothrombin *on page 219*
U.S. Brand Names Estratab® [DSC]; Menest®
Canadian Brand Names Estratab®
Synonyms Esterified Estrogens
Pharmacologic Class Estrogen Derivative

Estropipate (ES troe pih pate)
Gene(s) of Interest
CYP1A2 *on page 181*
Factor V *on page 194*
Prothrombin *on page 219*
U.S. Brand Names Ogen®; Ortho-Est®
Synonyms Ortho Est; Piperazine Estrone Sulfate
Pharmacologic Class Estrogen Derivative

♦ **Estrostep® 21 [DSC]** *see* Ethinyl Estradiol and Norethindrone *on page 84*
♦ **Estrostep® Fe** *see* Ethinyl Estradiol and Norethindrone *on page 84*

Ethinyl Estradiol and Desogestrel
(ETH in il es tra DYE ole & des oh JES trel)
Gene(s) of Interest
BRCA Genes *on page 176*
Factor V *on page 194*
Prothrombin *on page 219*
U.S. Brand Names Apri®; Cyclessa®; Desogen®; Kariva™; Mircette®; Ortho-Cept®
Canadian Brand Names Marvelon®
Synonyms Desogestrel and Ethinyl Estradiol
Pharmacologic Class Contraceptive; Estrogen and Progestin Combination

Ethinyl Estradiol and Drospirenone
(ETH in il es tra DYE ole & droh SPYE re none)
Gene(s) of Interest
BRCA Genes *on page 176*

ETHINYL ESTRADIOL AND NORELGESTROMIN

Factor V *on page 194*
Prothrombin *on page 219*
U.S. Brand Names Yasmin®
Synonyms Drospirenone and Ethinyl Estradiol
Pharmacologic Class Contraceptive

Ethinyl Estradiol and Ethynodiol Diacetate
(ETH in il es tra DYE ole & e thye noe DYE ole dye AS e tate)
Gene(s) of Interest
BRCA Genes *on page 176*
Factor V *on page 194*
Prothrombin *on page 219*
U.S. Brand Names Demulen®; Zovia™
Canadian Brand Names Demulen® 30
Synonyms Ethynodiol Diacetate and Ethinyl Estradiol
Pharmacologic Class Contraceptive; Estrogen and Progestin Combination

Ethinyl Estradiol and Etonogestrel
(ETH in il es tra DYE ole & et oh noe JES trel)
Gene(s) of Interest
BRCA Genes *on page 176*
Factor V *on page 194*
Prothrombin *on page 219*
U.S. Brand Names NuvaRing®
Synonyms Etonogestrel and Ethinyl Estradiol
Pharmacologic Class Contraceptive; Estrogen and Progestin Combination

Ethinyl Estradiol and Levonorgestrel
(ETH in il es tra DYE ole & LEE voe nor jes trel)
Gene(s) of Interest
BRCA Genes *on page 176*
Factor V *on page 194*
Prothrombin *on page 219*
U.S. Brand Names Alesse®; Aviane™; Enpresse™; Lessina™; Levlen®; Levlite™; Levora®; Nordette®; Portia™; PREVEN®; Tri-Levlen®; Triphasil®; Trivora®
Canadian Brand Names Min-Ovral®; Triquilar®
Synonyms Levonorgestrel and Ethinyl Estradiol
Pharmacologic Class Contraceptive

♦ **Ethinyl Estradiol and NGM** *see* Ethinyl Estradiol and Norgestimate *on page 84*

Ethinyl Estradiol and Norelgestromin
(ETH in il es tra DYE ole & nor el JES troe min)
Gene(s) of Interest
BRCA Genes *on page 176*
Factor V *on page 194*
Prothrombin *on page 219*
(Continued)

Ethinyl Estradiol and Norelgestromin
(Continued)

U.S. Brand Names Ortho Evra™

Canadian Brand Names Evra™

Synonyms Norelgestromin and Ethinyl Estradiol

Pharmacologic Class Contraceptive; Estrogen and Progestin Combination

Ethinyl Estradiol and Norethindrone
(ETH in il es tra DYE ole & nor eth IN drone)

Gene(s) of Interest
BRCA Genes *on page 176*
Factor V *on page 194*
Prothrombin *on page 219*

U.S. Brand Names Brevicon®; Estrostep® 21 [DSC]; Estrostep® Fe; femhrt®; Loestrin®; Loestrin® Fe; Microgestin™ Fe; Modicon®; Necon® 0.5/35; Necon® 1/35; Necon® 7/7/7; Necon® 10/11; Norinyl® 1+35; Nortrel™; Nortrel® 7/7/7; Ortho-Novum®; Ovcon®; Tri-Norinyl®

Canadian Brand Names Brevicon® 0.5/35; Brevicon® 1/35; FemHRT®; Loestrin™ 1.5.30; Minestrin™ 1/20; Ortho® 0.5/35; Ortho® 1/35; Ortho® 7/7/7; Select™ 1/35; Synphasic®

Synonyms Norethindrone Acetate and Ethinyl Estradiol

Pharmacologic Class Contraceptive; Estrogen and Progestin Combination

Ethinyl Estradiol and Norgestimate
(ETH in il es tra DYE ole & nor JES ti mate)

Gene(s) of Interest
BRCA Genes *on page 176*
Factor V *on page 194*
Prothrombin *on page 219*

U.S. Brand Names Ortho-Cyclen®; Ortho Tri-Cyclen®; Ortho Tri-Cyclen® Lo; Sprintec™

Canadian Brand Names Cyclen®; Tri-Cyclen®

Synonyms Ethinyl Estradiol and NGM; Norgestimate and Ethinyl Estradiol

Pharmacologic Class Contraceptive; Estrogen and Progestin Combination

Ethinyl Estradiol and Norgestrel
(ETH in il es tra DYE ole & nor JES trel)

Gene(s) of Interest
BRCA Genes *on page 176*
Factor V *on page 194*
Prothrombin *on page 219*

U.S. Brand Names Cryselle™; Lo/Ovral®; Low-Ogestrel®; Ogestrel®; Ovral®

Synonyms Morning After Pill; Norgestrel and Ethinyl Estradiol

FELBAMATE

Pharmacologic Class Contraceptive; Estrogen and Progestin Combination

♦ **Ethmozine®** *see Moricizine on page 115*

Ethosuximide (eth oh SUKS i mide)
Gene(s) of Interest
CYP3A4 *on page 189*
U.S. Brand Names Zarontin®
Pharmacologic Class Anticonvulsant, Succinimide

♦ **Ethynodiol Diacetate and Ethinyl Estradiol** *see Ethinyl Estradiol and Ethynodiol Diacetate on page 83*

Etodolac (ee toe DOE lak)
Gene(s) of Interest
Leukotriene C4 Synthase *on page 206*
U.S. Brand Names Lodine®; Lodine® XL
Canadian Brand Names Apo®-Etodolac; Utradol™
Pharmacologic Class Nonsteroidal Anti-inflammatory Drug (NSAID)

♦ **Etonogestrel and Ethinyl Estradiol** *see Ethinyl Estradiol and Etonogestrel on page 83*

Etoposide (e toe POE side)
Gene(s) of Interest
CYP3A4 *on page 189*
U.S. Brand Names Toposar®; VePesid®
Synonyms Epipodophyllotoxin; VP-16; VP-16-213
Pharmacologic Class Antineoplastic Agent, Podophyllotoxin Derivative

♦ **Etrafon®** *see Amitriptyline and Perphenazine on page 49*
♦ **Eulexin®** *see Flutamide on page 89*
♦ **Evista®** *see Raloxifene on page 134*
♦ **Exelon®** *see Rivastigmine on page 137*

Famotidine (fa MOE ti deen)
Gene(s) of Interest None known
U.S. Brand Names Pepcid®; Pepcid® AC [OTC]
Canadian Brand Names Apo®-Famotidine; Gen-Famotidine; Novo-Famotidine; Nu-Famotidine; Pepcid® I.V.; ratio-Famotidine; Rhoxal-famotidine; Riva-Famotidine
Pharmacologic Class Histamine H_2 Antagonist

♦ **Fansidar®** *see Sulfadoxine and Pyrimethamine on page 143*

Felbamate (FEL ba mate)
Gene(s) of Interest
CYP3A4 *on page 189*
U.S. Brand Names Felbatol®
Pharmacologic Class Anticonvulsant, Miscellaneous

♦ **Felbatol®** *see Felbamate on page 85*

- ♦ **Feldene®** *see Piroxicam on page 128*

Felodipine (fe LOE di peen)
Gene(s) of Interest
CYP3A4 *on page 189*
P-Glycoprotein *on page 213*
U.S. Brand Names Plendil®
Canadian Brand Names Renedil®
Pharmacologic Class Calcium Channel Blocker

- ♦ **femhrt®** *see Ethinyl Estradiol and Norethindrone on page 84*
- ♦ **Femring™** *see Estradiol on page 80*

Fenofibrate (fen oh FYE brate)
Gene(s) of Interest
Angiotensin-Converting Enzyme *on page 163*
Cholesteryl Ester Transfer Protein *on page 179*
U.S. Brand Names TriCor®
Canadian Brand Names Apo®-Fenofibrate; Apo®-Feno-Micro; Gen-Fenofibrate Micro; Lipidil Micro®; Lipidil Supra®; Novo-Fenofibrate; Nu-Fenofibrate; PMS-Fenofibrate Micro
Synonyms Procetofene; Proctofene
Pharmacologic Class Antilipemic Agent, Fibric Acid

Fenoprofen (fen oh PROE fen)
Gene(s) of Interest
Leukotriene C4 Synthase *on page 206*
U.S. Brand Names Nalfon®
Pharmacologic Class Nonsteroidal Anti-inflammatory Drug (NSAID)

Fenoterol (fen oh TER ole)
Gene(s) of Interest
Beta-2 Adrenergic Receptor *on page 171*
Canadian Brand Names Berotec®
Pharmacologic Class Beta$_2$ Agonist

Fentanyl (FEN ta nil)
Gene(s) of Interest
COMT *on page 180*
CYP3A4 *on page 189*
U.S. Brand Names Actiq®; Duragesic®; Sublimaze®
Pharmacologic Class Analgesic, Narcotic; General Anesthetic

- ♦ **Feratab® [OTC]** *see Ferrous Sulfate on page 87*
- ♦ **Fer-Gen-Sol [OTC]** *see Ferrous Sulfate on page 87*
- ♦ **Fer-In-Sol® [OTC]** *see Ferrous Sulfate on page 87*
- ♦ **Fer-Iron® [OTC]** *see Ferrous Sulfate on page 87*

FLUOROURACIL

Ferrous Sulfate (FER us SUL fate)
Gene(s) of Interest None known
U.S. Brand Names Feratab® [OTC]; Fer-Gen-Sol [OTC]; Fer-In-Sol® [OTC]; Fer-Iron® [OTC]; Slow FE® [OTC]
Canadian Brand Names Apo®-Ferrous Sulfate; Ferodan™
Synonyms FeSO$_4$; Iron Sulfate
Pharmacologic Class Iron Salt

♦ **FeSO$_4$** see Ferrous Sulfate on page 87

Fexofenadine (feks oh FEN a deen)
Gene(s) of Interest
  P-Glycoprotein on page 213
U.S. Brand Names Allegra®
Pharmacologic Class Antihistamine, Nonsedating

♦ **Fioricet® with Codeine** see Butalbital, Acetaminophen, Caffeine, and Codeine on page 58
♦ **Fiorinal® With Codeine** see Butalbital, Aspirin, Caffeine, and Codeine on page 59
♦ **FK506** see Tacrolimus on page 144
♦ **Flagyl®** see Metronidazole on page 112
♦ **Flagyl ER®** see Metronidazole on page 112

Flecainide (fle KAY nide)
Gene(s) of Interest
  Cardiac Potassium Ion Channel on page 177
  Cardiac Sodium Channel on page 178
  CYP2D6 on page 186
U.S. Brand Names Tambocor™
Pharmacologic Class Antiarrhythmic Agent, Class Ic

♦ **Flexeril®** see Cyclobenzaprine on page 69
♦ **Flomax®** see Tamsulosin on page 145
♦ **Flonase®** see Fluticasone on page 89
♦ **Flovent®** see Fluticasone on page 89
♦ **Flovent® Rotadisk®** see Fluticasone on page 89
♦ **Floxin®** see Ofloxacin on page 121

Fluconazole (floo KOE na zole)
Gene(s) of Interest None known
U.S. Brand Names Diflucan®
Canadian Brand Names Apo®-Fluconazole
Pharmacologic Class Antifungal Agent, Oral; Antifungal Agent, Parenteral

♦ **Fluoroplex®** see Fluorouracil on page 87

Fluorouracil (flure oh YOOR a sil)
Gene(s) of Interest
  Dihydropyrimidine Dehydrogenase on page 193
  (Continued)

Fluorouracil *(Continued)*
Methylenetetrahydrofolate Reductase *on page 210*
Thymydilate Synthetase *on page 221*
U.S. Brand Names Adrucil®; Carac™; Efudex®; Fluoroplex®
Synonyms 5-Fluorouracil; FU; 5-FU
Pharmacologic Class Antineoplastic Agent, Antimetabolite

♦ **5-Fluorouracil** *see* Fluorouracil *on page 87*

Fluoxetine (floo OKS e teen)
Gene(s) of Interest
Cardiac Potassium Ion Channel *on page 177*
Cardiac Sodium Channel *on page 178*
CYP2C9 *on page 183*
CYP2D6 *on page 186*
G-Protein Beta-3 Subunit *on page 197*
Gs Protein Alpha-Subunit *on page 198*
5HT Transporter *on page 204*

U.S. Brand Names Prozac®; Prozac® Weekly™; Sarafem™
Canadian Brand Names Alti-Fluoxetine; Apo®-Fluoxetine; CO Fluoxetine; Gen-Fluoxetine; Novo-Fluoxetine; Nu-Fluoxetine; PMS-Fluoxetine; Rhoxal-fluoxetine
Pharmacologic Class Antidepressant, Selective Serotonin Reuptake Inhibitor

Flupenthixol (floo pen THIKS ol)
Gene(s) of Interest
Alpha-1 Adrenergic Receptor *on page 161*
Cardiac Potassium Ion Channel *on page 177*
Cardiac Sodium Channel *on page 178*
D2 Receptor *on page 190*

Canadian Brand Names Fluanxol®
Pharmacologic Class Antipsychotic Agent, Thioxanthene Derivative

Fluphenazine (floo FEN a zeen)
Gene(s) of Interest
Alpha-1 Adrenergic Receptor *on page 161*
D2 Receptor *on page 190*
P-Glycoprotein *on page 213*

U.S. Brand Names Prolixin®; Prolixin Decanoate®; Prolixin Enanthate® [DSC]
Canadian Brand Names Apo®-Fluphenazine; Apo®-Fluphenazine Decanoate; Modecate®; Moditen® Enanthate; Moditen® HCl; PMS-Fluphenazine Decanoate
Pharmacologic Class Antipsychotic Agent, Phenothiazine, Piperazine

Flurazepam (flure AZ e pam)
Gene(s) of Interest
CYP3A4 *on page 189*

U.S. Brand Names Dalmane®
Canadian Brand Names Apo®-Flurazepam
Pharmacologic Class Benzodiazepine

Flurbiprofen (flure BI proe fen)
Gene(s) of Interest
Leukotriene C4 Synthase *on page 206*
U.S. Brand Names Ansaid®; Ocufen®
Canadian Brand Names Alti-Flurbiprofen; Apo®-Flurbiprofen; Froben®; Froben-SR®; Novo-Flurprofen; Nu-Flurprofen
Pharmacologic Class Nonsteroidal Anti-inflammatory Drug (NSAID)

Flutamide (FLOO ta mide)
Gene(s) of Interest
CYP1A2 *on page 181*
CYP3A4 *on page 189*
U.S. Brand Names Eulexin®
Canadian Brand Names Apo®-Flutamide; Euflex®; Novo-Flutamide; PMS-Flutamide
Synonyms Niftolid; 4'-Nitro-3'-Trifluoromethylisobutyrantide; NSC-147834; SCH 13521
Pharmacologic Class Antineoplastic Agent, Antiandrogen

Fluticasone (floo TIK a sone)
Gene(s) of Interest None known
U.S. Brand Names Cutivate®; Flonase®; Flovent®; Flovent® Rotadisk®
Canadian Brand Names Flovent® HFA
Pharmacologic Class Corticosteroid, Inhalant (Oral); Corticosteroid, Nasal; Corticosteroid, Topical; Corticosteroid, Topical (Medium Potency)

Fluticasone and Salmeterol
(floo TIK a sone & sal ME te role)
Gene(s) of Interest Beta-2 Adrenergic Receptor *on page 171*
U.S. Brand Names Advair™ Diskus®
Synonyms Salmeterol and Fluticasone
Pharmacologic Class Beta$_2$ Agonist; Corticosteroid, Inhalant (Oral)

Fluvastatin (FLOO va sta tin)
Gene(s) of Interest
Angiotensin-Converting Enzyme *on page 163*
Apolipoprotein E *on page 168*
Beta-Fibrinogen *on page 174*
Cholesteryl Ester Transfer Protein *on page 179*
Glycoprotein IIIa Receptor *on page 196*
Low-Density Lipoprotein Receptor *on page 209*
Stromelysin-1 *on page 219*
U.S. Brand Names Lescol®; Lescol® XL
Pharmacologic Class Antilipemic Agent, HMG-CoA Reductase Inhibitor

FLUVOXAMINE

Fluvoxamine (floo VOKS a meen)
Gene(s) of Interest
CYP1A2 *on page 181*
G-Protein Beta-3 Subunit *on page 197*
Gs Protein Alpha-Subunit *on page 198*
5HT Transporter *on page 204*
U.S. Brand Names Luvox® [DSC]
Canadian Brand Names Alti-Fluvoxamine; Apo®-Fluvoxamine; Novo-Fluvoxamine; Nu-Fluvoxamine; PMS-Fluvoxamine
Pharmacologic Class Antidepressant, Selective Serotonin Reuptake Inhibitor

♦ **Foradil® Aerolizer™** *see* Formoterol *on page 90*

Formoterol (for MOH te rol)
Gene(s) of Interest
Beta-2 Adrenergic Receptor *on page 171*
U.S. Brand Names Foradil® Aerolizer™
Canadian Brand Names Foradil®; Oxeze® Turbuhaler®
Pharmacologic Class Beta$_2$ Agonist

♦ **Fortovase®** *see* Saquinavir *on page 139*
♦ **Fosamax®** *see* Alendronate *on page 46*

Foscarnet (fos KAR net)
Gene(s) of Interest
Cardiac Potassium Ion Channel *on page 177*
Cardiac Sodium Channel *on page 178*
U.S. Brand Names Foscavir®
Synonyms PFA; Phosphonoformate; Phosphonoformic Acid
Pharmacologic Class Antiviral Agent

♦ **Foscavir®** *see* Foscarnet *on page 90*

Fosinopril (foe SIN oh pril)
Gene(s) of Interest
Aldosterone Synthase *on page 160*
Angiotensin-Converting Enzyme *on page 163*
Angiotensin II Type I Receptor *on page 166*
Angiotensinogen *on page 167*
Bradykinin B2 Receptor *on page 175*
U.S. Brand Names Monopril®
Pharmacologic Class Angiotensin-Converting Enzyme (ACE) Inhibitor

Fosphenytoin (FOS fen i toyn)
Gene(s) of Interest
CYP2C9 *on page 183*
CYP2C19 *on page 185*
U.S. Brand Names Cerebyx®
Pharmacologic Class Anticonvulsant, Hydantoin

♦ **Frusemide** *see* Furosemide *on page 91*

GEMFIBROZIL

- **FU** *see* Fluorouracil *on page 87*
- **5-FU** *see* Fluorouracil *on page 87*
- **Furadantin®** *see* Nitrofurantoin *on page 119*

Furazolidone (fyoor a ZOE li done)
Gene(s) of Interest
Glucose-6-Phosphate Dehydrogenase *on page 195*
Canadian Brand Names Furoxone®
Pharmacologic Class Antiprotozoal

Furosemide (fyoor OH se mide)
Gene(s) of Interest
Alpha-Adducin *on page 162*
U.S. Brand Names Lasix®
Canadian Brand Names Apo®-Furosemide; Lasix® Special
Synonyms Frusemide
Pharmacologic Class Diuretic, Loop

Gabapentin (GA ba pen tin)
Gene(s) of Interest None known
U.S. Brand Names Neurontin®
Canadian Brand Names Apo®-Gabapentin; Novo-Gabapentin; PMS-Gabapentin
Pharmacologic Class Anticonvulsant, Miscellaneous

- **Gabitril®** *see* Tiagabine *on page 148*

Galantamine (ga LAN ta meen)
Gene(s) of Interest
Apolipoprotein E *on page 168*
U.S. Brand Names Reminyl®
Pharmacologic Class Acetylcholinesterase Inhibitor (Central)

- **Gantrisin®** *see* SulfiSOXAZOLE *on page 144*

Gatifloxacin (gat i FLOKS a sin)
Gene(s) of Interest
Cardiac Potassium Ion Channel *on page 177*
Cardiac Sodium Channel *on page 178*
U.S. Brand Names Tequin®; Zymar™
Pharmacologic Class Antibiotic, Ophthalmic; Antibiotic, Quinolone

Gemfibrozil (jem FI broe zil)
Gene(s) of Interest
Angiotensin-Converting Enzyme *on page 163*
Cholesteryl Ester Transfer Protein *on page 179*
U.S. Brand Names Lopid®
Canadian Brand Names Apo®-Gemfibrozil; Gen-Gemfibrozil; Novo-Gemfibrozil; Nu-Gemfibrozil; PMS-Gemfibrozil
Synonyms Cl-719
Pharmacologic Class Antilipemic Agent, Fibric Acid

GLIMEPIRIDE

- **Genesec® [OTC]** *see* Acetaminophen and Phenyltoloxamine *on page 45*
- **Gengraf™** *see* CycloSPORINE *on page 69*
- **Genpril® [OTC]** *see* Ibuprofen *on page 96*
- **Geodon®** *see* Ziprasidone *on page 157*
- **GI87084B** *see* Remifentanil *on page 135*
- **Gleevec™** *see* Imatinib *on page 97*
- **Glibenclamide** *see* GlyBURIDE *on page 92*

Glimepiride (GLYE me pye ride)
Gene(s) of Interest
CYP2C9 *on page 183*
U.S. Brand Names Amaryl®
Pharmacologic Class Antidiabetic Agent, Sulfonylurea

GlipiZIDE (GLIP i zide)
Gene(s) of Interest
CYP2C9 *on page 183*
U.S. Brand Names Glucotrol®; Glucotrol® XL
Synonyms Glydiazinamide
Pharmacologic Class Antidiabetic Agent, Sulfonylurea

- **Glivec** *see* Imatinib *on page 97*
- **Glucophage®** *see* Metformin *on page 109*
- **Glucophage® XR** *see* Metformin *on page 109*
- **Glucotrol®** *see* GlipiZIDE *on page 92*
- **Glucotrol® XL** *see* GlipiZIDE *on page 92*
- **Glucovance®** *see* Glyburide and Metformin *on page 92*
- **Glybenclamide** *see* GlyBURIDE *on page 92*
- **Glybenzcyclamide** *see* GlyBURIDE *on page 92*

GlyBURIDE (GLYE byoor ide)
Gene(s) of Interest None known
U.S. Brand Names Diaβeta®; Glynase® PresTab®; Micronase®
Canadian Brand Names Albert® Glyburide; Apo®-Glyburide; Euglucon®; Gen-Glybe; Novo-Glyburide; Nu-Glyburide; PMS-Glyburide; ratio-Glyburide
Synonyms Diabeta; Glibenclamide; Glybenclamide; Glybenzcyclamide
Pharmacologic Class Antidiabetic Agent, Sulfonylurea

Glyburide and Metformin (GLYE byoor ide & met FOR min)
Gene(s) of Interest None known
U.S. Brand Names Glucovance®
Synonyms Metformin and Glyburide
Pharmacologic Class Antidiabetic Agent, Biguanide; Antidiabetic Agent, Sulfonylurea

- **Glydiazinamide** *see* GlipiZIDE *on page 92*
- **Glynase® PresTab®** *see* GlyBURIDE *on page 92*

Guanabenz (GWAHN a benz)
Gene(s) of Interest
CYP1A2 *on page 181*
U.S. Brand Names Wytensin® [DSC]
Pharmacologic Class Alpha$_2$-Adrenergic Agonist

- **Gynodiol®** *see* Estradiol *on page 80*
- **Halcion®** *see* Triazolam *on page 151*
- **Haldol®** *see* Haloperidol *on page 93*
- **Haldol® Decanoate** *see* Haloperidol *on page 93*
- **Halfprin® [OTC]** *see* Aspirin *on page 51*

Halofantrine (ha loe FAN trin)
Gene(s) of Interest
Cardiac Potassium Ion Channel *on page 177*
Cardiac Sodium Channel *on page 178*
CYP3A4 *on page 189*
Pharmacologic Class Antimalarial Agent

Haloperidol (ha loe PER i dole)
Gene(s) of Interest
Alpha-1 Adrenergic Receptor *on page 161*
Cardiac Potassium Ion Channel *on page 177*
Cardiac Sodium Channel *on page 178*
CYP2D6 *on page 186*
CYP3A4 *on page 189*
D2 Receptor *on page 190*
D3 Receptor *on page 191*
D4 Receptor *on page 192*
P-Glycoprotein *on page 213*
U.S. Brand Names Haldol®; Haldol® Decanoate
Canadian Brand Names Apo®-Haloperidol; Apo®-Haloperidol LA; Haloperidol-LA Omega; Haloperidol Long Acting; Novo-Peridol; Peridol; PMS-Haloperidol LA
Pharmacologic Class Antipsychotic Agent, Butyrophenone

- **Haltran® [OTC]** *see* Ibuprofen *on page 96*
- **HCTZ** *see* Hydrochlorothiazide *on page 94*
- **Hemril-HC®** *see* Hydrocortisone *on page 95*

Heparin (HEP a rin)
Gene(s) of Interest
Platelet Fc Gamma Receptor *on page 216*
U.S. Brand Names Hep-Lock®
Canadian Brand Names Hepalean®; Hepalean® Leo; Hepalean®-LOK
Pharmacologic Class Anticoagulant

- **Hep-Lock®** *see* Heparin *on page 93*
- **Humalog®** *see* Insulin Preparations *on page 98*
- **Humalog® Mix 75/25™** *see* Insulin Preparations *on page 98*

HYDRALAZINE

- **Humulin® 50/50** *see* Insulin Preparations *on page 98*
- **Humulin® 70/30** *see* Insulin Preparations *on page 98*
- **Humulin® L** *see* Insulin Preparations *on page 98*
- **Humulin® N** *see* Insulin Preparations *on page 98*
- **Humulin® R** *see* Insulin Preparations *on page 98*
- **Humulin® R (Concentrated) U-500** *see* Insulin Preparations *on page 98*
- **Humulin® U** *see* Insulin Preparations *on page 98*
- **Hydergine [DSC]** *see* Ergoloid Mesylates *on page 79*

HydrALAZINE (hye DRAL a zeen)
Gene(s) of Interest
N-Acetyltransferase 2 Enzyme *on page 211*
Canadian Brand Names Apo®-Hydralazine; Apresoline®; Novo-Hylazin; Nu-Hydral
Synonyms Apresoline [DSC]
Pharmacologic Class Vasodilator

- **Hydrocet®** *see* Hydrocodone and Acetaminophen *on page 94*

Hydrochlorothiazide (hye droe klor oh THYE a zide)
Gene(s) of Interest
Alpha-Adducin *on page 162*
G-Protein Beta-3 Subunit *on page 197*
U.S. Brand Names Aquazide® H; Microzide™; Oretic®
Canadian Brand Names Apo®-Hydro; Novo-Hydrazide
Synonyms HCTZ
Pharmacologic Class Diuretic, Thiazide

- **Hydrochlorothiazide and Lisinopril** *see* Lisinopril and Hydrochlorothiazide *on page 104*
- **Hydrochlorothiazide and Losartan** *see* Losartan and Hydrochlorothiazide *on page 105*

Hydrocodone and Acetaminophen
(hye droe KOE done & a seet a MIN oh fen)
Gene(s) of Interest
COMT *on page 180*
U.S. Brand Names Anexsia®; Bancap HC®; Ceta-Plus®; Co-Gesic®; Hydrocet®; Hydrogesic® [DSC]; Lorcet® 10/650; Lorcet®-HD; Lorcet® Plus; Lortab®; Margesic® H; Maxidone™; Norco®; Stagesic®; Vicodin®; Vicodin® ES; Vicodin® HP; Zydone®
Synonyms Acetaminophen and Hydrocodone
Pharmacologic Class Analgesic Combination (Narcotic)

Hydrocodone and Aspirin
(hye droe KOE done & AS pir in)
Gene(s) of Interest
COMT *on page 180*
Glycoprotein IIIa Receptor *on page 196*
Leukotriene C4 Synthase *on page 206*

U.S. Brand Names Damason-P®
Synonyms Aspirin and Hydrocodone
Pharmacologic Class Analgesic Combination (Narcotic)

Hydrocodone and Ibuprofen
(hye droe KOE done & eye byoo PROE fen)
Gene(s) of Interest
COMT *on page 180*
Leukotriene C4 Synthase *on page 206*
U.S. Brand Names Vicoprofen®
Synonyms Ibuprofen and Hydrocodone
Pharmacologic Class Analgesic, Narcotic

Hydrocortisone (hye droe KOR ti sone)
Gene(s) of Interest
P-Glycoprotein *on page 213*
U.S. Brand Names A-hydroCort®; Anucort-HC®; Anusol-HC®; Anusol® HC-1 [OTC]; Aquanil™ HC [OTC]; CaldeCORT® [OTC]; Cetacort®; Colocort™; CortaGel® Maximum Strength [OTC]; Cortaid® Intensive Therapy [OTC]; Cortaid® Maximum Strength [OTC]; Cortaid® Sensitive Skin With Aloe [OTC]; Cortef®; Corticool® [OTC]; Cortifoam®; Cortizone®-5 [OTC]; Cortizone®-10 Maximum Strength [OTC]; Cortizone®-10 Plus Maximum Strength [OTC]; Cortizone® 10 Quick Shot [OTC]; Cortizone® for Kids [OTC]; Dermarest Dricort® [OTC]; Dermtex® HC [OTC]; EarSol® HC; Hemril-HC®; Hydrocortone®; Hydrocortone® Phosphate; Hytone®; LactiCare-HC®; Locoid®; Locoid Lipocream®; Nupercainal® Hydrocortisone Cream [OTC]; Nutracort®; Pandel®; Post Peel Healing Balm [OTC]; Preparation H® Hydrocortisone [OTC]; Proctocort®; ProctoCream® HC; Proctosol-HC®; Sarnol®-HC [OTC]; Solu-Cortef®; Summer's Eve® SpecialCare™ Medicated Anti-Itch Cream [OTC]; Texacort®; Theracort® [OTC]; Westcort®

Canadian Brand Names Aquacort®; Cortamed®; Cortate®; Cortenema®; Cortoderm; Emo-Cort®; Hycort™; Hyderm; HydroVal®; Locoid®; Prevex® HC; Sarna® HC
Synonyms Compound F; Cortisol
Pharmacologic Class Corticosteroid, Rectal; Corticosteroid, Systemic; Corticosteroid, Topical

♦ **Hydrocortone®** *see* Hydrocortisone *on page 95*
♦ **Hydrocortone® Phosphate** *see* Hydrocortisone *on page 95*

Hydroflumethiazide (hye droe floo meth EYE a zide)
Gene(s) of Interest
Alpha-Adducin *on page 162*
G-Protein Beta-3 Subunit *on page 197*
U.S. Brand Names Diucardin® [DSC]; Saluron® [DSC]
Pharmacologic Class Diuretic, Thiazide

♦ **Hydrogesic® [DSC]** *see* Hydrocodone and Acetaminophen *on page 94*

Hydromorphone (hye droe MOR fone)
Gene(s) of Interest
COMT *on page 180*

U.S. Brand Names Dilaudid®; Dilaudid-HP®

Canadian Brand Names Dilaudid-HP-Plus®; Dilaudid® Sterile Powder; Dilaudid-XP®; Hydromorph Contin®; Hydromorphone HP; PMS-Hydromorphone

Synonyms Dihydromorphinone

Pharmacologic Class Analgesic, Narcotic

Hydroxychloroquine (hye droks ee KLOR oh kwin)
Gene(s) of Interest
Glucose-6-Phosphate Dehydrogenase *on page 195*

U.S. Brand Names Plaquenil®

Pharmacologic Class Aminoquinoline (Antimalarial)

◆ **Hydroxydaunomycin Hydrochloride** *see* DOXOrubicin *on page 76*

HydrOXYzine (hye DROKS i zeen)
Gene(s) of Interest
P-Glycoprotein *on page 213*

U.S. Brand Names Atarax®; Vistaril®

Canadian Brand Names Apo®-Hydroxyzine; Novo-Hydroxyzin; PMS-Hydroxyzine

Pharmacologic Class Antiemetic; Antihistamine

◆ **Hygroton [DSC]** *see* Chlorthalidone *on page 63*
◆ **Hytone®** *see* Hydrocortisone *on page 95*
◆ **Hytrin®** *see* Terazosin *on page 146*
◆ **Hyzaar®** *see* Losartan and Hydrochlorothiazide *on page 105*

Ibuprofen (eye byoo PROE fen)
Gene(s) of Interest
Leukotriene C4 Synthase *on page 206*

U.S. Brand Names Advil® [OTC]; Advil® Children's [OTC]; Advil® Infants' Concentrated Drops [OTC]; Advil® Junior [OTC]; Advil® Migraine [OTC]; Genpril® [OTC]; Haltran® [OTC]; Ibu-Tab®; I-Prin [OTC]; Menadol® [OTC]; Midol® Maximum Strength Cramp Formula [OTC]; Motrin®; Motrin® Children's [OTC]; Motrin® IB [OTC]; Motrin® Infants' [OTC]; Motrin® Junior Strength [OTC]; Motrin® Migraine Pain [OTC]

Canadian Brand Names Apo®-Ibuprofen; Novo-Profen®; Nu-Ibuprofen

Synonyms *p*-Isobutylhydratropic Acid

Pharmacologic Class Nonsteroidal Anti-inflammatory Drug (NSAID)

◆ **Ibuprofen and Hydrocodone** *see* Hydrocodone and Ibuprofen *on page 95*
◆ **Ibu-Tab®** *see* Ibuprofen *on page 96*

IMIPRAMINE

Ibutilide (i BYOO ti lide)
Gene(s) of Interest
  Cardiac Potassium Ion Channel *on page 177*
  Cardiac Sodium Channel *on page 178*
U.S. Brand Names Corvert®
Pharmacologic Class Antiarrhythmic Agent, Class III

- **ICI 204, 219** *see* Zafirlukast *on page 156*
- **ICI-46474** *see* Tamoxifen *on page 145*
- **ICI-D1694** *see* Raltitrexed *on page 135*
- **ICRF-187** *see* Dexrazoxane *on page 71*
- **Ifex®** *see* Ifosfamide *on page 97*

Ifosfamide (eye FOSS fa mide)
Gene(s) of Interest
  CYP2C9 *on page 183*
  CYP2C19 *on page 185*
  CYP3A4 *on page 189*
U.S. Brand Names Ifex®
Synonyms Isophosphamide; NSC-109724; Z4942
Pharmacologic Class Antineoplastic Agent, Alkylating Agent; Antineoplastic Agent, Alkylating Agent (Nitrogen Mustard)

Imatinib (eye MAT eh nib)
Gene(s) of Interest
  CYP3A4 *on page 189*
U.S. Brand Names Gleevec™
Synonyms CGP 57148B; Glivec; STI571
Pharmacologic Class Antineoplastic, Tyrosine Kinase Inhibitor

- **Imidazol Carboxamide Dimethyltriazene** *see* Dacarbazine *on page 69*
- **Imidazole Carboxamide** *see* Dacarbazine *on page 69*

Imipramine (im IP ra meen)
Gene(s) of Interest
  Alpha-1 Adrenergic Receptor *on page 161*
  Cardiac Potassium Ion Channel *on page 177*
  Cardiac Sodium Channel *on page 178*
  CYP2C19 *on page 185*
  G-Protein Beta-3 Subunit *on page 197*
  Gs Protein Alpha-Subunit *on page 198*
  P-Glycoprotein *on page 213*
U.S. Brand Names Tofranil®; Tofranil-PM®
Canadian Brand Names Apo®-Imipramine
Pharmacologic Class Antidepressant, Tricyclic (Tertiary Amine)

- **Imitrex®** *see* Sumatriptan *on page 144*
- **Imuran®** *see* Azathioprine *on page 54*
- **Inapsine®** *see* Droperidol *on page 76*

Indapamide (in DAP a mide)
Gene(s) of Interest
Alpha-Adducin *on page 162*
Cardiac Potassium Ion Channel *on page 177*
Cardiac Sodium Channel *on page 178*
G-Protein Beta-3 Subunit *on page 197*

U.S. Brand Names Lozol®
Canadian Brand Names Apo®-Indapamide; Gen-Indapamide; Lozide®; Novo-Indapamide; Nu-Indapamide; PMS-Indapamide
Pharmacologic Class Diuretic, Thiazide-Related

- **Inderal®** *see* Propranolol *on page 132*
- **Inderal® LA** *see* Propranolol *on page 132*
- **Indocin®** *see* Indomethacin *on page 98*
- **Indocin® I.V.** *see* Indomethacin *on page 98*
- **Indocin® SR** *see* Indomethacin *on page 98*
- **Indometacin** *see* Indomethacin *on page 98*

Indomethacin (in doe METH a sin)
Gene(s) of Interest
Leukotriene C4 Synthase *on page 206*

U.S. Brand Names Indocin®; Indocin® I.V.; Indocin® SR
Canadian Brand Names Apo®-Indomethacin; Indocid®; Indocid® P.D.A.; Indo-Lemmon; Indotec; Novo-Methacin; Nu-Indo; Rhodacine®
Synonyms Indometacin
Pharmacologic Class Nonsteroidal Anti-inflammatory Drug (NSAID)

- **Infumorph®** *see* Morphine Sulfate *on page 115*
- **INH** *see* Isoniazid *on page 99*
- **Inspra™** *see* Eplerenone *on page 78*

Insulin Preparations (IN su lin prep a RAY shuns)
Gene(s) of Interest None known

U.S. Brand Names Humalog®; Humalog® Mix 75/25™; Humulin® 50/50; Humulin® 70/30; Humulin® L; Humulin® N; Humulin® R; Humulin® R (Concentrated) U-500; Humulin® U; Lantus®; Lente® Iletin® II; Novolin® 70/30; Novolin® L; Novolin® N; Novolin® R; NovoLog®; NovoLog® Mix 70/30; NPH Iletin® II; Regular Iletin® II; Velosulin® BR (Buffered)
Canadian Brand Names Humalog®; Humalog® Mix 25™; Humulin®; Iletin® II Pork; Novolin® ge; NovoRapid®
Pharmacologic Class Antidiabetic Agent, Insulin; Antidote

- **Integrilin®** *see* Eptifibatide *on page 78*
- **Intrifiban** *see* Eptifibatide *on page 78*
- **Invirase®** *see* Saquinavir *on page 139*

Ipratropium and Albuterol
(i pra TROE pee um & al BYOO ter ole)
Gene(s) of Interest
Beta-2 Adrenergic Receptor *on page 171*

ISOPROTERENOL

   Glycoprotein IIIa Receptor *on page 196*
   Leukotriene C4 Synthase *on page 206*
 U.S. Brand Names Combivent®; DuoNeb™
 Synonyms Albuterol and Ipratropium
 Pharmacologic Class Bronchodilator

- **I-Prin [OTC]** *see* Ibuprofen *on page 96*
- **Iproveratril Hydrochloride** *see* Verapamil *on page 154*

Irbesartan (ir be SAR tan)
 Gene(s) of Interest
   Aldosterone Synthase *on page 160*
   Angiotensin-Converting Enzyme *on page 163*
   Angiotensin II Type I Receptor *on page 166*
   Angiotensinogen *on page 167*
 U.S. Brand Names Avapro®
 Pharmacologic Class Angiotensin II Receptor Blocker

Irinotecan (eye rye no TEE kan)
 Gene(s) of Interest
   CYP3A4 *on page 189*
   UDP-Glucuronosyltransferase *on page 224*
 U.S. Brand Names Camptosar®
 Synonyms Camptothecin-11; CPT-11
 Pharmacologic Class Antineoplastic Agent, Natural Source (Plant) Derivative

- **Iron Sulfate** *see* Ferrous Sulfate *on page 87*
- **ISD** *see* Isosorbide Dinitrate *on page 100*
- **ISDN** *see* Isosorbide Dinitrate *on page 100*
- **Isobamate** *see* Carisoprodol *on page 61*

Isoniazid (eye soe NYE a zid)
 Gene(s) of Interest
   N-Acetyltransferase 2 Enzyme *on page 211*
 U.S. Brand Names Nydrazid®
 Canadian Brand Names Isotamine®; PMS-Isoniazid
 Synonyms INH; Isonicotinic Acid Hydrazide
 Pharmacologic Class Antitubercular Agent

- **Isonicotinic Acid Hydrazide** *see* Isoniazid *on page 99*
- **Isonipecaine Hydrochloride** *see* Meperidine *on page 108*
- **Isophosphamide** *see* Ifosfamide *on page 97*

Isoproterenol (eye soe proe TER e nole)
 Gene(s) of Interest
   Beta-2 Adrenergic Receptor *on page 171*
 U.S. Brand Names Isuprel®
 Pharmacologic Class Beta$_1$/Beta$_2$ Agonist

- **Isoptin® SR** *see* Verapamil *on page 154*
- **Isordil®** *see* Isosorbide Dinitrate *on page 100*

Isosorbide Dinitrate (eye soe SOR bide dye NYE trate)
Gene(s) of Interest
CYP3A4 *on page 189*
U.S. Brand Names Dilatrate®-SR; Isordil®
Canadian Brand Names Apo®-ISDN; Cedocard®-SR; Coronex®; Novo-Sorbide; PMS-Isosorbide
Synonyms ISD; ISDN
Pharmacologic Class Vasodilator

Isradipine (iz RA di peen)
Gene(s) of Interest
Cardiac Potassium Ion Channel *on page 177*
Cardiac Sodium Channel *on page 178*
CYP3A4 *on page 189*
U.S. Brand Names DynaCirc®; DynaCirc® CR
Pharmacologic Class Calcium Channel Blocker

♦ **Isuprel®** *see* Isoproterenol *on page 99*

Itraconazole (i tra KOE na zole)
Gene(s) of Interest
P-Glycoprotein *on page 213*
U.S. Brand Names Sporanox®
Pharmacologic Class Antifungal Agent, Oral

Ivermectin (eye ver MEK tin)
Gene(s) of Interest
P-Glycoprotein *on page 213*
U.S. Brand Names Stromectol®
Pharmacologic Class Anthelmintic

♦ **K+8** *see* Potassium Chloride *on page 128*
♦ **K+10** *see* Potassium Chloride *on page 128*
♦ **Kadian®** *see* Morphine Sulfate *on page 115*
♦ **Kaon-Cl-10®** *see* Potassium Chloride *on page 128*
♦ **Kaon-Cl® 20** *see* Potassium Chloride *on page 128*
♦ **Kariva™** *see* Ethinyl Estradiol and Desogestrel *on page 82*
♦ **Kay Ciel®** *see* Potassium Chloride *on page 128*
♦ **K+ Care®** *see* Potassium Chloride *on page 128*
♦ **KCl** *see* Potassium Chloride *on page 128*
♦ **K-Dur® 10** *see* Potassium Chloride *on page 128*
♦ **K-Dur® 20** *see* Potassium Chloride *on page 128*
♦ **Keflex®** *see* Cephalexin *on page 62*
♦ **Keftab®** *see* Cephalexin *on page 62*
♦ **Kenalog®** *see* Triamcinolone *on page 151*
♦ **Kenalog-10®** *see* Triamcinolone *on page 151*
♦ **Kenalog-40®** *see* Triamcinolone *on page 151*
♦ **Kenalog® in Orabase®** *see* Triamcinolone *on page 151*
♦ **Keoxifene Hydrochloride** *see* Raloxifene *on page 134*

- **Kerlone®** *see Betaxolol on page 56*
- **Ketalar®** *see Ketamine on page 101*

Ketamine (KEET a meen)
Gene(s) of Interest
CYP2C9 *on page 183*
CYP3A4 *on page 189*
U.S. Brand Names Ketalar®
Pharmacologic Class General Anesthetic

Ketoconazole (kee toe KOE na zole)
Gene(s) of Interest
P-Glycoprotein *on page 213*
U.S. Brand Names Nizoral®; Nizoral® A-D [OTC]
Canadian Brand Names Apo®-Ketoconazole; Ketoderm®; Novo-Ketoconazole
Pharmacologic Class Antifungal Agent, Oral; Antifungal Agent, Topical

Ketoprofen (kee toe PROE fen)
Gene(s) of Interest
Leukotriene C4 Synthase *on page 206*
U.S. Brand Names Orudis® [DSC]; Orudis® KT [OTC]; Oruvail®
Canadian Brand Names Apo®-Keto; Apo®-Keto-E; Apo®-Keto SR; Novo-Keto; Novo-Keto-EC; Nu-Ketoprofen; Nu-Ketoprofen-E; Orudis® SR; Rhodis™; Rhodis-EC™; Rhodis SR™
Pharmacologic Class Nonsteroidal Anti-inflammatory Drug (NSAID)

Ketorolac (KEE toe role ak)
Gene(s) of Interest
Leukotriene C4 Synthase *on page 206*
U.S. Brand Names Acular®; Acular® PF; Toradol®
Canadian Brand Names Apo®-Ketorolac; Apo®-Ketorolac Injectable; Novo-Ketorolac; Toradol® IM
Pharmacologic Class Nonsteroidal Anti-inflammatory Drug (NSAID)

- **Klaron®** *see Sulfacetamide on page 142*
- **Klonopin™** *see Clonazepam on page 66*
- **K-Lor™** *see Potassium Chloride on page 128*
- **Klor-Con®** *see Potassium Chloride on page 128*
- **Klor-Con® 8** *see Potassium Chloride on page 128*
- **Klor-Con® 10** *see Potassium Chloride on page 128*
- **Klor-Con®/25** *see Potassium Chloride on page 128*
- **Klor-Con® M10** *see Potassium Chloride on page 128*
- **Klor-Con® M20** *see Potassium Chloride on page 128*
- **Klotrix®** *see Potassium Chloride on page 128*
- **K-Tab®** *see Potassium Chloride on page 128*
- **L 754030** *see Aprepitant on page 50*
- **LactiCare-HC®** *see Hydrocortisone on page 95*
- **Lanoxicaps®** *see Digoxin on page 73*

LANSOPRAZOLE

- **Lanoxin®** *see* Digoxin *on page 73*

Lansoprazole (lan SOE pra zole)
Gene(s) of Interest
CYP2C19 *on page 185*
U.S. Brand Names Prevacid®
Pharmacologic Class Proton Pump Inhibitor

- **Lantus®** *see* Insulin Preparations *on page 98*
- **Lariam®** *see* Mefloquine *on page 108*
- **Lasix®** *see* Furosemide *on page 91*

Latanoprost (la TA noe prost)
Gene(s) of Interest None known
U.S. Brand Names Xalatan®
Pharmacologic Class Ophthalmic Agent, Antiglaucoma; Prostaglandin, Ophthalmic

- **LCR** *see* VinCRIstine *on page 155*
- **L-Deprenyl** *see* Selegiline *on page 139*
- **Lente® Iletin® II** *see* Insulin Preparations *on page 98*
- **Lescol®** *see* Fluvastatin *on page 89*
- **Lescol® XL** *see* Fluvastatin *on page 89*
- **Lessina™** *see* Ethinyl Estradiol and Levonorgestrel *on page 83*
- **Leurocristine** *see* VinCRIstine *on page 155*
- **Leurocristine Sulfate** *see* VinCRIstine *on page 155*

Levalbuterol (leve al BYOO ter ole)
Gene(s) of Interest
Beta-2 Adrenergic Receptor *on page 171*
U.S. Brand Names Xopenex®
Synonyms R-albuterol
Pharmacologic Class Beta$_2$ Agonist

- **Levaquin®** *see* Levofloxacin *on page 102*
- **Levlen®** *see* Ethinyl Estradiol and Levonorgestrel *on page 83*
- **Levlite™** *see* Ethinyl Estradiol and Levonorgestrel *on page 83*
- **Levo-Dromoran®** *see* Levorphanol *on page 103*

Levofloxacin (lee voe FLOKS a sin)
Gene(s) of Interest
Cardiac Potassium Ion Channel *on page 177*
Cardiac Sodium Channel *on page 178*
U.S. Brand Names Levaquin®; Quixin™
Pharmacologic Class Antibiotic, Quinolone

- **Levomepromazine** *see* Methotrimeprazine *on page 110*

Levomethadyl Acetate Hydrochloride
(lee voe METH a dil AS e tate hye droe KLOR ide)
Gene(s) of Interest
Cardiac Potassium Ion Channel *on page 177*

LIDOCAINE

Cardiac Sodium Channel *on page 178*
COMT *on page 180*
CYP3A4 *on page 189*
U.S. Brand Names ORLAAM®
Pharmacologic Class Analgesic, Narcotic

Levonorgestrel (LEE voe nor jes trel)
Gene(s) of Interest
BRCA Genes *on page 176*
Prothrombin *on page 219*
U.S. Brand Names Mirena®; Norplant® Implant [DSC]; Plan B®
Synonyms LNg 20
Pharmacologic Class Contraceptive

- **Levonorgestrel and Ethinyl Estradiol** *see* Ethinyl Estradiol and Levonorgestrel *on page 83*
- **Levora®** *see* Ethinyl Estradiol and Levonorgestrel *on page 83*

Levorphanol (lee VOR fa nole)
Gene(s) of Interest
COMT *on page 180*
U.S. Brand Names Levo-Dromoran®
Pharmacologic Class Analgesic, Narcotic

- **Levothroid®** *see* Levothyroxine *on page 103*

Levothyroxine (lee voe thye ROKS een)
Gene(s) of Interest None known
U.S. Brand Names Levothroid®; Levoxyl®; Novothyrox; Synthroid®; Unithroid®
Canadian Brand Names Eltroxin®
Synonyms *L*-Thyroxine Sodium; T_4
Pharmacologic Class Thyroid Product

- **Levoxyl®** *see* Levothyroxine *on page 103*
- **Lexapro™** *see* Escitalopram *on page 80*
- **Librium®** *see* Chlordiazepoxide *on page 62*
- **LidaMantle®** *see* Lidocaine *on page 103*

Lidocaine (LYE doe kane)
Gene(s) of Interest
CYP3A4 *on page 189*
P-Glycoprotein *on page 213*
U.S. Brand Names Anestacon®; Band-Aid® Hurt-Free™ Antiseptic Wash [OTC]; Burnamycin [OTC]; Burn Jel [OTC]; Burn-O-Jel [OTC]; ELA-Max® [OTC]; ELA-Max® 5 [OTC]; LidaMantle®; Lidoderm®; Premjact® [OTC]; Solarcaine® Aloe Extra Burn Relief [OTC]; Topicaine® [OTC]; Xylocaine®; Xylocaine® MPF; Xylocaine® Viscous; Zilactin-L® [OTC]
Canadian Brand Names Lidodan™; Xylocard®; Zilactin®
Synonyms Lignocaine Hydrochloride
(Continued)

LIDOCAINE AND PRILOCAINE

Lidocaine *(Continued)*
Pharmacologic Class Analgesic, Topical; Antiarrhythmic Agent, Class Ib; Local Anesthetic

Lidocaine and Prilocaine (LYE doe kane & PRIL oh kane)
Gene(s) of Interest
CYP3A4 *on page 189*
Glucose-6-Phosphate Dehydrogenase *on page 195*
P-Glycoprotein *on page 213*
U.S. Brand Names EMLA®
Synonyms Prilocaine and Lidocaine
Pharmacologic Class Local Anesthetic

- **Lidoderm®** *see* Lidocaine *on page 103*
- **Lignocaine Hydrochloride** *see* Lidocaine *on page 103*
- **Limbitrol®** *see* Amitriptyline and Chlordiazepoxide *on page 48*
- **Limbitrol® DS** *see* Amitriptyline and Chlordiazepoxide *on page 48*
- **Lipitor®** *see* Atorvastatin *on page 53*

Lisinopril (lyse IN oh pril)
Gene(s) of Interest
Aldosterone Synthase *on page 160*
Angiotensin-Converting Enzyme *on page 163*
Angiotensin II Type I Receptor *on page 166*
Angiotensinogen *on page 167*
Bradykinin B2 Receptor *on page 175*
U.S. Brand Names Prinivil®; Zestril®
Canadian Brand Names Apo®-Lisinopril
Pharmacologic Class Angiotensin-Converting Enzyme (ACE) Inhibitor

Lisinopril and Hydrochlorothiazide
(lyse IN oh pril & hye droe klor oh THYE a zide)
Gene(s) of Interest
Aldosterone Synthase *on page 160*
Alpha-Adducin *on page 162*
Angiotensin-Converting Enzyme *on page 163*
Angiotensin II Type I Receptor *on page 166*
Angiotensinogen *on page 167*
Bradykinin B2 Receptor *on page 175*
G-Protein Beta-3 Subunit *on page 197*
U.S. Brand Names Prinzide®; Zestoretic®
Synonyms Hydrochlorothiazide and Lisinopril
Pharmacologic Class Antihypertensive Agent Combination

- **LNg 20** *see* Levonorgestrel *on page 103*
- **Locoid®** *see* Hydrocortisone *on page 95*
- **Locoid Lipocream®** *see* Hydrocortisone *on page 95*
- **Lodine®** *see* Etodolac *on page 85*
- **Lodine® XL** *see* Etodolac *on page 85*

LOSARTAN AND HYDROCHLOROTHIAZIDE

- **Loestrin®** see Ethinyl Estradiol and Norethindrone on page 84
- **Loestrin® Fe** see Ethinyl Estradiol and Norethindrone on page 84
- **Lo/Ovral®** see Ethinyl Estradiol and Norgestrel on page 84
- **Lopid®** see Gemfibrozil on page 91
- **Lopressor®** see Metoprolol on page 112

Loratadine (lor AT a deen)
Gene(s) of Interest None known
U.S. Brand Names Alavert™ [OTC]; Claritin® [OTC]
Canadian Brand Names Apo®-Loratadine; Claritin® Kids
Pharmacologic Class Antihistamine

Lorazepam (lor A ze pam)
Gene(s) of Interest None known
U.S. Brand Names Ativan®; Lorazepam Intensol®
Canadian Brand Names Apo®-Lorazepam; Novo-Lorazepam®; Nu-Loraz; Riva-Lorazepam
Pharmacologic Class Benzodiazepine

- **Lorazepam Intensol®** see Lorazepam on page 105
- **Lorcet® 10/650** see Hydrocodone and Acetaminophen on page 94
- **Lorcet®-HD** see Hydrocodone and Acetaminophen on page 94
- **Lorcet® Plus** see Hydrocodone and Acetaminophen on page 94
- **Lortab®** see Hydrocodone and Acetaminophen on page 94

Losartan (loe SAR tan)
Gene(s) of Interest
Aldosterone Synthase on page 160
Angiotensin-Converting Enzyme on page 163
Angiotensin II Type I Receptor on page 166
Angiotensinogen on page 167
CYP2C9 on page 183
U.S. Brand Names Cozaar®
Synonyms DuP 753; MK594
Pharmacologic Class Angiotensin II Receptor Blocker

Losartan and Hydrochlorothiazide
(loe SAR tan & hye droe klor oh THYE a zide)
Gene(s) of Interest
Aldosterone Synthase on page 160
Alpha-Adducin on page 162
Angiotensin-Converting Enzyme on page 163
Angiotensin II Type I Receptor on page 166
Angiotensinogen on page 167
CYP2C9 on page 183
G-Protein Beta-3 Subunit on page 197
U.S. Brand Names Hyzaar®
Canadian Brand Names Hyzaar® DS
Synonyms Hydrochlorothiazide and Losartan
Pharmacologic Class Antihypertensive Agent Combination

LOVASTATIN

- **Lotensin®** *see* Benazepril *on page 55*
- **Lotrel®** *see* Amlodipine and Benazepril *on page 49*

Lovastatin (LOE va sta tin)
Gene(s) of Interest
Angiotensin-Converting Enzyme *on page 163*
Apolipoprotein E *on page 168*
Beta-Fibrinogen *on page 174*
Cholesteryl Ester Transfer Protein *on page 179*
CYP3A4 *on page 189*
Glycoprotein IIIa Receptor *on page 196*
Low-Density Lipoprotein Receptor *on page 209*
P-Glycoprotein *on page 213*
Stromelysin-1 *on page 219*

U.S. Brand Names Altocor™; Mevacor®

Canadian Brand Names Apo®-Lovastatin; Gen-Lovastatin; ratio-Lovastatin

Synonyms Mevinolin; Monacolin K

Pharmacologic Class Antilipemic Agent, HMG-CoA Reductase Inhibitor

- **Low-Ogestrel®** *see* Ethinyl Estradiol and Norgestrel *on page 84*

Loxapine (LOKS a peen)
Gene(s) of Interest
Alpha-1 Adrenergic Receptor *on page 161*
Cardiac Potassium Ion Channel *on page 177*
Cardiac Sodium Channel *on page 178*
D2 Receptor *on page 190*

U.S. Brand Names Loxitane®; Loxitane® C

Canadian Brand Names Apo®-Loxapine; Nu-Loxapine; PMS-Loxapine

Synonyms Oxilapine Succinate

Pharmacologic Class Antipsychotic Agent, Dibenzoxazepine

- **Loxitane®** *see* Loxapine *on page 106*
- **Loxitane® C** *see* Loxapine *on page 106*
- **Lozol®** *see* Indapamide *on page 98*
- **L-Thyroxine Sodium** *see* Levothyroxine *on page 103*
- **Lu-26-054** *see* Escitalopram *on page 80*
- **Ludiomil** *see* Maprotiline *on page 107*
- **Luminal® Sodium** *see* Phenobarbital *on page 127*
- **Lunelle™** *see* Estradiol and Medroxyprogesterone *on page 81*
- **Luvox® [DSC]** *see* Fluvoxamine *on page 90*
- **LY139603** *see* Atomoxetine *on page 53*
- **LY170053** *see* Olanzapine *on page 121*
- **Macrobid®** *see* Nitrofurantoin *on page 119*
- **Macrodantin®** *see* Nitrofurantoin *on page 119*

Mafenide (MA fe nide)
Gene(s) of Interest
Glucose-6-Phosphate Dehydrogenase *on page 195*
U.S. Brand Names Sulfamylon®
Pharmacologic Class Antibiotic, Topical

Maprotiline (ma PROE ti leen)
Gene(s) of Interest
P-Glycoprotein *on page 213*
Canadian Brand Names Novo-Maprotiline
Synonyms Ludiomil
Pharmacologic Class Antidepressant, Tetracyclic

- **Margesic® H** *see* Hydrocodone and Acetaminophen *on page 94*
- **Mavik®** *see* Trandolapril *on page 150*
- **Maxair™** *see* Pirbuterol *on page 128*
- **Maxair™ Autohaler™** *see* Pirbuterol *on page 128*
- **Maxidone™** *see* Hydrocodone and Acetaminophen *on page 94*
- **Mebaral®** *see* Mephobarbital *on page 108*

Meclizine (MEK li zeen)
Gene(s) of Interest None known
U.S. Brand Names Antivert®; Bonine® [OTC]; Dramamine® Less Drowsy Formula [OTC]
Canadian Brand Names Bonamine™
Pharmacologic Class Antiemetic; Antihistamine

Meclofenamate (me kloe fen AM ate)
Gene(s) of Interest
Leukotriene C4 Synthase *on page 206*
Canadian Brand Names Meclomen®
Pharmacologic Class Nonsteroidal Anti-inflammatory Drug (NSAID)

- **Medrol®** *see* MethylPREDNISolone *on page 111*

MedroxyPROGESTERone
(me DROKS ee proe JES te rone)
Gene(s) of Interest
BRCA Genes *on page 176*
Prothrombin *on page 219*
U.S. Brand Names Depo-Provera®; Depo-Provera® Contraceptive; Provera®
Canadian Brand Names Alti-MPA; Gen-Medroxy; Novo-Medrone
Synonyms Acetoxymethylprogesterone; Medroxyprogesterone Acetate; Methylacetoxyprogesterone
Pharmacologic Class Contraceptive; Progestin

- **Medroxyprogesterone Acetate** *see* MedroxyPROGESTERone *on page 107*
- **Medroxyprogesterone Acetate and Estradiol Cypionate** *see* Estradiol and Medroxyprogesterone *on page 81*

MEFENAMIC ACID

- **Medroxyprogesterone and Estradiol** *see* Estradiol and Medroxyprogesterone *on page 81*
- **Medroxyprogesterone and Estrogens (Conjugated)** *see* Estrogens (Conjugated/Equine) and Medroxyprogesterone *on page 81*

Mefenamic Acid (me fe NAM ik AS id)
Gene(s) of Interest
Leukotriene C4 Synthase *on page 206*
U.S. Brand Names Ponstel®
Canadian Brand Names Apo®-Mefenamic; Nu-Mefenamic; PMS-Mefenamic Acid; Ponstan®
Pharmacologic Class Nonsteroidal Anti-inflammatory Drug (NSAID)

Mefloquine (ME floe kwin)
Gene(s) of Interest
CYP3A4 *on page 189*
P-Glycoprotein *on page 213*
U.S. Brand Names Lariam®
Pharmacologic Class Antimalarial Agent

- **Mellaril® [DSC]** *see* Thioridazine *on page 147*

Meloxicam (mel OKS i kam)
Gene(s) of Interest
Leukotriene C4 Synthase *on page 206*
U.S. Brand Names MOBIC®
Canadian Brand Names Mobicox®
Pharmacologic Class Nonsteroidal Anti-inflammatory Drug (NSAID)

- **Menadol® [OTC]** *see* Ibuprofen *on page 96*
- **Menest®** *see* Estrogens (Esterified) *on page 82*
- **Mepergan** *see* Meperidine and Promethazine *on page 108*

Meperidine (me PER i deen)
Gene(s) of Interest
COMT *on page 180*
U.S. Brand Names Demerol®; Meperitab®
Synonyms Isonipecaine Hydrochloride; Pethidine Hydrochloride
Pharmacologic Class Analgesic, Narcotic

Meperidine and Promethazine
(me PER i deen & proe METH a zeen)
Gene(s) of Interest
COMT *on page 180*
Synonyms Mepergan; Promethazine and Meperidine
Pharmacologic Class Analgesic Combination (Narcotic)

- **Meperitab®** *see* Meperidine *on page 108*

Mephobarbital (me foe BAR bi tal)
Gene(s) of Interest
CYP2C19 *on page 185*

U.S. Brand Names Mebaral®
Synonyms Methylphenobarbital
Pharmacologic Class Barbiturate

Mercaptopurine (mer kap toe PYOOR een)
Gene(s) of Interest
Thiopurine Methyltransferase *on page 220*
U.S. Brand Names Purinethol®
Synonyms 6-Mercaptopurine; 6-MP; NSC-755
Pharmacologic Class Antineoplastic Agent, Antimetabolite

- **6-Mercaptopurine** *see Mercaptopurine on page 109*
- **Meridia®** *see Sibutramine on page 140*

Mesoridazine (mez oh RID a zeen)
Gene(s) of Interest
Alpha-1 Adrenergic Receptor *on page 161*
Cardiac Potassium Ion Channel *on page 177*
Cardiac Sodium Channel *on page 178*
D2 Receptor *on page 190*
U.S. Brand Names Serentil®
Pharmacologic Class Antipsychotic Agent, Phenothiazine, Piperidine

Mestranol and Norethindrone
(MES tra nole & nor eth IN drone)
Gene(s) of Interest
BRCA Genes *on page 176*
Prothrombin *on page 219*
U.S. Brand Names Necon® 1/50; Norinyl® 1+50; Ortho-Novum® 1/50
Synonyms Norethindrone and Mestranol
Pharmacologic Class Contraceptive; Estrogen and Progestin Combination

- **Metadate® CD** *see Methylphenidate on page 111*
- **Metadate™ ER** *see Methylphenidate on page 111*

Metaproterenol (met a proe TER e nol)
Gene(s) of Interest
Beta-2 Adrenergic Receptor *on page 171*
U.S. Brand Names Alupent®
Synonyms Orciprenaline Sulfate
Pharmacologic Class Beta$_2$ Agonist

Metaxalone (me TAKS a lone)
Gene(s) of Interest None known
U.S. Brand Names Skelaxin®
Pharmacologic Class Skeletal Muscle Relaxant

Metformin (met FOR min)
Gene(s) of Interest None known
U.S. Brand Names Glucophage®; Glucophage® XR
(Continued)

Metformin *(Continued)*
Canadian Brand Names Alti-Metformin; Apo®-Metformin; Gen-Metformin; Glycon; Novo-Metformin; Nu-Metformin; PMS-Metformin; Rho®-Metformin; Rhoxal-metformin FC

Pharmacologic Class Antidiabetic Agent, Biguanide

♦ **Metformin and Glyburide** *see* Glyburide and Metformin *on page 92*

Methadone (METH a done)
Gene(s) of Interest
COMT *on page 180*
CYP2D6 *on page 186*
CYP3A4 *on page 189*

U.S. Brand Names Dolophine®; Methadone Intensol™; Methadose®

Canadian Brand Names Metadol™

Pharmacologic Class Analgesic, Narcotic

♦ **Methadone Intensol™** *see* Methadone *on page 110*
♦ **Methadose®** *see* Methadone *on page 110*
♦ **Methaminodiazepoxide Hydrochloride** *see* Chlordiazepoxide *on page 62*
♦ **Methergine®** *see* Methylergonovine *on page 111*

Methotrimeprazine (meth oh trye MEP ra zeen)
Gene(s) of Interest
COMT *on page 180*

Canadian Brand Names Apo®-Methoprazine; Novo-Meprazine; Nozinan®

Synonyms Levomepromazine

Pharmacologic Class Analgesic, Non-narcotic

Methsuximide (meth SUKS i mide)
Gene(s) of Interest
CYP2C19 *on page 185*

U.S. Brand Names Celontin®

Pharmacologic Class Anticonvulsant, Succinimide

Methyclothiazide (meth i kloe THYE a zide)
Gene(s) of Interest
Alpha-Adducin *on page 162*
G-Protein Beta-3 Subunit *on page 197*

U.S. Brand Names Aquatensen®; Enduron®

Pharmacologic Class Diuretic, Thiazide

♦ **Methylacetoxyprogesterone** *see* MedroxyPROGESTERone *on page 107*

Methylene Blue (METH i leen bloo)
Gene(s) of Interest
Glucose-6-Phosphate Dehydrogenase *on page 195*

METOLAZONE

U.S. Brand Names Urolene Blue®
Pharmacologic Class Antidote

Methylergonovine (meth il er goe NOE veen)
Gene(s) of Interest
CYP3A4 on page 189
U.S. Brand Names Methergine®
Pharmacologic Class Ergot Derivative

- **Methylin™** see Methylphenidate on page 111
- **Methylin™ ER** see Methylphenidate on page 111
- **Methylmorphine** see Codeine on page 67

Methylphenidate (meth il FEN i date)
Gene(s) of Interest None known
U.S. Brand Names Concerta®; Metadate® CD; Metadate™ ER; Methylin™; Methylin™ ER; Ritalin®; Ritalin® LA; Ritalin-SR®
Canadian Brand Names PMS-Methylphenidate; Riphenidate
Pharmacologic Class Central Nervous System Stimulant

- **Methylphenobarbital** see Mephobarbital on page 108

MethylPREDNISolone (meth il pred NIS oh lone)
Gene(s) of Interest None known
U.S. Brand Names A-Methapred®; Depo-Medrol®; Medrol®; Solu-Medrol®
Synonyms 6-α-Methylprednisolone
Pharmacologic Class Corticosteroid, Systemic

- **6-α-Methylprednisolone** see MethylPREDNISolone on page 111

Methysergide (meth i SER jide)
Gene(s) of Interest
CYP3A4 on page 189
U.S. Brand Names Sansert® [DSC]
Pharmacologic Class Ergot Derivative

Metoclopramide (met oh kloe PRA mide)
Gene(s) of Interest
D2 Receptor on page 190
U.S. Brand Names Reglan®
Canadian Brand Names Apo®-Metoclop; Nu-Metoclopramide
Pharmacologic Class Antiemetic; Gastrointestinal Agent, Prokinetic

Metolazone (me TOLE a zone)
Gene(s) of Interest
Alpha-Adducin on page 162
G-Protein Beta-3 Subunit on page 197
U.S. Brand Names Mykrox®; Zaroxolyn®
Pharmacologic Class Diuretic, Thiazide-Related

Metoprolol (me toe PROE lole)
Gene(s) of Interest
Angiotensin-Converting Enzyme *on page 163*
Beta-1 Adrenergic Receptor *on page 171*
CYP2D6 *on page 186*
Gs Protein Alpha-Subunit *on page 198*
U.S. Brand Names Lopressor®; Toprol-XL®
Canadian Brand Names Apo®-Metoprolol; Betaloc®; Betaloc® Durules®; Novo-Metoprolol; Nu-Metop; PMS-Metoprolol
Pharmacologic Class Beta Blocker, Beta₁ Selective

- **MetroCream®** *see* Metronidazole *on page 112*
- **MetroGel®** *see* Metronidazole *on page 112*
- **MetroGel-Vaginal®** *see* Metronidazole *on page 112*
- **MetroLotion®** *see* Metronidazole *on page 112*

Metronidazole (me troe NI da zole)
Gene(s) of Interest None known
U.S. Brand Names Flagyl®; Flagyl ER®; MetroCream®; MetroGel®; MetroGel-Vaginal®; MetroLotion®; Noritate™
Canadian Brand Names Apo®-Metronidazole; Florazole® ER; Nidagel™; Novo-Nidazol
Pharmacologic Class Amebicide; Antibiotic, Topical; Antibiotic, Miscellaneous; Antiprotozoal

- **Mevacor®** *see* Lovastatin *on page 106*
- **Mevinolin** *see* Lovastatin *on page 106*

Mexiletine (MEKS i le teen)
Gene(s) of Interest
CYP1A2 *on page 181*
CYP2D6 *on page 186*
U.S. Brand Names Mexitil®
Canadian Brand Names Novo-Mexiletine
Pharmacologic Class Antiarrhythmic Agent, Class Ib

- **Mexitil®** *see* Mexiletine *on page 112*
- **Micardis®** *see* Telmisartan *on page 145*
- **Microgestin™ Fe** *see* Ethinyl Estradiol and Norethindrone *on page 84*
- **microK®** *see* Potassium Chloride *on page 128*
- **microK® 10** *see* Potassium Chloride *on page 128*
- **Micronase®** *see* GlyBURIDE *on page 92*
- **Micronor®** *see* Norethindrone *on page 119*
- **Microzide™** *see* Hydrochlorothiazide *on page 94*
- **Midamor®** *see* Amiloride *on page 47*

Midazolam (MID aye zoe lam)
Gene(s) of Interest
CYP3A4 *on page 189*

P-Glycoprotein *on page 213*
U.S. Brand Names Versed® [DSC]
Canadian Brand Names Apo®-Midazolam
Pharmacologic Class Benzodiazepine

- **Midol® Maximum Strength Cramp Formula [OTC]** *see* Ibuprofen *on page 96*
- **Mifeprex®** *see* Mifepristone *on page 113*

Mifepristone (mi FE pris tone)
Gene(s) of Interest
P-Glycoprotein *on page 213*
U.S. Brand Names Mifeprex®
Synonyms RU-486; RU-38486
Pharmacologic Class Abortifacient; Antineoplastic Agent, Hormone Antagonist; Antiprogestin

- **Migranal®** *see* Dihydroergotamine *on page 73*
- **Minocin®** *see* Minocycline *on page 113*

Minocycline (mi noe SYE kleen)
Gene(s) of Interest None known
U.S. Brand Names Dynacin®; Minocin®
Canadian Brand Names Alti-Minocycline; Apo®-Minocycline; Gen-Minocycline; Novo-Minocycline; PMS-Minocycline; Rhoxal-minocycline
Pharmacologic Class Antibiotic, Tetracycline Derivative

- **Mircette®** *see* Ethinyl Estradiol and Desogestrel *on page 82*
- **Mirena®** *see* Levonorgestrel *on page 103*

Mirtazapine (mir TAZ a peen)
Gene(s) of Interest
Alpha-1 Adrenergic Receptor *on page 161*
CYP1A2 *on page 181*
CYP3A4 *on page 189*
G-Protein Beta-3 Subunit *on page 197*
Gs Protein Alpha-Subunit *on page 198*
U.S. Brand Names Remeron®; Remeron SolTab®
Pharmacologic Class Antidepressant, Alpha-2 Antagonist

- **Misoprostol and Diclofenac** *see* Diclofenac and Misoprostol *on page 72*

Mitomycin (mye toe MYE sin)
Gene(s) of Interest
NAD(P)H Quinone Oxidoreductase *on page 212*
P-Glycoprotein *on page 213*
U.S. Brand Names Mutamycin®
Synonyms Mitomycin-C; Mitomycin-X; MTC; NSC-26980
Pharmacologic Class Antineoplastic Agent, Antibiotic

- **Mitomycin-C** *see* Mitomycin *on page 113*

MOCLOBEMIDE

- **Mitomycin-X** *see Mitomycin on page 113*
- **MK383** *see Tirofiban on page 149*
- **MK594** *see Losartan on page 105*
- **MK869** *see Aprepitant on page 50*
- **Moban®** *see Molindone on page 114*
- **MOBIC®** *see Meloxicam on page 108*

Moclobemide (moe KLOE be mide)
Gene(s) of Interest
CYP2C19 *on page 185*

Canadian Brand Names Alti-Moclobemide; Apo®-Moclobemide; Manerix®; Novo-Moclobemide; Nu-Moclobemide; PMS-Moclobemide

Synonyms Ro 11-1163

Pharmacologic Class Antidepressant, Monoamine Oxidase Inhibitor, Reversible

Modafinil (moe DAF i nil)
Gene(s) of Interest
CYP3A4 *on page 189*

U.S. Brand Names Provigil®

Canadian Brand Names Alertec®

Pharmacologic Class Stimulant

- **Modicon®** *see Ethinyl Estradiol and Norethindrone on page 84*

Moexipril (mo EKS i pril)
Gene(s) of Interest
Aldosterone Synthase *on page 160*
Angiotensin-Converting Enzyme *on page 163*
Angiotensin II Type I Receptor *on page 166*
Angiotensinogen *on page 167*
Bradykinin B2 Receptor *on page 175*

U.S. Brand Names Univasc®

Pharmacologic Class Angiotensin-Converting Enzyme (ACE) Inhibitor

Molindone (moe LIN done)
Gene(s) of Interest
Alpha-1 Adrenergic Receptor *on page 161*
D2 Receptor *on page 190*

U.S. Brand Names Moban®

Pharmacologic Class Antipsychotic Agent, Dihydroindoline

Mometasone Furoate (moe MET a sone FYOOR oh ate)
Gene(s) of Interest None known

U.S. Brand Names Elocon®; Nasonex®

Pharmacologic Class Corticosteroid, Nasal; Corticosteroid, Topical

- **Monacolin K** *see Lovastatin on page 106*
- **Monodox®** *see Doxycycline on page 76*
- **Monopril®** *see Fosinopril on page 90*

Montelukast (mon te LOO kast)
Gene(s) of Interest
CYP2C9 *on page 183*
Leukotriene C4 Synthase *on page 206*
5-Lipoxygenase *on page 208*
U.S. Brand Names Singulair®
Pharmacologic Class Leukotriene Receptor Antagonist

Moricizine (mor I siz een)
Gene(s) of Interest
CYP3A4 *on page 189*
U.S. Brand Names Ethmozine®
Pharmacologic Class Antiarrhythmic Agent, Class I

- **Morning After Pill** *see* Ethinyl Estradiol and Norgestrel *on page 84*

Morphine Sulfate (MOR feen SUL fate)
Gene(s) of Interest
COMT *on page 180*
U.S. Brand Names Astramorph/PF™; Avinza™; Duramorph®; Infumorph®; Kadian®; MS Contin®; MSIR®; Oramorph SR®; RMS®; Roxanol®; Roxanol 100®; Roxanol®-T
Canadian Brand Names Kadian®; M-Eslon®; Morphine HP®; Morphine LP® Epidural; M.O.S.-Sulfate®; MS-IR®; ratio-Morphine SR; Statex®
Synonyms MS
Pharmacologic Class Analgesic, Narcotic

- **Motrin®** *see* Ibuprofen *on page 96*
- **Motrin® Children's [OTC]** *see* Ibuprofen *on page 96*
- **Motrin® IB [OTC]** *see* Ibuprofen *on page 96*
- **Motrin® Infants' [OTC]** *see* Ibuprofen *on page 96*
- **Motrin® Junior Strength [OTC]** *see* Ibuprofen *on page 96*
- **Motrin® Migraine Pain [OTC]** *see* Ibuprofen *on page 96*

Moxifloxacin (moxs i FLOKS a sin)
Gene(s) of Interest
Cardiac Potassium Ion Channel *on page 177*
Cardiac Sodium Channel *on page 178*
U.S. Brand Names Avelox®; Avelox® I.V.; Vigamox™
Pharmacologic Class Antibiotic, Ophthalmic; Antibiotic, Quinolone

- **Moxilin®** *see* Amoxicillin *on page 49*
- **6-MP** *see* Mercaptopurine *on page 109*
- **MPA and Estrogens (Conjugated)** *see* Estrogens (Conjugated/Equine) and Medroxyprogesterone *on page 81*
- **MS** *see* Morphine Sulfate *on page 115*
- **MS Contin®** *see* Morphine Sulfate *on page 115*
- **MSIR®** *see* Morphine Sulfate *on page 115*
- **MTC** *see* Mitomycin *on page 113*

Mupirocin (myoo PEER oh sin)
Gene(s) of Interest None known
U.S. Brand Names Bactroban®; Bactroban® Nasal
Synonyms Pseudomonic Acid A
Pharmacologic Class Antibiotic, Topical

- **Mutamycin®** *see Mitomycin on page 113*
- **Mycobutin®** *see Rifabutin on page 136*
- **Mykrox®** *see Metolazone on page 111*
- **Myleran®** *see Busulfan on page 58*

Nabumetone (na BYOO me tone)
Gene(s) of Interest
  Leukotriene C4 Synthase *on page 206*
U.S. Brand Names Relafen®
Canadian Brand Names Apo®-Nabumetone; Gen-Nabumetone; Rhoxal-nabumetone
Pharmacologic Class Nonsteroidal Anti-inflammatory Drug (NSAID)

Nadolol (nay DOE lole)
Gene(s) of Interest
  Beta-1 Adrenergic Receptor *on page 171*
  Gs Protein Alpha-Subunit *on page 198*
U.S. Brand Names Corgard®
Canadian Brand Names Alti-Nadolol; Apo®-Nadol; Novo-Nadolol
Pharmacologic Class Beta Blocker, Nonselective

Nalbuphine (NAL byoo feen)
Gene(s) of Interest
  COMT *on page 180*
U.S. Brand Names Nubain®
Pharmacologic Class Analgesic, Narcotic

- **Nalfon®** *see Fenoprofen on page 86*

Nalidixic Acid (nal i DIKS ik AS id)
Gene(s) of Interest
  Glucose-6-Phosphate Dehydrogenase *on page 195*
U.S. Brand Names NegGram®
Synonyms Nalidixinic Acid
Pharmacologic Class Antibiotic, Quinolone

- **Nalidixinic Acid** *see Nalidixic Acid on page 116*
- **Naloxone and Buprenorphine** *see Buprenorphine and Naloxone on page 58*
- **Naloxone Hydrochloride Dihydrate and Buprenorphine Hydrochloride** *see Buprenorphine and Naloxone on page 58*
- **Naprelan®** *see Naproxen on page 117*
- **Naprosyn®** *see Naproxen on page 117*

Naproxen (na PROKS en)

Gene(s) of Interest
Leukotriene C4 Synthase *on page 206*

U.S. Brand Names Aleve® [OTC]; Anaprox®; Anaprox® DS; EC-Naprosyn®; Naprelan®; Naprosyn®

Canadian Brand Names Apo®-Napro-Na; Apo®-Napro-Na DS; Apo®-Naproxen; Apo®-Naproxen SR; Gen-Naproxen EC; Naxen®; Novo-Naproc EC; Novo-Naprox; Novo-Naprox Sodium; Novo-Naprox Sodium DS; Novo-Naprox SR; Nu-Naprox; Riva-Naproxen

Pharmacologic Class Nonsteroidal Anti-inflammatory Drug (NSAID)

- **Naqua®** *see* Trichlormethiazide *on page 151*
- **Nasacort®** *see* Triamcinolone *on page 151*
- **Nasacort® AQ** *see* Triamcinolone *on page 151*
- **Nasonex®** *see* Mometasone Furoate *on page 114*

Nateglinide (na te GLYE nide)

Gene(s) of Interest
CYP2C9 *on page 183*
CYP3A4 *on page 189*

U.S. Brand Names Starlix®

Pharmacologic Class Antidiabetic Agent, Miscellaneous

- **Naturetin®** *see* Bendroflumethiazide *on page 55*
- **Navane®** *see* Thiothixene *on page 148*
- **Navelbine®** *see* Vinorelbine *on page 155*
- **NebuPent®** *see* Pentamidine *on page 125*
- **Necon® 0.5/35** *see* Ethinyl Estradiol and Norethindrone *on page 84*
- **Necon® 1/35** *see* Ethinyl Estradiol and Norethindrone *on page 84*
- **Necon® 1/50** *see* Mestranol and Norethindrone *on page 109*
- **Necon® 7/7/7** *see* Ethinyl Estradiol and Norethindrone *on page 84*
- **Necon® 10/11** *see* Ethinyl Estradiol and Norethindrone *on page 84*

Nefazodone (nef AY zoe done)

Gene(s) of Interest
Alpha-1 Adrenergic Receptor *on page 161*
CYP3A4 *on page 189*
G-Protein Beta-3 Subunit *on page 197*
Gs Protein Alpha-Subunit *on page 198*
P-Glycoprotein *on page 213*

U.S. Brand Names Serzone®

Canadian Brand Names Apo®-Nefazodone; Lin-Nefazodone; Serzone-5HT$_2$®

Pharmacologic Class Antidepressant, Serotonin Reuptake Inhibitor/Antagonist

- **NegGram®** *see* Nalidixic Acid *on page 116*

Nelfinavir (nel FIN a veer)
Gene(s) of Interest
P-Glycoprotein *on page 213*
U.S. Brand Names Viracept®
Pharmacologic Class Antiretroviral Agent, Protease Inhibitor

- **Neoral®** *see* CycloSPORINE *on page 69*
- **Neosar®** *see* Cyclophosphamide *on page 69*
- **Neurontin®** *see* Gabapentin *on page 91*
- **Nexium®** *see* Esomeprazole *on page 80*

NiCARdipine (nye KAR de peen)
Gene(s) of Interest
CYP3A4 *on page 189*
P-Glycoprotein *on page 213*
U.S. Brand Names Cardene®; Cardene® I.V.; Cardene® SR
Pharmacologic Class Calcium Channel Blocker

- **Nifedical™ XL** *see* NIFEdipine *on page 118*

NIFEdipine (nye FED i peen)
Gene(s) of Interest
CYP3A4 *on page 189*
P-Glycoprotein *on page 213*
U.S. Brand Names Adalat® CC; Nifedical™ XL; Procardia®; Procardia XL®
Canadian Brand Names Adalat® XL®; Apo®-Nifed; Apo®-Nifed PA; Novo-Nifedin; Nu-Nifed
Pharmacologic Class Calcium Channel Blocker

- **Niftolid** *see* Flutamide *on page 89*
- **Nilandron®** *see* Nilutamide *on page 118*

Nilutamide (ni LOO ta mide)
Gene(s) of Interest
CYP2C19 *on page 185*
U.S. Brand Names Nilandron®
Canadian Brand Names Anandron®
Synonyms RU-23908
Pharmacologic Class Antiandrogen; Antineoplastic Agent, Antiandrogen

Nimodipine (nye MOE di peen)
Gene(s) of Interest
CYP3A4 *on page 189*
U.S. Brand Names Nimotop®
Pharmacologic Class Calcium Channel Blocker

- **Nimotop®** *see* Nimodipine *on page 118*

Nisoldipine (NYE sole di peen)
Gene(s) of Interest
CYP3A4 *on page 189*
U.S. Brand Names Sular®
Pharmacologic Class Calcium Channel Blocker

♦ **Nitalapram** *see* Citalopram *on page 64*

Nitrendipine (NYE tren di peen)
Gene(s) of Interest
CYP3A4 *on page 189*
P-Glycoprotein *on page 213*
Pharmacologic Class Calcium Channel Blocker

♦ **4'-Nitro-3'-Trifluoromethylisobutyrantide** *see* Flutamide *on page 89*

Nitrofurantoin (nye troe fyoor AN toyn)
Gene(s) of Interest
Glucose-6-Phosphate Dehydrogenase *on page 195*
U.S. Brand Names Furadantin®; Macrobid®; Macrodantin®
Canadian Brand Names Apo®-Nitrofurantoin; Novo-Furantoin
Pharmacologic Class Antibiotic, Miscellaneous

♦ **Nizoral®** *see* Ketoconazole *on page 101*
♦ **Nizoral® A-D [OTC]** *see* Ketoconazole *on page 101*
♦ **Nolvadex®** *see* Tamoxifen *on page 145*
♦ **Norco®** *see* Hydrocodone and Acetaminophen *on page 94*
♦ **Nordette®** *see* Ethinyl Estradiol and Levonorgestrel *on page 83*
♦ **Norelgestromin and Ethinyl Estradiol** *see* Ethinyl Estradiol and Norelgestromin *on page 83*

Norethindrone (nor eth IN drone)
Gene(s) of Interest
BRCA Genes *on page 176*
Prothrombin *on page 219*
U.S. Brand Names Aygestin®; Camila™; Errin™; Micronor®; Nor-QD®
Canadian Brand Names Norlutate®
Synonyms Norethisterone
Pharmacologic Class Contraceptive; Progestin

♦ **Norethindrone Acetate and Ethinyl Estradiol** *see* Ethinyl Estradiol and Norethindrone *on page 84*
♦ **Norethindrone and Mestranol** *see* Mestranol and Norethindrone *on page 109*
♦ **Norethisterone** *see* Norethindrone *on page 119*
♦ **Norgestimate and Ethinyl Estradiol** *see* Ethinyl Estradiol and Norgestimate *on page 84*

Norgestrel (nor JES trel)
Gene(s) of Interest
BRCA Genes *on page 176*
(Continued)

Norgestrel *(Continued)*
Prothrombin *on page 219*
U.S. Brand Names Ovrette®
Pharmacologic Class Contraceptive

- **Norgestrel and Ethinyl Estradiol** *see* Ethinyl Estradiol and Norgestrel *on page 84*
- **Norinyl® 1+35** *see* Ethinyl Estradiol and Norethindrone *on page 84*
- **Norinyl® 1+50** *see* Mestranol and Norethindrone *on page 109*
- **Noritate™** *see* Metronidazole *on page 112*
- **Norpace®** *see* Disopyramide *on page 74*
- **Norpace® CR** *see* Disopyramide *on page 74*
- **Norplant® Implant [DSC]** *see* Levonorgestrel *on page 103*
- **Norpramin®** *see* Desipramine *on page 71*
- **Nor-QD®** *see* Norethindrone *on page 119*
- **Nortrel™** *see* Ethinyl Estradiol and Norethindrone *on page 84*
- **Nortrel™ 7/7/7** *see* Ethinyl Estradiol and Norethindrone *on page 84*

Nortriptyline (nor TRIP ti leen)
Gene(s) of Interest
Alpha-1 Adrenergic Receptor *on page 161*
G-Protein Beta-3 Subunit *on page 197*
Gs Protein Alpha-Subunit *on page 198*
P-Glycoprotein *on page 213*
U.S. Brand Names Aventyl® HCl; Pamelor®
Canadian Brand Names Alti-Nortriptyline; Apo®-Nortriptyline; Aventyl®; Gen-Nortriptyline; Norventyl; Novo-Nortriptyline; Nu-Nortriptyline; PMS-Nortriptyline
Pharmacologic Class Antidepressant, Tricyclic (Secondary Amine)

- **Norvasc®** *see* Amlodipine *on page 49*
- **Norvir®** *see* Ritonavir *on page 137*
- **Novolin® 70/30** *see* Insulin Preparations *on page 98*
- **Novolin® L** *see* Insulin Preparations *on page 98*
- **Novolin® N** *see* Insulin Preparations *on page 98*
- **Novolin® R** *see* Insulin Preparations *on page 98*
- **NovoLog®** *see* Insulin Preparations *on page 98*
- **NovoLog® Mix 70/30** *see* Insulin Preparations *on page 98*
- **Novothyrox** *see* Levothyroxine *on page 103*
- **NPH Iletin® II** *see* Insulin Preparations *on page 98*
- **NSC-752** *see* Thioguanine *on page 147*
- **NSC-755** *see* Mercaptopurine *on page 109*
- **NSC-26271** *see* Cyclophosphamide *on page 69*
- **NSC-26980** *see* Mitomycin *on page 113*
- **NSC-49842** *see* VinBLAStine *on page 154*
- **NSC-67574** *see* VinCRIStine *on page 155*
- **NSC-109724** *see* Ifosfamide *on page 97*
- **NSC-123127** *see* DOXOrubicin *on page 76*

OLANZAPINE

- **NSC-125973** *see* Paclitaxel *on page 124*
- **NSC-147834** *see* Flutamide *on page 89*
- **NSC-180973** *see* Tamoxifen *on page 145*
- **NSC-628503** *see* Docetaxel *on page 75*
- **NSC-639186** *see* Raltitrexed *on page 135*
- **NSC-706363** *see* Arsenic Trioxide *on page 51*
- **Nubain®** *see* Nalbuphine *on page 116*
- **Numorphan®** *see* Oxymorphone *on page 124*
- **Nupercainal® Hydrocortisone Cream [OTC]** *see* Hydrocortisone *on page 95*
- **Nutracort®** *see* Hydrocortisone *on page 95*
- **NuvaRing®** *see* Ethinyl Estradiol and Etonogestrel *on page 83*
- **NVB** *see* Vinorelbine *on page 155*
- **Nydrazid®** *see* Isoniazid *on page 99*

Octreotide (ok TREE oh tide)
Gene(s) of Interest
Cardiac Potassium Ion Channel *on page 177*
Cardiac Sodium Channel *on page 178*
U.S. Brand Names Sandostatin®; Sandostatin LAR®
Pharmacologic Class Antidiarrheal; Somatostatin Analog

- **Ocu-Chlor®** *see* Chloramphenicol *on page 62*
- **Ocufen®** *see* Flurbiprofen *on page 89*
- **Ocuflox®** *see* Ofloxacin *on page 121*
- **Ocusulf-10** *see* Sulfacetamide *on page 142*

Ofloxacin (oh FLOKS a sin)
Gene(s) of Interest
P-Glycoprotein *on page 213*
U.S. Brand Names Floxin®; Ocuflox®
Canadian Brand Names Apo®-Oflox
Pharmacologic Class Antibiotic, Quinolone

- **Ogen®** *see* Estropipate *on page 82*
- **Ogestrel®** *see* Ethinyl Estradiol and Norgestrel *on page 84*

Olanzapine (oh LAN za peen)
Gene(s) of Interest
Alpha-1 Adrenergic Receptor *on page 161*
D2 Receptor *on page 190*
D3 Receptor *on page 191*
Histamine 1 and 2 Receptors *on page 199*
5HT2A Receptor *on page 201*
5HT2C Receptor *on page 202*
5HT6 Receptor *on page 203*
TNF-Alpha *on page 222*
U.S. Brand Names Zyprexa®; Zyprexa® Zydis®
Synonyms LY170053
Pharmacologic Class Antipsychotic Agent, Thienobenzodiazepine

Olmesartan (ole me SAR tan)
Gene(s) of Interest
Aldosterone Synthase *on page 160*
Angiotensin-Converting Enzyme *on page 163*
Angiotensin II Type I Receptor *on page 166*
Angiotensinogen *on page 167*
U.S. Brand Names Benicar™
Pharmacologic Class Angiotensin II Receptor Blocker

Olopatadine (oh loe pa TA deen)
Gene(s) of Interest None known
U.S. Brand Names Patanol®
Pharmacologic Class Antihistamine; Ophthalmic Agent, Miscellaneous

Omeprazole (oh ME pray zol)
Gene(s) of Interest
CYP2C19 *on page 185*
U.S. Brand Names Prilosec®
Canadian Brand Names Losec®
Pharmacologic Class Proton Pump Inhibitor

- **Omnicef®** *see* Cefdinir *on page 61*
- **Oncovin® [DSC]** *see* VinCRIStine *on page 155*
- **Onxol™** *see* Paclitaxel *on page 124*
- **OPC13013** *see* Cilostazol *on page 64*
- **OPC14597** *see* Aripiprazole *on page 51*
- **Opium and Belladonna** *see* Belladonna and Opium *on page 55*

Opium Tincture (OH pee um TING chur)
Gene(s) of Interest
COMT *on page 180*
Synonyms DTO; Opium Tincture, Deodorized
Pharmacologic Class Analgesic, Narcotic; Antidiarrheal

- **Opium Tincture, Deodorized** *see* Opium Tincture *on page 122*
- **Optivar™** *see* Azelastine *on page 54*
- **Oramorph SR®** *see* Morphine Sulfate *on page 115*
- **Orap®** *see* Pimozide *on page 127*
- **Orciprenaline Sulfate** *see* Metaproterenol *on page 109*
- **Oretic®** *see* Hydrochlorothiazide *on page 94*
- **Orinase Diagnostic® [DSC]** *see* TOLBUTamide *on page 149*
- **ORLAAM®** *see* Levomethadyl Acetate Hydrochloride *on page 102*
- **Ortho-Cept®** *see* Ethinyl Estradiol and Desogestrel *on page 82*
- **Ortho-Cyclen®** *see* Ethinyl Estradiol and Norgestimate *on page 84*
- **Ortho-Est®** *see* Estropipate *on page 82*
- **Ortho Evra™** *see* Ethinyl Estradiol and Norelgestromin *on page 83*
- **Ortho-Novum®** *see* Ethinyl Estradiol and Norethindrone *on page 84*

OXYCODONE AND ASPIRIN

- **Ortho-Novum® 1/50** see Mestranol and Norethindrone on page 109
- **Ortho Tri-Cyclen®** see Ethinyl Estradiol and Norgestimate on page 84
- **Ortho Tri-Cyclen® Lo** see Ethinyl Estradiol and Norgestimate on page 84
- **Orudis® [DSC]** see Ketoprofen on page 101
- **Orudis® KT [OTC]** see Ketoprofen on page 101
- **Oruvail®** see Ketoprofen on page 101
- **Ovace™** see Sulfacetamide on page 142
- **Ovcon®** see Ethinyl Estradiol and Norethindrone on page 84
- **Ovral®** see Ethinyl Estradiol and Norgestrel on page 84
- **Ovrette®** see Norgestrel on page 119

Oxaprozin (oks a PROE zin)
Gene(s) of Interest
Leukotriene C4 Synthase on page 206
U.S. Brand Names Daypro®
Canadian Brand Names Apo®-Oxaprozin; Rhoxal-oxaprozin
Pharmacologic Class Nonsteroidal Anti-inflammatory Drug (NSAID)

- **Oxilapine Succinate** see Loxapine on page 106

Oxycodone (oks i KOE done)
Gene(s) of Interest
COMT on page 180
CYP2D6 on page 186
U.S. Brand Names OxyContin®; Oxydose™; OxyFast®; OxyIR®; Percolone® [DSC]; Roxicodone™; Roxicodone™ Intensol™
Canadian Brand Names Oxy.IR®; Supeudol®
Synonyms Dihydrohydroxycodeinone
Pharmacologic Class Analgesic, Narcotic

Oxycodone and Acetaminophen
(oks i KOE done & a seet a MIN oh fen)
Gene(s) of Interest
COMT on page 180
CYP2D6 on page 186
U.S. Brand Names Endocet®; Percocet® 2.5/325; Percocet® 5/325; Percocet® 7.5/325; Percocet® 7.5/500; Percocet® 10/325; Percocet® 10/650; Roxicet®; Roxicet® 5/500; Tylox®
Canadian Brand Names Oxycocet®; Percocet®; Percocet®-Demi
Synonyms Acetaminophen and Oxycodone
Pharmacologic Class Analgesic, Narcotic

Oxycodone and Aspirin (oks i KOE done & AS pir in)
Gene(s) of Interest
COMT on page 180
CYP2D6 on page 186
Glycoprotein IIIa Receptor on page 196
Leukotriene C4 Synthase on page 206
(Continued)

Oxycodone and Aspirin *(Continued)*
U.S. Brand Names Endodan®; Percodan®; Percodan®-Demi [DSC]
Canadian Brand Names Endodan®; Oxycodan®
Synonyms Aspirin and Oxycodone
Pharmacologic Class Analgesic, Narcotic

- **OxyContin®** *see* Oxycodone *on page 123*
- **Oxydose™** *see* Oxycodone *on page 123*
- **OxyFast®** *see* Oxycodone *on page 123*
- **OxyIR®** *see* Oxycodone *on page 123*

Oxymorphone (oks i MOR fone)
Gene(s) of Interest
COMT *on page 180*
U.S. Brand Names Numorphan®
Pharmacologic Class Analgesic, Narcotic

- **P-071** *see* Cetirizine *on page 62*
- **Pacerone®** *see* Amiodarone *on page 48*

Paclitaxel (PAK li taks el)
Gene(s) of Interest
CYP2C9 *on page 183*
CYP3A4 *on page 189*
P-Glycoprotein *on page 213*
U.S. Brand Names Onxol™; Taxol®
Synonyms NSC-125973
Pharmacologic Class Antineoplastic Agent, Antimicrotubular; Antineoplastic Agent, Natural Source (Plant) Derivative

- **Pamelor®** *see* Nortriptyline *on page 120*
- **Pandel®** *see* Hydrocortisone *on page 95*

Pantoprazole (pan TOE pra zole)
Gene(s) of Interest None known
U.S. Brand Names Protonix®
Canadian Brand Names Panto™ IV; Pantoloc™
Pharmacologic Class Proton Pump Inhibitor

Paregoric (par e GOR ik)
Gene(s) of Interest
COMT *on page 180*
Synonyms Camphorated Tincture of Opium
Pharmacologic Class Analgesic, Narcotic

- **Pariprazole** *see* Rabeprazole *on page 134*
- **Parlodel®** *see* Bromocriptine *on page 57*

Paroxetine (pa ROKS e teen)
Gene(s) of Interest
CYP2D6 *on page 186*

PENTAZOCINE COMBINATIONS

G-Protein Beta-3 Subunit *on page 197*
Gs Protein Alpha-Subunit *on page 198*
5HT Transporter *on page 204*
TNF-Alpha *on page 222*
Tryptophan Hydroxylase *on page 223*
U.S. Brand Names Paxil®; Paxil® CR™
Pharmacologic Class Antidepressant, Selective Serotonin Reuptake Inhibitor

- **Patanol®** *see* Olopatadine *on page 122*
- **Paxil®** *see* Paroxetine *on page 124*
- **Paxil® CR™** *see* Paroxetine *on page 124*
- **PCA** *see* Procainamide *on page 130*
- **PCE®** *see* Erythromycin *on page 79*
- **PCP** *see* Phencyclidine *on page 127*
- **Pediazole®** *see* Erythromycin and Sulfisoxazole *on page 80*

Penicillin V Potassium (pen i SIL in vee poe TASS ee um)
Gene(s) of Interest None known
U.S. Brand Names Veetids®
Canadian Brand Names Apo®-Pen VK; Nadopen-V®; Novo-Pen-VK®; Nu-Pen-VK®; PVF® K
Synonyms Pen VK; Phenoxymethyl Penicillin
Pharmacologic Class Antibiotic, Penicillin

- **Pentam-300®** *see* Pentamidine *on page 125*

Pentamidine (pen TAM i deen)
Gene(s) of Interest
Cardiac Potassium Ion Channel *on page 177*
Cardiac Sodium Channel *on page 178*
CYP2C19 *on page 185*
U.S. Brand Names NebuPent®; Pentam-300®
Canadian Brand Names Pentacarinat®
Pharmacologic Class Antibiotic, Miscellaneous

Pentazocine (pen TAZ oh seen)
Gene(s) of Interest
COMT *on page 180*
U.S. Brand Names Talwin®; Talwin® NX
Pharmacologic Class Analgesic, Narcotic

Pentazocine Combinations
(pen TAZ oh seen kom bi NAY shuns)
Gene(s) of Interest
COMT *on page 180*
U.S. Brand Names Talacen®
Pharmacologic Class Analgesic Combination (Narcotic)

- **Pen VK** *see* Penicillin V Potassium *on page 125*
- **Pepcid®** *see* Famotidine *on page 85*
- **Pepcid® AC [OTC]** *see* Famotidine *on page 85*

PERGOLIDE

- **Percocet® 2.5/325** *see* Oxycodone and Acetaminophen *on page 123*
- **Percocet® 5/325** *see* Oxycodone and Acetaminophen *on page 123*
- **Percocet® 7.5/325** *see* Oxycodone and Acetaminophen *on page 123*
- **Percocet® 7.5/500** *see* Oxycodone and Acetaminophen *on page 123*
- **Percocet® 10/325** *see* Oxycodone and Acetaminophen *on page 123*
- **Percocet® 10/650** *see* Oxycodone and Acetaminophen *on page 123*
- **Percodan®** *see* Oxycodone and Aspirin *on page 123*
- **Percodan®-Demi [DSC]** *see* Oxycodone and Aspirin *on page 123*
- **Percogesic® [OTC]** *see* Acetaminophen and Phenyltoloxamine *on page 45*
- **Percolone® [DSC]** *see* Oxycodone *on page 123*

Pergolide (PER go lide)
Gene(s) of Interest
CYP2D6 *on page 186*
CYP3A4 *on page 189*

U.S. Brand Names Permax®

Pharmacologic Class Anti-Parkinson's Agent, Dopamine Agonist; Ergot Derivative

Perindopril Erbumine (per IN doe pril er BYOO meen)
Gene(s) of Interest
Aldosterone Synthase *on page 160*
Angiotensin-Converting Enzyme *on page 163*
Angiotensin II Type I Receptor *on page 166*
Angiotensinogen *on page 167*
Bradykinin B2 Receptor *on page 175*

U.S. Brand Names Aceon®

Canadian Brand Names Coversyl®

Pharmacologic Class Angiotensin-Converting Enzyme (ACE) Inhibitor

- **Periostat®** *see* Doxycycline *on page 76*
- **Permax®** *see* Pergolide *on page 126*

Perphenazine (per FEN a zeen)
Gene(s) of Interest
Alpha-1 Adrenergic Receptor *on page 161*
CYP2D6 *on page 186*
D2 Receptor *on page 190*

U.S. Brand Names Trilafon® [DSC]

Canadian Brand Names Apo®-Perphenazine

Pharmacologic Class Antipsychotic Agent, Phenothiazine, Piperazine

- **Perphenazine and Amitriptyline** *see* Amitriptyline and Perphenazine *on page 49*

PIMOZIDE

- **Persantine®** *see* Dipyridamole *on page 74*
- **Pethidine Hydrochloride** *see* Meperidine *on page 108*
- **PFA** *see* Foscarnet *on page 90*
- **Phenaphen® With Codeine** *see* Acetaminophen and Codeine *on page 44*

Phencyclidine (fen SYE kli deen)
Gene(s) of Interest
CYP3A4 *on page 189*
Synonyms PCP
Pharmacologic Class General Anesthetic

- **Phenergan® With Codeine** *see* Promethazine and Codeine *on page 131*

Phenobarbital (fee noe BAR bi tal)
Gene(s) of Interest
CYP2C19 *on page 185*
U.S. Brand Names Luminal® Sodium
Synonyms Phenobarbitone; Phenylethylmalonylurea
Pharmacologic Class Anticonvulsant, Barbiturate; Barbiturate

- **Phenobarbitone** *see* Phenobarbital *on page 127*
- **Phenoxymethyl Penicillin** *see* Penicillin V Potassium *on page 125*
- **Phenylethylmalonylurea** *see* Phenobarbital *on page 127*
- **Phenylgesic® [OTC]** *see* Acetaminophen and Phenyltoloxamine *on page 45*
- **Phenyltoloxamine and Acetaminophen** *see* Acetaminophen and Phenyltoloxamine *on page 45*
- **Phenytek™** *see* Phenytoin *on page 127*

Phenytoin (FEN i toyn)
Gene(s) of Interest
CYP2C9 *on page 183*
CYP2C19 *on page 185*
P-Glycoprotein *on page 213*
U.S. Brand Names Dilantin®; Phenytek™
Synonyms Diphenylhydantoin; DPH
Pharmacologic Class Antiarrhythmic Agent, Class Ib; Anticonvulsant, Hydantoin

- **Phosphonoformate** *see* Foscarnet *on page 90*
- **Phosphonoformic Acid** *see* Foscarnet *on page 90*
- ***p*-Hydroxyampicillin** *see* Amoxicillin *on page 49*

Pimozide (PI moe zide)
Gene(s) of Interest
Alpha-1 Adrenergic Receptor *on page 161*
Cardiac Potassium Ion Channel *on page 177*
Cardiac Sodium Channel *on page 178*
CYP1A2 *on page 181*
CYP2D6 *on page 186*
(Continued)

Pimozide *(Continued)*
CYP3A4 *on page 189*
D2 Receptor *on page 190*
U.S. Brand Names Orap®
Pharmacologic Class Antipsychotic Agent, Diphenylbutylperidine

Pioglitazone (pye oh GLI ta zone)
Gene(s) of Interest
CYP2C9 *on page 183*
CYP3A4 *on page 189*
U.S. Brand Names Actos®
Pharmacologic Class Antidiabetic Agent, Thiazolidinedione

♦ **Piperazine Estrone Sulfate** *see* Estropipate *on page 82*

Pirbuterol (peer BYOO ter ole)
Gene(s) of Interest
Beta-2 Adrenergic Receptor *on page 171*
U.S. Brand Names Maxair™; Maxair™ Autohaler™
Pharmacologic Class Beta$_2$ Agonist

Piroxicam (peer OKS i kam)
Gene(s) of Interest
Leukotriene C4 Synthase *on page 206*
U.S. Brand Names Feldene®
Canadian Brand Names Apo®-Piroxicam; Gen-Piroxicam; Novo-Pirocam®; Nu-Pirox; Pexicam®
Pharmacologic Class Nonsteroidal Anti-inflammatory Drug (NSAID)

♦ *p*-Isobutylhydratropic Acid *see* Ibuprofen *on page 96*
♦ **Plan B**® *see* Levonorgestrel *on page 103*
♦ **Plaquenil**® *see* Hydroxychloroquine *on page 96*
♦ **Plavix**® *see* Clopidogrel *on page 66*
♦ **Plendil**® *see* Felodipine *on page 86*
♦ **Pletal**® *see* Cilostazol *on page 64*

Polythiazide (pol i THYE a zide)
Gene(s) of Interest
Alpha-Adducin *on page 162*
G-Protein Beta-3 Subunit *on page 197*
U.S. Brand Names Renese®
Pharmacologic Class Diuretic, Thiazide

♦ **Ponstel**® *see* Mefenamic Acid *on page 108*
♦ **Portia**™ *see* Ethinyl Estradiol and Levonorgestrel *on page 83*
♦ **Post Peel Healing Balm [OTC]** *see* Hydrocortisone *on page 95*

Potassium Chloride (poe TASS ee um KLOR ide)
Gene(s) of Interest None known
U.S. Brand Names K+8; K+10; Kaon-Cl-10®; Kaon-Cl® 20; Kay Ciel®; K+ Care®; K-Dur® 10; K-Dur® 20; K-Lor™; Klor-Con®; Klor-Con® 8;

PREDNISONE

Klor-Con® 10; Klor-Con®/25; Klor-Con® M10; Klor-Con® M20; Klotrix®; K-Tab®; microK®; microK® 10; Rum-K®

Canadian Brand Names Apo®-K; K-10®; K-Lyte®/Cl; Micro-K Extencaps®; Roychlor®; Slow-K®

Synonyms KCl

Pharmacologic Class Electrolyte Supplement, Oral; Electrolyte Supplement, Parenteral

- **Prandin®** see Repaglinide on page 136
- **Pravachol®** see Pravastatin on page 129

Pravastatin (PRA va stat in)

Gene(s) of Interest
Angiotensin-Converting Enzyme on page 163
Apolipoprotein E on page 168
Beta-Fibrinogen on page 174
Cholesteryl Ester Transfer Protein on page 179
Glycoprotein IIIa Receptor on page 196
Low-Density Lipoprotein Receptor on page 209
Stromelysin-1 on page 219

U.S. Brand Names Pravachol®

Canadian Brand Names Apo®-Pravastatin; Lin-Pravastatin; Novo-Pravastatin

Pharmacologic Class Antilipemic Agent, HMG-CoA Reductase Inhibitor

- **Precedex™** see Dexmedetomidine on page 71

PredniSONE (PRED ni sone)

Gene(s) of Interest None known

U.S. Brand Names Deltasone®; Prednisone Intensol™; Sterapred®; Sterapred® DS

Canadian Brand Names Apo®-Prednisone; Winpred™

Synonyms Deltacortisone; Deltadehydrocortisone

Pharmacologic Class Corticosteroid, Systemic

- **Prednisone Intensol™** see PredniSONE on page 129
- **Pregnenedione** see Progesterone on page 131
- **Premarin®** see Estrogens (Conjugated/Equine) on page 81
- **Premject® [OTC]** see Lidocaine on page 103
- **Premphase®** see Estrogens (Conjugated/Equine) and Medroxyprogesterone on page 81
- **Prempro™** see Estrogens (Conjugated/Equine) and Medroxyprogesterone on page 81
- **Preparation H® Hydrocortisone [OTC]** see Hydrocortisone on page 95
- **Prevacid®** see Lansoprazole on page 102
- **PREVEN®** see Ethinyl Estradiol and Levonorgestrel on page 83
- **Prilocaine and Lidocaine** see Lidocaine and Prilocaine on page 104
- **Prilosec®** see Omeprazole on page 122

PRIMAQUINE

Primaquine (PRIM a kween)
Gene(s) of Interest
　Glucose-6-Phosphate Dehydrogenase *on page 195*
Synonyms Prymaccone
Pharmacologic Class Aminoquinoline (Antimalarial)

◆ **Primsol®** *see* Trimethoprim *on page 152*
◆ **Prinivil®** *see* Lisinopril *on page 104*
◆ **Prinzide®** *see* Lisinopril and Hydrochlorothiazide *on page 104*

Probenecid (proe BEN e sid)
Gene(s) of Interest
　Glucose-6-Phosphate Dehydrogenase *on page 195*
　P-Glycoprotein *on page 213*
Canadian Brand Names Benuryl™
Synonyms Benemid [DSC]
Pharmacologic Class Uricosuric Agent

Procainamide (proe kane A mide)
Gene(s) of Interest
　Cardiac Potassium Ion Channel *on page 177*
　Cardiac Sodium Channel *on page 178*
　N-Acetyltransferase 2 Enzyme *on page 211*
U.S. Brand Names Procanbid®; Pronestyl®; Pronestyl-SR®
Canadian Brand Names Apo®-Procainamide; Procan® SR
Synonyms PCA; Procaine Amide Hydrochloride
Pharmacologic Class Antiarrhythmic Agent, Class Ia

◆ **Procaine Amide Hydrochloride** *see* Procainamide *on page 130*
◆ **Procanbid®** *see* Procainamide *on page 130*
◆ **Procardia®** *see* NIFEdipine *on page 118*
◆ **Procardia XL®** *see* NIFEdipine *on page 118*
◆ **Procetofene** *see* Fenofibrate *on page 86*
◆ **Prochieve™** *see* Progesterone *on page 131*

Prochlorperazine (proe klor PER a zeen)
Gene(s) of Interest
　Alpha-1 Adrenergic Receptor *on page 161*
　D2 Receptor *on page 190*
　P-Glycoprotein *on page 213*
U.S. Brand Names Compazine®; Compro™
Canadian Brand Names Apo®-Prochlorperazine; Nu-Prochlor; Stemetil®
Synonyms Chlormeprazine
Pharmacologic Class Antiemetic; Antipsychotic Agent, Phenothiazine, Piperazine

◆ **Proctocort®** *see* Hydrocortisone *on page 95*
◆ **ProctoCream® HC** *see* Hydrocortisone *on page 95*
◆ **Proctofene** *see* Fenofibrate *on page 86*
◆ **Proctosol-HC®** *see* Hydrocortisone *on page 95*

- **Progestasert®** *see Progesterone on page 131*

Progesterone (proe JES ter one)
Gene(s) of Interest
P-Glycoprotein *on page 213*
U.S. Brand Names Crinone®; Prochieve™; Progestasert®; Prometrium®
Synonyms Pregnenedione; Progestin
Pharmacologic Class Progestin

- **Progestin** *see Progesterone on page 131*
- **Prograf®** *see Tacrolimus on page 144*
- **Prolixin®** *see Fluphenazine on page 88*
- **Prolixin Decanoate®** *see Fluphenazine on page 88*
- **Prolixin Enanthate® [DSC]** *see Fluphenazine on page 88*
- **Proloprim®** *see Trimethoprim on page 152*

Promethazine (proe METH a zeen)
Gene(s) of Interest None known
Canadian Brand Names Phenergan®
Pharmacologic Class Antiemetic; Antihistamine; Phenothiazine Derivative; Sedative

Promethazine and Codeine
(proe METH a zeen & KOE deen)
Gene(s) of Interest
COMT *on page 180*
CYP2D6 *on page 186*
U.S. Brand Names Phenergan® With Codeine
Synonyms Codeine and Promethazine
Pharmacologic Class Antihistamine/Antitussive

- **Promethazine and Meperidine** *see Meperidine and Promethazine on page 108*
- **Prometrium®** *see Progesterone on page 131*
- **Pronap-100®** *see Propoxyphene and Acetaminophen on page 132*
- **Pronestyl®** *see Procainamide on page 130*
- **Pronestyl-SR®** *see Procainamide on page 130*

Propafenone (proe pa FEEN one)
Gene(s) of Interest
CYP2D6 *on page 186*
P-Glycoprotein *on page 213*
U.S. Brand Names Rythmol®
Canadian Brand Names Apo®-Propafenone
Pharmacologic Class Antiarrhythmic Agent, Class Ic

Propofol (PROE po fole)
Gene(s) of Interest
CYP2C9 *on page 183*
(Continued)

PROPOXYPHENE

Propofol *(Continued)*
U.S. Brand Names Diprivan®
Pharmacologic Class General Anesthetic

Propoxyphene (proe POKS i feen)
Gene(s) of Interest
  COMT *on page 180*
U.S. Brand Names Darvon®; Darvon-N®
Canadian Brand Names 642® Tablet
Synonyms Dextropropoxyphene
Pharmacologic Class Analgesic, Narcotic

Propoxyphene and Acetaminophen
(proe POKS i feen & a seet a MIN oh fen)
Gene(s) of Interest
  COMT *on page 180*
U.S. Brand Names Darvocet-N® 50; Darvocet-N® 100; Pronap-100®
Synonyms Acetaminophen and Propoxyphene; Propoxyphene Hydrochloride and Acetaminophen; Propoxyphene Napsylate and Acetaminophen
Pharmacologic Class Analgesic Combination (Narcotic)

Propoxyphene and Aspirin (proe POKS i feen & AS pir in)
Gene(s) of Interest
  COMT *on page 180*
U.S. Brand Names Darvon® Compound-65 Pulvules®
Synonyms Aspirin and Propoxyphene; Propoxyphene Hydrochloride and Aspirin; Propoxyphene Napsylate and Aspirin
Pharmacologic Class Analgesic Combination (Narcotic)

- **Propoxyphene Hydrochloride and Acetaminophen** *see* Propoxyphene and Acetaminophen *on page 132*
- **Propoxyphene Hydrochloride and Aspirin** *see* Propoxyphene and Aspirin *on page 132*
- **Propoxyphene Napsylate and Acetaminophen** *see* Propoxyphene and Acetaminophen *on page 132*
- **Propoxyphene Napsylate and Aspirin** *see* Propoxyphene and Aspirin *on page 132*

Propranolol (proe PRAN oh lole)
Gene(s) of Interest
  Beta-1 Adrenergic Receptor *on page 171*
  CYP1A2 *on page 181*
  CYP2C19 *on page 185*
  Gs Protein Alpha-Subunit *on page 198*
  P-Glycoprotein *on page 213*
U.S. Brand Names Inderal®; Inderal® LA; Propranolol Intensol™
Canadian Brand Names Apo®-Propranolol; Nu-Propranolol
Pharmacologic Class Antiarrhythmic Agent, Class II; Beta Blocker, Nonselective

- **Propranolol Intensol™** *see* Propranolol *on page 132*
- **Propulsid®** *see* Cisapride *on page 64*
- **2-Propylpentanoic Acid** *see* Valproic Acid and Derivatives *on page 153*
- **2-Propylvaleric Acid** *see* Valproic Acid and Derivatives *on page 153*
- **Protonix®** *see* Pantoprazole *on page 124*
- **Protopic®** *see* Tacrolimus *on page 144*

Protriptyline (proe TRIP ti leen)
Gene(s) of Interest
Alpha-1 Adrenergic Receptor *on page 161*
G-Protein Beta-3 Subunit *on page 197*
Gs Protein Alpha-Subunit *on page 198*
U.S. Brand Names Vivactil®
Pharmacologic Class Antidepressant, Tricyclic (Secondary Amine)

- **Proventil®** *see* Albuterol *on page 46*
- **Proventil® HFA** *see* Albuterol *on page 46*
- **Proventil® Repetabs®** *see* Albuterol *on page 46*
- **Provera®** *see* MedroxyPROGESTERone *on page 107*
- **Provigil®** *see* Modafinil *on page 114*
- **Prozac®** *see* Fluoxetine *on page 88*
- **Prozac® Weekly™** *see* Fluoxetine *on page 88*
- **Prudoxin™** *see* Doxepin *on page 76*
- **Prymaccone** *see* Primaquine *on page 130*
- **Pseudomonic Acid A** *see* Mupirocin *on page 116*
- **Pulmicort Respules®** *see* Budesonide *on page 57*
- **Pulmicort Turbuhaler®** *see* Budesonide *on page 57*
- **Purinethol®** *see* Mercaptopurine *on page 109*
- **Pyrimethamine and Sulfadoxine** *see* Sulfadoxine and Pyrimethamine *on page 143*

Quetiapine (kwe TYE a peen)
Gene(s) of Interest
Alpha-1 Adrenergic Receptor *on page 161*
Cardiac Potassium Ion Channel *on page 177*
Cardiac Sodium Channel *on page 178*
CYP3A4 *on page 189*
D2 Receptor *on page 190*
U.S. Brand Names Seroquel®
Pharmacologic Class Antipsychotic Agent, Dibenzothiazepine

- **Quibron®-T** *see* Theophylline *on page 147*
- **Quibron®-T/SR** *see* Theophylline *on page 147*
- **Quinaglute® Dura-Tabs®** *see* Quinidine *on page 134*

Quinapril (KWIN a pril)
Gene(s) of Interest
Aldosterone Synthase *on page 160*
(Continued)

Quinapril *(Continued)*
Angiotensin-Converting Enzyme *on page 163*
Angiotensin II Type I Receptor *on page 166*
Angiotensinogen *on page 167*
Bradykinin B2 Receptor *on page 175*

U.S. Brand Names Accupril®

Pharmacologic Class Angiotensin-Converting Enzyme (ACE) Inhibitor

♦ **Quinidex® Extentabs®** *see* Quinidine *on page 134*

Quinidine (KWIN i deen)
Gene(s) of Interest
Cardiac Potassium Ion Channel *on page 177*
Cardiac Sodium Channel *on page 178*
CYP2D6 *on page 186*
CYP3A4 *on page 189*
Glucose-6-Phosphate Dehydrogenase *on page 195*
P-Glycoprotein *on page 213*

U.S. Brand Names Quinaglute® Dura-Tabs®; Quinidex® Extentabs®

Canadian Brand Names Apo®-Quin-G; Apo®-Quinidine; BioQuin® Durules™; Novo-Quinidin; Quinate®

Pharmacologic Class Antiarrhythmic Agent, Class Ia

Quinine (KWYE nine)
Gene(s) of Interest
CYP2D6 *on page 186*
Glucose-6-Phosphate Dehydrogenase *on page 195*
P-Glycoprotein *on page 213*

Canadian Brand Names Quinine-Odan™

Pharmacologic Class Antimalarial Agent

♦ **Quixin™** *see* Levofloxacin *on page 102*

Rabeprazole (ra BE pray zole)
Gene(s) of Interest
CYP2C19 *on page 185*

U.S. Brand Names Aciphex®

Canadian Brand Names Pariet®

Synonyms Pariprazole

Pharmacologic Class Proton Pump Inhibitor

♦ **R-albuterol** *see* Levalbuterol *on page 102*

Raloxifene (ral OKS i feen)
Gene(s) of Interest None known

U.S. Brand Names Evista®

Synonyms Keoxifene Hydrochloride

Pharmacologic Class Selective Estrogen Receptor Modulator (SERM)

Raltitrexed (ral ti TREX ed)
Gene(s) of Interest
Methylenetetrahydrofolate Reductase *on page 210*
Canadian Brand Names Tomudex®
Synonyms ICI-D1694; NSC-639186; ZD1694
Pharmacologic Class Antineoplastic Agent, Antimetabolite

Ramipril (ra MI pril)
Gene(s) of Interest
Aldosterone Synthase *on page 160*
Angiotensin-Converting Enzyme *on page 163*
Angiotensin II Type I Receptor *on page 166*
Angiotensinogen *on page 167*
Bradykinin B2 Receptor *on page 175*
U.S. Brand Names Altace®
Pharmacologic Class Angiotensin-Converting Enzyme (ACE) Inhibitor

Ranitidine (ra NI ti deen)
Gene(s) of Interest
P-Glycoprotein *on page 213*
U.S. Brand Names Zantac®; Zantac® 75 [OTC]
Canadian Brand Names Alti-Ranitidine; Apo®-Ranitidine; Gen-Ranidine; Novo-Ranidine; Nu-Ranit; PMS-Ranitidine; Rhoxal-ranitidine
Pharmacologic Class Histamine H_2 Antagonist

♦ **Rapamune®** *see* Sirolimus *on page 141*

Rasburicase (ras BYOOR i kayse)
Gene(s) of Interest
Glucose-6-Phosphate Dehydrogenase *on page 195*
U.S. Brand Names Elitek™
Pharmacologic Class Enzyme; Enzyme, Urate-Oxidase (Recombinant)

♦ **Reglan®** *see* Metoclopramide *on page 111*
♦ **Regular Iletin® II** *see* Insulin Preparations *on page 98*
♦ **Relafen®** *see* Nabumetone *on page 116*
♦ **Relpax®** *see* Eletriptan *on page 77*
♦ **Remeron®** *see* Mirtazapine *on page 113*
♦ **Remeron SolTab®** *see* Mirtazapine *on page 113*

Remifentanil (rem i FEN ta nil)
Gene(s) of Interest
COMT *on page 180*
U.S. Brand Names Ultiva®
Synonyms GI87084B
Pharmacologic Class Analgesic, Narcotic

♦ **Reminyl®** *see* Galantamine *on page 91*
♦ **Renese®** *see* Polythiazide *on page 128*

+ **ReoPro®** *see Abciximab on page 44*

Repaglinide (re pa GLI nide)
Gene(s) of Interest
CYP3A4 *on page 189*
U.S. Brand Names Prandin®
Canadian Brand Names GlucoNorm®
Pharmacologic Class Antidiabetic Agent, Miscellaneous

+ **Requip®** *see Ropinirole on page 138*

Reserpine (re SER peen)
Gene(s) of Interest
P-Glycoprotein *on page 213*
Pharmacologic Class Rauwolfia Alkaloid

+ **Restasis™** *see CycloSPORINE on page 69*
+ **Restoril®** *see Temazepam on page 145*
+ **Rhinocort® [DSC]** *see Budesonide on page 57*
+ **Rhinocort® Aqua™** *see Budesonide on page 57*

Rifabutin (rif a BYOO tin)
Gene(s) of Interest
CYP1A2 *on page 181*
U.S. Brand Names Mycobutin®
Synonyms Ansamycin
Pharmacologic Class Antibiotic, Miscellaneous; Antitubercular Agent

+ **Rifadin®** *see Rifampin on page 136*
+ **Rifampicin** *see Rifampin on page 136*

Rifampin (RIF am pin)
Gene(s) of Interest
CYP2C9 *on page 183*
P-Glycoprotein *on page 213*
U.S. Brand Names Rifadin®; Rimactane®
Canadian Brand Names Rofact™
Synonyms Rifampicin
Pharmacologic Class Antibiotic, Miscellaneous; Antitubercular Agent

+ **Rilutek®** *see Riluzole on page 136*

Riluzole (RIL yoo zole)
Gene(s) of Interest
CYP1A2 *on page 181*
U.S. Brand Names Rilutek®
Synonyms 2-Amino-6-Trifluoromethoxy-Benzothiazole; RP54274
Pharmacologic Class Glutamate Inhibitor

+ **Rimactane®** *see Rifampin on page 136*

Risedronate (ris ED roe nate)
Gene(s) of Interest None known
U.S. Brand Names Actonel®
Pharmacologic Class Bisphosphonate Derivative

- **Risperdal®** see Risperidone on page 137
- **Risperdal Consta™ [Investigational]** see Risperidone on page 137
- **Risperdal M-Tab™** see Risperidone on page 137

Risperidone (ris PER i done)
Gene(s) of Interest
Alpha-1 Adrenergic Receptor on page 161
Cardiac Potassium Ion Channel on page 177
Cardiac Sodium Channel on page 178
D2 Receptor on page 190
D3 Receptor on page 191
D4 Receptor on page 192
5HT2A Receptor on page 201
5HT2C Receptor on page 202

U.S. Brand Names Risperdal®; Risperdal Consta™ [Investigational]
Synonyms Risperdal M-Tab™
Pharmacologic Class Antipsychotic Agent, Benzisoxazole

- **Ritalin®** see Methylphenidate on page 111
- **Ritalin® LA** see Methylphenidate on page 111
- **Ritalin-SR®** see Methylphenidate on page 111

Ritonavir (ri TOE na veer)
Gene(s) of Interest
CYP2D6 on page 186
P-Glycoprotein on page 213
U.S. Brand Names Norvir®
Canadian Brand Names Norvir® SEC
Pharmacologic Class Antiretroviral Agent, Protease Inhibitor

Rivastigmine (ri va STIG meen)
Gene(s) of Interest
Apolipoprotein E on page 168
U.S. Brand Names Exelon®
Synonyms ENA 713; SDZ ENA 713
Pharmacologic Class Acetylcholinesterase Inhibitor (Central)

- **RMS®** see Morphine Sulfate on page 115
- **Ro 11-1163** see Moclobemide on page 114

Rofecoxib (roe fe COX ib)
Gene(s) of Interest
Leukotriene C4 Synthase on page 206
U.S. Brand Names Vioxx®
Pharmacologic Class Nonsteroidal Anti-inflammatory Drug (NSAID), COX-2 Selective

ROPINIROLE

♦ **Romycin®** see Erythromycin *on page 79*

Ropinirole (roe PIN i role)
Gene(s) of Interest
CYP1A2 *on page 181*
CYP2D6 *on page 186*
U.S. Brand Names Requip®
Pharmacologic Class Anti-Parkinson's Agent, Dopamine Agonist

Rosiglitazone (roh si GLI ta zone)
Gene(s) of Interest
CYP2C9 *on page 183*
U.S. Brand Names Avandia®
Pharmacologic Class Antidiabetic Agent, Thiazolidinedione

Rosuvastatin (roe SOO va sta tin)
Gene(s) of Interest
Angiotensin-Converting Enzyme *on page 163*
Apolipoprotein E *on page 168*
Beta-Fibrinogen *on page 174*
Cholesteryl Ester Transfer Protein *on page 179*
Glycoprotein IIIa Receptor *on page 196*
Low-Density Lipoprotein Receptor *on page 209*
Stromelysin-1 *on page 219*

Canadian Brand Names Crestor®
Pharmacologic Class Antilipemic Agent, HMG-CoA Reductase Inhibitor

♦ **Roxanol®** see Morphine Sulfate *on page 115*
♦ **Roxanol 100®** see Morphine Sulfate *on page 115*
♦ **Roxanol®-T** see Morphine Sulfate *on page 115*
♦ **Roxicet®** see Oxycodone and Acetaminophen *on page 123*
♦ **Roxicet® 5/500** see Oxycodone and Acetaminophen *on page 123*
♦ **Roxicodone™** see Oxycodone *on page 123*
♦ **Roxicodone™ Intensol™** see Oxycodone *on page 123*
♦ **RP-6976** see Docetaxel *on page 75*
♦ **RP54274** see Riluzole *on page 136*
♦ **RU-486** see Mifepristone *on page 113*
♦ **RU-23908** see Nilutamide *on page 118*
♦ **RU-38486** see Mifepristone *on page 113*
♦ **Rubex®** see DOXOrubicin *on page 76*
♦ **Rum-K®** see Potassium Chloride *on page 128*
♦ **Rythmol®** see Propafenone *on page 131*
♦ **Salbutamol** see Albuterol *on page 46*
♦ **Salicylazosulfapyridine** see Sulfasalazine *on page 143*

Salmeterol (sal ME te role)
Gene(s) of Interest
Beta-2 Adrenergic Receptor *on page 171*

SERTRALINE

U.S. Brand Names Serevent®; Serevent® Diskus®
Pharmacologic Class Beta$_2$ Agonist

- **Salmeterol and Fluticasone** *see* Fluticasone and Salmeterol *on page 89*
- **Saluron® [DSC]** *see* Hydroflumethiazide *on page 95*
- **Sandimmune®** *see* CycloSPORINE *on page 69*
- **Sandostatin®** *see* Octreotide *on page 121*
- **Sandostatin LAR®** *see* Octreotide *on page 121*
- **Sansert® [DSC]** *see* Methysergide *on page 111*

Saquinavir (sa KWIN a veer)
Gene(s) of Interest
P-Glycoprotein *on page 213*
U.S. Brand Names Fortovase®; Invirase®
Pharmacologic Class Antiretroviral Agent, Protease Inhibitor

- **Sarafem™** *see* Fluoxetine *on page 88*
- **Sarnol®-HC [OTC]** *see* Hydrocortisone *on page 95*
- **SCH 13521** *see* Flutamide *on page 89*
- **S-Citalopram** *see* Escitalopram *on page 80*
- **SDZ ENA 713** *see* Rivastigmine *on page 137*
- **Sectral®** *see* Acebutolol *on page 44*

Selegiline (se LE ji leen)
Gene(s) of Interest
CYP2C9 *on page 183*
U.S. Brand Names Eldepryl®
Canadian Brand Names Apo®-Selegiline; Gen-Selegiline; Novo-Selegiline; Nu-Selegiline
Synonyms Deprenyl; L-Deprenyl
Pharmacologic Class Antidepressant, Monoamine Oxidase Inhibitor; Anti-Parkinson's Agent, MAO Type B Inhibitor

- **Septra®** *see* Sulfamethoxazole and Trimethoprim *on page 143*
- **Septra® DS** *see* Sulfamethoxazole and Trimethoprim *on page 143*
- **Serentil®** *see* Mesoridazine *on page 109*
- **Serevent®** *see* Salmeterol *on page 138*
- **Serevent® Diskus®** *see* Salmeterol *on page 138*
- **Seroquel®** *see* Quetiapine *on page 133*

Sertraline (SER tra leen)
Gene(s) of Interest
CYP2C9 *on page 183*
CYP2C19 *on page 185*
CYP3A4 *on page 189*
G-Protein Beta-3 Subunit *on page 197*
Gs Protein Alpha-Subunit *on page 198*
5HT Transporter *on page 204*
U.S. Brand Names Zoloft®
(Continued)

Sertraline *(Continued)*
Canadian Brand Names Apo®-Sertraline; Gen-Sertraline; Novo-Sertraline; ratio-Sertraline; Rhoxal-sertraline
Pharmacologic Class Antidepressant, Selective Serotonin Reuptake Inhibitor

♦ **Serzone®** *see* Nefazodone *on page 117*

Sibutramine (si BYOO tra meen)
Gene(s) of Interest
Beta-3 Adrenergic Receptor *on page 174*
CYP3A4 *on page 189*
U.S. Brand Names Meridia®
Pharmacologic Class Anorexiant

Sildenafil (sil DEN a fil)
Gene(s) of Interest
CYP3A4 *on page 189*
U.S. Brand Names Viagra®
Synonyms UK 92480UK-92480
Pharmacologic Class Phosphodiesterase Enzyme Inhibitor

♦ **Silvadene®** *see* Silver Sulfadiazine *on page 140*

Silver Sulfadiazine (SIL ver sul fa DYE a zeen)
Gene(s) of Interest
Glucose-6-Phosphate Dehydrogenase *on page 195*
U.S. Brand Names Silvadene®; SSD®; SSD® AF; Thermazene®
Canadian Brand Names Dermazin™; Flamazine®
Pharmacologic Class Antibiotic, Topical

Simvastatin (SIM va stat in)
Gene(s) of Interest
Angiotensin-Converting Enzyme *on page 163*
Apolipoprotein E *on page 168*
Beta-Fibrinogen *on page 174*
Cholesteryl Ester Transfer Protein *on page 179*
CYP3A4 *on page 189*
Glycoprotein IIIa Receptor *on page 196*
Low-Density Lipoprotein Receptor *on page 209*
P-Glycoprotein *on page 213*
Stromelysin-1 *on page 219*
U.S. Brand Names Zocor®
Canadian Brand Names Apo®-Simvastatin; Gen-Simvastatin; Riva-Simvastatin
Pharmacologic Class Antilipemic Agent, HMG-CoA Reductase Inhibitor

♦ **Sinequan®** *see* Doxepin *on page 76*
♦ **Singulair®** *see* Montelukast *on page 115*
♦ **Sirdalud®** *see* Tizanidine *on page 149*

Sirolimus (sir OH li mus)
Gene(s) of Interest
CYP3A4 *on page 189*
U.S. Brand Names Rapamune®
Pharmacologic Class Immunosuppressant Agent

- **Skelaxin®** *see* Metaxalone *on page 109*
- **Slow FE® [OTC]** *see* Ferrous Sulfate *on page 87*
- **SMZ-TMP** *see* Sulfamethoxazole and Trimethoprim *on page 143*
- **Solaraze™** *see* Diclofenac *on page 72*
- **Solarcaine® Aloe Extra Burn Relief [OTC]** *see* Lidocaine *on page 103*
- **Solu-Cortef®** *see* Hydrocortisone *on page 95*
- **Solu-Medrol®** *see* MethylPREDNISolone *on page 111*
- **Soma®** *see* Carisoprodol *on page 61*
- **Sorine®** *see* Sotalol *on page 141*

Sotalol (SOE ta lole)
Gene(s) of Interest
Beta-1 Adrenergic Receptor *on page 171*
Cardiac Potassium Ion Channel *on page 177*
Cardiac Sodium Channel *on page 178*
Gs Protein Alpha-Subunit *on page 198*
U.S. Brand Names Betapace®; Betapace AF®; Sorine®
Canadian Brand Names Alti-Sotalol; Apo®-Sotalol; Gen-Sotalol; Lin-Sotalol; Novo-Sotalol; Nu-Sotalol; PMS-Sotalol; Rho®-Sotalol; Sotacor®
Pharmacologic Class Antiarrhythmic Agent, Class II; Antiarrhythmic Agent, Class III; Beta Blocker, Nonselective

Sparfloxacin (spar FLOKS a sin)
Gene(s) of Interest
Cardiac Potassium Ion Channel *on page 177*
Cardiac Sodium Channel *on page 178*
U.S. Brand Names Zagam®
Pharmacologic Class Antibiotic, Quinolone

Spiramycin (speer a MYE sin)
Gene(s) of Interest
CYP3A4 *on page 189*
Canadian Brand Names Rovamycine®
Pharmacologic Class Antibiotic, Macrolide

Spirapril (SPYE ra pril)
Gene(s) of Interest
Aldosterone Synthase *on page 160*
Angiotensin-Converting Enzyme *on page 163*
Angiotensin II Type I Receptor *on page 166*
Angiotensinogen *on page 167*
Bradykinin B2 Receptor *on page 175*
(Continued)

Spirapril *(Continued)*
Pharmacologic Class Angiotensin-Converting Enzyme (ACE) Inhibitor

Spironolactone (speer on oh LAK tone)
Gene(s) of Interest None known
U.S. Brand Names Aldactone®
Canadian Brand Names Novo-Spiroton
Pharmacologic Class Diuretic, Potassium Sparing

- **Sporanox®** *see* Itraconazole *on page 100*
- **Sprintec™** *see* Ethinyl Estradiol and Norgestimate *on page 84*
- **SSD®** *see* Silver Sulfadiazine *on page 140*
- **SSD® AF** *see* Silver Sulfadiazine *on page 140*
- **Stadol®** *see* Butorphanol *on page 59*
- **Stadol® NS** *see* Butorphanol *on page 59*
- **Stagesic®** *see* Hydrocodone and Acetaminophen *on page 94*
- **Starlix®** *see* Nateglinide *on page 117*
- **Staticin®** *see* Erythromycin *on page 79*
- **Stelazine®** *see* Trifluoperazine *on page 151*
- **Sterapred®** *see* PredniSONE *on page 129*
- **Sterapred® DS** *see* PredniSONE *on page 129*
- **STI571** *see* Imatinib *on page 97*
- **St. Joseph® Pain Reliever [OTC]** *see* Aspirin *on page 51*
- **Strattera™** *see* Atomoxetine *on page 53*
- **Stromectol®** *see* Ivermectin *on page 100*
- **Sublimaze®** *see* Fentanyl *on page 86*
- **Suboxone®** *see* Buprenorphine and Naloxone *on page 58*
- **Subutex®** *see* Buprenorphine *on page 57*
- **Sufenta®** *see* Sufentanil *on page 142*

Sufentanil (soo FEN ta nil)
Gene(s) of Interest
  COMT *on page 180*
  CYP3A4 *on page 189*
U.S. Brand Names Sufenta®
Pharmacologic Class Analgesic, Narcotic; General Anesthetic

- **Sular®** *see* Nisoldipine *on page 119*
- **Sulf-10®** *see* Sulfacetamide *on page 142*

Sulfacetamide (sul fa SEE ta mide)
Gene(s) of Interest
  Glucose-6-Phosphate Dehydrogenase *on page 195*
  N-Acetyltransferase 2 Enzyme *on page 211*
U.S. Brand Names AK-Sulf®; Bleph®-10; Carmol® Scalp; Klaron®; Ocusulf-10; Ovace™; Sulf-10®
Canadian Brand Names Cetamide™; Diosulf™; Sodium Sulamyd®

Pharmacologic Class Antibiotic, Ophthalmic; Antibiotic, Sulfonamide Derivative

SulfaDIAZINE (sul fa DYE a zeen)
Gene(s) of Interest
CYP2C9 *on page 183*
Glucose-6-Phosphate Dehydrogenase *on page 195*
N-Acetyltransferase 2 Enzyme *on page 211*
Pharmacologic Class Antibiotic, Sulfonamide Derivative

Sulfadoxine and Pyrimethamine
(sul fa DOKS een & peer i METH a meen)
Gene(s) of Interest
Glucose-6-Phosphate Dehydrogenase *on page 195*
U.S. Brand Names Fansidar®
Synonyms Pyrimethamine and Sulfadoxine
Pharmacologic Class Antimalarial Agent

Sulfamethoxazole and Trimethoprim
(sul fa meth OKS a zole & trye METH oh prim)
Gene(s) of Interest
CYP2C9 *on page 183*
Glucose-6-Phosphate Dehydrogenase *on page 195*
N-Acetyltransferase 2 Enzyme *on page 211*
U.S. Brand Names Bactrim™; Bactrim™ DS; Septra®; Septra® DS
Canadian Brand Names Apo®-Sulfatrim; Novo-Trimel; Novo-Trimel D.S.; Nu-Cotrimox®; Septra® Injection
Synonyms Co-Trimoxazole; SMZ-TMP; Sulfatrim; TMP-SMZ; Trimethoprim and Sulfamethoxazole
Pharmacologic Class Antibiotic, Sulfonamide Derivative; Antibiotic, Miscellaneous

♦ **Sulfamylon®** *see* Mafenide *on page 107*

Sulfasalazine (sul fa SAL a zeen)
Gene(s) of Interest
Glucose-6-Phosphate Dehydrogenase *on page 195*
U.S. Brand Names Azulfidine®; Azulfidine® EN-tabs®
Canadian Brand Names Alti-Sulfasalazine; Salazopyrin®; Salazopyrin En-Tabs®
Synonyms Salicylazosulfapyridine
Pharmacologic Class 5-Aminosalicylic Acid Derivative

♦ **Sulfatrim** *see* Sulfamethoxazole and Trimethoprim *on page 143*

Sulfinpyrazone (sul fin PEER a zone)
Gene(s) of Interest
CYP2C9 *on page 183*
Canadian Brand Names Apo®-Sulfinpyrazone; Nu-Sulfinpyrazone
Synonyms Anturane
Pharmacologic Class Uricosuric Agent

SULFISOXAZOLE

SulfiSOXAZOLE (sul fi SOKS a zole)
Gene(s) of Interest
CYP2C9 *on page 183*
Glucose-6-Phosphate Dehydrogenase *on page 195*
N-Acetyltransferase 2 Enzyme *on page 211*
U.S. Brand Names Gantrisin®
Canadian Brand Names Novo-Soxazole®; Sulfizole®
Synonyms Sulphafurazole
Pharmacologic Class Antibiotic, Sulfonamide Derivative

♦ **Sulfisoxazole and Erythromycin** *see* Erythromycin and Sulfisoxazole *on page 80*

Sulindac (sul IN dak)
Gene(s) of Interest
Leukotriene C4 Synthase *on page 206*
U.S. Brand Names Clinoril®
Canadian Brand Names Apo®-Sulin; Novo-Sundac; Nu-Sundac
Pharmacologic Class Nonsteroidal Anti-inflammatory Drug (NSAID)

♦ **Sulphafurazole** *see* SulfiSOXAZOLE *on page 144*

Sumatriptan (soo ma TRIP tan)
Gene(s) of Interest None known
U.S. Brand Names Imitrex®
Pharmacologic Class Serotonin 5-HT$_{1D}$ Receptor Agonist

♦ **Summer's Eve® SpecialCare™ Medicated Anti-Itch Cream [OTC]** *see* Hydrocortisone *on page 95*
♦ **Sumycin®** *see* Tetracycline *on page 146*
♦ **Sureprin 81™ [OTC]** *see* Aspirin *on page 51*
♦ **Surmontil®** *see* Trimipramine *on page 152*
♦ **Synalgos®-DC** *see* Dihydrocodeine, Aspirin, and Caffeine *on page 73*
♦ **Synthroid®** *see* Levothyroxine *on page 103*
♦ **T$_4$** *see* Levothyroxine *on page 103*
♦ **Tac™-3 [DSC]** *see* Triamcinolone *on page 151*

Tacrine (TAK reen)
Gene(s) of Interest
Apolipoprotein E *on page 168*
CYP1A2 *on page 181*
U.S. Brand Names Cognex®
Synonyms Tetrahydroaminoacrine; THA
Pharmacologic Class Acetylcholinesterase Inhibitor (Central)

Tacrolimus (ta KROE li mus)
Gene(s) of Interest
CYP3A4 *on page 189*
P-Glycoprotein *on page 213*
U.S. Brand Names Prograf®; Protopic®

TEMAZEPAM

Synonyms FK506
Pharmacologic Class Immunosuppressant Agent; Topical Skin Product

- **Tagamet®** see Cimetidine on page 64
- **Tagamet® HB 200 [OTC]** see Cimetidine on page 64
- **Talacen®** see Pentazocine Combinations on page 125
- **Talwin®** see Pentazocine on page 125
- **Talwin® NX** see Pentazocine on page 125
- **TAM** see Tamoxifen on page 145
- **Tambocor™** see Flecainide on page 87

Tamoxifen (ta MOKS i fen)
Gene(s) of Interest
CYP2C9 on page 183
P-Glycoprotein on page 213
U.S. Brand Names Nolvadex®
Canadian Brand Names Apo®-Tamox; Gen-Tamoxifen; Nolvadex®-D; Novo-Tamoxifen; PMS-Tamoxifen; Tamofen®
Synonyms ICI-46474; NSC-180973; TAM
Pharmacologic Class Antineoplastic Agent, Estrogen Receptor Antagonist

Tamsulosin (tam SOO loe sin)
Gene(s) of Interest
CYP3A4 on page 189
U.S. Brand Names Flomax®
Pharmacologic Class Alpha$_1$ Blocker

- **Tavist®** see Clemastine on page 65
- **Tavist®-1 [OTC]** see Clemastine on page 65
- **Taxol®** see Paclitaxel on page 124
- **Taxotere®** see Docetaxel on page 75
- **TCN** see Tetracycline on page 146
- **Tegretol®** see Carbamazepine on page 60
- **Tegretol®-XR** see Carbamazepine on page 60

Telmisartan (tel mi SAR tan)
Gene(s) of Interest
Aldosterone Synthase on page 160
Angiotensin-Converting Enzyme on page 163
Angiotensin II Type I Receptor on page 166
Angiotensinogen on page 167
U.S. Brand Names Micardis®
Pharmacologic Class Angiotensin II Receptor Blocker

Temazepam (te MAZ e pam)
Gene(s) of Interest None known
U.S. Brand Names Restoril®
Canadian Brand Names Apo®-Temazepam; Gen-Temazepam; Novo-Temazepam; Nu-Temazepam; PMS-Temazepam
(Continued)

Temazepam *(Continued)*
Pharmacologic Class Benzodiazepine

Teniposide (ten i POE side)
Gene(s) of Interest
CYP3A4 *on page 189*
U.S. Brand Names Vumon
Synonyms EPT; VM-26
Pharmacologic Class Antineoplastic Agent, Miscellaneous

- **Tenormin®** *see Atenolol on page 53*
- **Tequin®** *see Gatifloxacin on page 91*

Terazosin (ter AY zoe sin)
Gene(s) of Interest None known
U.S. Brand Names Hytrin®
Canadian Brand Names Alti-Terazosin; Apo®-Terazosin; Novo-Terazosin; Nu-Terazosin; PMS-Terazosin
Pharmacologic Class Alpha$_1$ Blocker

Terbutaline (ter BYOO ta leen)
Gene(s) of Interest
Beta-2 Adrenergic Receptor *on page 171*
U.S. Brand Names Brethine®
Canadian Brand Names Bricanyl® [DSC]
Pharmacologic Class Beta$_2$ Agonist

- **Tessalon®** *see Benzonatate on page 55*
- **Testim™** *see Testosterone on page 146*
- **Testoderm®** *see Testosterone on page 146*
- **Testoderm® TTS [DSC]** *see Testosterone on page 146*
- **Testoderm® with Adhesive** *see Testosterone on page 146*
- **Testopel®** *see Testosterone on page 146*

Testosterone (tes TOS ter one)
Gene(s) of Interest
P-Glycoprotein *on page 213*
U.S. Brand Names Androderm®; AndroGel®; Delatestryl®; Depo®-Testosterone; Testim™; Testoderm®; Testoderm® TTS [DSC]; Testoderm® with Adhesive; Testopel®
Canadian Brand Names Andriol®; Andropository; Depotest® 100; Everone® 200; Virilon® IM
Pharmacologic Class Androgen

Tetracycline (tet ra SYE kleen)
Gene(s) of Interest None known
U.S. Brand Names Sumycin®; Wesmycin®
Canadian Brand Names Apo®-Tetra; Novo-Tetra; Nu-Tetra
Synonyms Achromycin; TCN
Pharmacologic Class Antibiotic, Tetracycline Derivative

- **Tetrahydroaminoacrine** see Tacrine on page 144
- **Teveten®** see Eprosartan on page 78
- **Texacort®** see Hydrocortisone on page 95
- **TG** see Thioguanine on page 147
- **6-TG** see Thioguanine on page 147
- **THA** see Tacrine on page 144
- **Thalitone®** see Chlorthalidone on page 63
- **Theo-24®** see Theophylline on page 147
- **Theochron®** see Theophylline on page 147
- **Theolair™** see Theophylline on page 147
- **Theolair-SR® [DSC]** see Theophylline on page 147

Theophylline (thee OFF i lin)
Gene(s) of Interest
CYP1A2 on page 181
CYP3A4 on page 189

U.S. Brand Names Elixophyllin®; Quibron®-T; Quibron®-T/SR; Theo-24®; Theochron®; Theolair™; Theolair-SR® [DSC]; T-Phyl®; Uniphyl®

Canadian Brand Names Apo®-Theo LA; Novo-Theophyl SR; PMS-Theophylline; Pulmophylline; ratio-Theo-Bronc; Theochron® SR; Theo-Dur®; Uniphyl® SRT

Pharmacologic Class Theophylline Derivative

- **Theophylline Ethylenediamine** see Aminophylline on page 48
- **Theracort® [OTC]** see Hydrocortisone on page 95
- **Theramycin Z®** see Erythromycin on page 79
- **Thermazene®** see Silver Sulfadiazine on page 140

Thioguanine (thye oh GWAH neen)
Gene(s) of Interest
Thiopurine Methyltransferase on page 220

Canadian Brand Names Lanvis®

Synonyms 2-Amino-6-Mercaptopurine; NSC-752; TG; 6-TG; 6-Thioguanine; Tioguanine

Pharmacologic Class Antineoplastic Agent, Antimetabolite (Purine Antagonist)

- **6-Thioguanine** see Thioguanine on page 147

Thioridazine (thye oh RID a zeen)
Gene(s) of Interest
Alpha-1 Adrenergic Receptor on page 161
Cardiac Potassium Ion Channel on page 177
Cardiac Sodium Channel on page 178
CYP2D6 on page 186
D2 Receptor on page 190

U.S. Brand Names Mellaril® [DSC]; Thioridazine Intensol™

Canadian Brand Names Apo®-Thioridazine

Pharmacologic Class Antipsychotic Agent, Phenothiazine, Piperidine

THIOTHIXENE

- **Thioridazine Intensol™** *see Thioridazine on page 147*

Thiothixene (thye oh THIKS een)
Gene(s) of Interest
Alpha-1 Adrenergic Receptor *on page 161*
Cardiac Potassium Ion Channel *on page 177*
Cardiac Sodium Channel *on page 178*
CYP1A2 *on page 181*
D2 Receptor *on page 190*
U.S. Brand Names Navane®
Synonyms Tiotixene
Pharmacologic Class Antipsychotic Agent, Thioxanthene Derivative

- **Thorazine®** *see ChlorproMAZINE on page 63*

Tiagabine (tye AG a been)
Gene(s) of Interest
CYP3A4 *on page 189*
U.S. Brand Names Gabitril®
Pharmacologic Class Anticonvulsant, Miscellaneous

Tiaprofenic Acid (tye ah PRO fen ik AS id)
Gene(s) of Interest
Leukotriene C4 Synthase *on page 206*
Canadian Brand Names Albert® Tiafen; Apo®-Tiaprofenic; Dom-Tiaprofenic®; Novo-Tiaprofenic; Nu-Tiaprofenic; PMS-Tiaprofenic; Surgam®; Surgam® SR; Tiaprofenic-200; Tiaprofenic-300
Pharmacologic Class Nonsteroidal Anti-inflammatory Drug (NSAID)

- **Tiazac®** *see Diltiazem on page 74*
- **Ticlid®** *see Ticlopidine on page 148*

Ticlopidine (tye KLOE pi deen)
Gene(s) of Interest
Glycoprotein IIIa Receptor *on page 196*
U.S. Brand Names Ticlid®
Canadian Brand Names Alti-Ticlopidine; Apo®-Ticlopidine; Gen-Ticlopidine; Nu-Ticlopidine; PMS-Ticlopidine; Rhoxal-ticlopidine
Pharmacologic Class Antiplatelet Agent

- **Tikosyn™** *see Dofetilide on page 75*

Timolol (TYE moe lole)
Gene(s) of Interest
Beta-1 Adrenergic Receptor *on page 171*
CYP2D6 *on page 186*
Gs Protein Alpha-Subunit *on page 198*
U.S. Brand Names Betimol®; Blocadren®; Timoptic®; Timoptic® OcuDose®; Timoptic-XE®
Canadian Brand Names Alti-Timolol; Apo®-Timol; Apo®-Timop; Gen-Timolol; Nu-Timolol; Phoxal-timolol; PMS-Timolol; Tim-AK

Pharmacologic Class Beta Blocker, Nonselective; Ophthalmic Agent, Antiglaucoma

- **Timoptic®** *see Timolol on page 148*
- **Timoptic® OcuDose®** *see Timolol on page 148*
- **Timoptic-XE®** *see Timolol on page 148*
- **Tioguanine** *see Thioguanine on page 147*
- **Tiotixene** *see Thiothixene on page 148*

Tirofiban (tye roe FYE ban)
Gene(s) of Interest
Glycoprotein IIIa Receptor *on page 196*
U.S. Brand Names Aggrastat®
Synonyms MK383
Pharmacologic Class Antiplatelet Agent, Glycoprotein IIb/IIIa Inhibitor

Tizanidine (tye ZAN i deen)
Gene(s) of Interest
Cardiac Potassium Ion Channel *on page 177*
Cardiac Sodium Channel *on page 178*
U.S. Brand Names Zanaflex®
Synonyms Sirdalud®
Pharmacologic Class Alpha$_2$-Adrenergic Agonist

- **TMP** *see Trimethoprim on page 152*
- **TMP-SMZ** *see Sulfamethoxazole and Trimethoprim on page 143*
- **Tofranil®** *see Imipramine on page 97*
- **Tofranil-PM®** *see Imipramine on page 97*

TOLBUTamide (tole BYOO ta mide)
Gene(s) of Interest
CYP2C9 *on page 183*
U.S. Brand Names Orinase Diagnostic® [DSC]; Tol-Tab®
Canadian Brand Names Apo®-Tolbutamide
Pharmacologic Class Antidiabetic Agent, Sulfonylurea

- **Tolectin®** *see Tolmetin on page 149*
- **Tolectin® DS** *see Tolmetin on page 149*

Tolmetin (TOLE met in)
Gene(s) of Interest
Leukotriene C4 Synthase *on page 206*
U.S. Brand Names Tolectin®; Tolectin® DS
Pharmacologic Class Nonsteroidal Anti-inflammatory Drug (NSAID)

- **Tol-Tab®** *see TOLBUTamide on page 149*

Tolterodine (tole TER oh deen)
Gene(s) of Interest
CYP3A4 *on page 189*
(Continued)

Tolterodine *(Continued)*
U.S. Brand Names Detrol®; Detrol® LA
Canadian Brand Names Unidet®
Pharmacologic Class Anticholinergic Agent

- **Tomoxetine** *see* Atomoxetine *on page 53*
- **Topamax®** *see* Topiramate *on page 150*
- **Topicaine® [OTC]** *see* Lidocaine *on page 103*

Topiramate (toe PYRE a mate)
Gene(s) of Interest None known
U.S. Brand Names Topamax®
Pharmacologic Class Anticonvulsant, Miscellaneous

- **Toposar®** *see* Etoposide *on page 85*
- **Toprol-XL®** *see* Metoprolol *on page 112*
- **Toradol®** *see* Ketorolac *on page 101*
- **Tornalate [DSC]** *see* Bitolterol *on page 56*

Torsemide (TORE se mide)
Gene(s) of Interest
Alpha-Adducin *on page 162*
CYP2C9 *on page 183*
U.S. Brand Names Demadex®
Pharmacologic Class Diuretic, Loop

- **T-Phyl®** *see* Theophylline *on page 147*
- **Tracleer™** *see* Bosentan *on page 56*

Tramadol (TRA ma dole)
Gene(s) of Interest
COMT *on page 180*
CYP2D6 *on page 186*
U.S. Brand Names Ultram®
Pharmacologic Class Analgesic, Non-narcotic

- **Tramadol Hydrochloride and Acetaminophen** *see* Acetaminophen and Tramadol *on page 45*

Trandolapril (tran DOE la pril)
Gene(s) of Interest
Aldosterone Synthase *on page 160*
Angiotensin-Converting Enzyme *on page 163*
Angiotensin II Type I Receptor *on page 166*
Angiotensinogen *on page 167*
Bradykinin B2 Receptor *on page 175*
U.S. Brand Names Mavik®
Pharmacologic Class Angiotensin-Converting Enzyme (ACE) Inhibitor

- **Tranxene®** *see* Clorazepate *on page 67*

Trazodone (TRAZ oh done)
Gene(s) of Interest
Alpha-1 Adrenergic Receptor *on page 161*
CYP3A4 *on page 189*
G-Protein Beta-3 Subunit *on page 197*
Gs Protein Alpha-Subunit *on page 198*

U.S. Brand Names Desyrel®

Canadian Brand Names Alti-Trazodone; Apo®-Trazodone; Apo®-Trazodone D; Gen-Trazodone; Novo-Trazodone; Nu-Trazodone; PMS-Trazodone

Pharmacologic Class Antidepressant, Serotonin Reuptake Inhibitor/Antagonist

Triamcinolone (trye am SIN oh lone)
Gene(s) of Interest None known

U.S. Brand Names Aristocort®; Aristocort® A; Aristocort® Forte; Aristospan®; Azmacort®; Kenalog®; Kenalog-10®; Kenalog-40®; Kenalog® in Orabase®; Nasacort®; Nasacort® AQ; Tac™-3 [DSC]; Triderm®; Tri-Nasal®

Canadian Brand Names Oracort; Triaderm; Trinasal®

Pharmacologic Class Corticosteroid, Adrenal; Corticosteroid, Inhalant (Oral); Corticosteroid, Nasal; Corticosteroid, Systemic; Corticosteroid, Topical

♦ **Triavil®** *see* Amitriptyline and Perphenazine *on page 49*

Triazolam (trye AY zoe lam)
Gene(s) of Interest
CYP3A4 *on page 189*

U.S. Brand Names Halcion®

Canadian Brand Names Apo®-Triazo; Gen-Triazolam

Pharmacologic Class Benzodiazepine

Trichlormethiazide (trye klor meth EYE a zide)
Gene(s) of Interest
Alpha-Adducin *on page 162*
G-Protein Beta-3 Subunit *on page 197*

U.S. Brand Names Naqua®

Canadian Brand Names Metahydrin®; Metatensin®; Trichlorex®

Pharmacologic Class Diuretic, Thiazide

♦ **TriCor®** *see* Fenofibrate *on page 86*
♦ **Triderm®** *see* Triamcinolone *on page 151*

Trifluoperazine (trye floo oh PER a zeen)
Gene(s) of Interest
Alpha-1 Adrenergic Receptor *on page 161*
CYP1A2 *on page 181*
D2 Receptor *on page 190*

U.S. Brand Names Stelazine®
(Continued)

Trifluoperazine *(Continued)*
Canadian Brand Names Apo®-Trifluoperazine; Novo-Trifluzine; PMS-Trifluoperazine; Terfluzine
Pharmacologic Class Antipsychotic Agent, Phenothiazine, Piperazine

- **Trilafon® [DSC]** *see Perphenazine on page 126*
- **Tri-Levlen®** *see Ethinyl Estradiol and Levonorgestrel on page 83*

Trimethoprim (trye METH oh prim)
Gene(s) of Interest
CYP2C9 *on page 183*
U.S. Brand Names Primsol®; Proloprim®
Canadian Brand Names Apo®-Trimethoprim
Synonyms TMP
Pharmacologic Class Antibiotic, Miscellaneous

- **Trimethoprim and Sulfamethoxazole** *see Sulfamethoxazole and Trimethoprim on page 143*

Trimipramine (trye MI pra meen)
Gene(s) of Interest
Alpha-1 Adrenergic Receptor *on page 161*
CYP2C19 *on page 185*
CYP3A4 *on page 189*
G-Protein Beta-3 Subunit *on page 197*
Gs Protein Alpha-Subunit *on page 198*
P-Glycoprotein *on page 213*
U.S. Brand Names Surmontil®
Canadian Brand Names Apo®-Trimip; Novo-Tripramine; Nu-Trimipramine; Rhotrimine®
Pharmacologic Class Antidepressant, Tricyclic (Tertiary Amine)

- **Trimox®** *see Amoxicillin on page 49*
- **Tri-Nasal®** *see Triamcinolone on page 151*
- **Tri-Norinyl®** *see Ethinyl Estradiol and Norethindrone on page 84*
- **Triphasil®** *see Ethinyl Estradiol and Levonorgestrel on page 83*
- **Trisenox™** *see Arsenic Trioxide on page 51*
- **Trivora®** *see Ethinyl Estradiol and Levonorgestrel on page 83*
- **T-Stat®** *see Erythromycin on page 79*
- **Tylenol® With Codeine** *see Acetaminophen and Codeine on page 44*
- **Tylox®** *see Oxycodone and Acetaminophen on page 123*
- **UCB-P071** *see Cetirizine on page 62*
- **UK-68-798** *see Dofetilide on page 75*
- **UK-92480** *see Sildenafil on page 140*
- **UK-109496** *see Voriconazole on page 155*
- **Ultiva®** *see Remifentanil on page 135*
- **Ultracet™** *see Acetaminophen and Tramadol on page 45*
- **Ultram®** *see Tramadol on page 150*

VALSARTAN

- **Uniphyl®** *see* Theophylline *on page 147*
- **Unithroid®** *see* Levothyroxine *on page 103*
- **Univasc®** *see* Moexipril *on page 114*
- **Urolene Blue®** *see* Methylene Blue *on page 110*
- **Vagifem®** *see* Estradiol *on page 80*

Valacyclovir (val ay SYE kloe veer)
Gene(s) of Interest None known
U.S. Brand Names Valtrex®
Pharmacologic Class Antiviral Agent, Oral

Valdecoxib (val de KOKS ib)
Gene(s) of Interest
  Leukotriene C4 Synthase *on page 206*
U.S. Brand Names Bextra®
Pharmacologic Class Nonsteroidal Anti-inflammatory Drug (NSAID), COX-2 Selective

- **Valium®** *see* Diazepam *on page 72*
- **Valproate Semisodium** *see* Valproic Acid and Derivatives *on page 153*
- **Valproate Sodium** *see* Valproic Acid and Derivatives *on page 153*
- **Valproic Acid** *see* Valproic Acid and Derivatives *on page 153*

Valproic Acid and Derivatives
(val PROE ik AS id & dah RIV ah tives)
Gene(s) of Interest None known
U.S. Brand Names Depacon®; Depakene®; Depakote® Delayed Release; Depakote® ER; Depakote® Sprinkle®
Canadian Brand Names Alti-Divalproex; Apo®-Divalproex; Epival® ER; Epival® I.V.; Gen-Divalproex; Novo-Divalproex; Nu-Divalproex; PMS-Valproic Acid; PMS-Valproic Acid E.C.; Rhoxal-valproic
Synonyms Dipropylacetic Acid; Divalproex Sodium; DPA; 2-Propylpentanoic Acid; 2-Propylvaleric Acid; Valproate Semisodium; Valproate Sodium; Valproic Acid
Pharmacologic Class Anticonvulsant, Miscellaneous

Valsartan (val SAR tan)
Gene(s) of Interest
  Aldosterone Synthase *on page 160*
  Angiotensin-Converting Enzyme *on page 163*
  Angiotensin II Type I Receptor *on page 166*
  Angiotensinogen *on page 167*
U.S. Brand Names Diovan®
Pharmacologic Class Angiotensin II Receptor Blocker

- **Valtrex®** *see* Valacyclovir *on page 153*
- **Vanatrip®** *see* Amitriptyline *on page 48*
- **Vascor®** *see* Bepridil *on page 55*
- **Vasotec®** *see* Enalapril *on page 78*
- **Vasotec® I.V.** *see* Enalapril *on page 78*

VENLAFAXINE

- **VCR** *see* VinCRIStine *on page 155*
- **Veetids®** *see* Penicillin V Potassium *on page 125*
- **Velban® [DSC]** *see* VinBLAStine *on page 154*
- **Velosulin® BR (Buffered)** *see* Insulin Preparations *on page 98*

Venlafaxine (VEN la faks een)
Gene(s) of Interest
CYP3A4 *on page 189*
U.S. Brand Names Effexor®; Effexor® XR
Pharmacologic Class Antidepressant, Serotonin/Norepinephrine Reuptake Inhibitor

- **Ventolin®** *see* Albuterol *on page 46*
- **Ventolin® HFA** *see* Albuterol *on page 46*
- **VePesid®** *see* Etoposide *on page 85*

Verapamil (ver AP a mil)
Gene(s) of Interest
CYP3A4 *on page 189*
P-Glycoprotein *on page 213*
U.S. Brand Names Calan®; Calan® SR; Covera-HS®; Isoptin® SR; Verelan®; Verelan® PM
Canadian Brand Names Alti-Verapamil; Apo®-Verap; Chronovera®; Covera®; Gen-Verapamil; Gen-Verapamil SR; Isoptin®; Isoptin® I.V.; Novo-Veramil; Novo-Veramil SR; Nu-Verap; Tarka®
Synonyms Iproveratril Hydrochloride
Pharmacologic Class Antiarrhythmic Agent, Class IV; Calcium Channel Blocker

- **Verelan®** *see* Verapamil *on page 154*
- **Verelan® PM** *see* Verapamil *on page 154*
- **Versed® [DSC]** *see* Midazolam *on page 112*
- **VFEND®** *see* Voriconazole *on page 155*
- **Viagra®** *see* Sildenafil *on page 140*
- **Vibramycin®** *see* Doxycycline *on page 76*
- **Vibra-Tabs®** *see* Doxycycline *on page 76*
- **Vicodin®** *see* Hydrocodone and Acetaminophen *on page 94*
- **Vicodin® ES** *see* Hydrocodone and Acetaminophen *on page 94*
- **Vicodin® HP** *see* Hydrocodone and Acetaminophen *on page 94*
- **Vicoprofen®** *see* Hydrocodone and Ibuprofen *on page 95*
- **Vigamox™** *see* Moxifloxacin *on page 115*

VinBLAStine (vin BLAS teen)
Gene(s) of Interest
CYP3A4 *on page 189*
P-Glycoprotein *on page 213*
U.S. Brand Names Velban® [DSC]
Synonyms NSC-49842; Vincaleucoblastine; Vincaleukoblastine; VLB
Pharmacologic Class Antineoplastic Agent, Natural Source (Plant) Derivative; Antineoplastic Agent, Vinca Alkaloid

- **Vincaleucoblastine** *see* VinBLAStine *on page 154*
- **Vincaleukoblastine** *see* VinBLAStine *on page 154*
- **Vincasar PFS®** *see* VinCRIStine *on page 155*

VinCRIStine (vin KRIS teen)
Gene(s) of Interest
CYP3A4 *on page 189*
U.S. Brand Names Oncovin® [DSC]; Vincasar PFS®
Synonyms LCR; Leurocristine; Leurocristine Sulfate; NSC-67574; VCR
Pharmacologic Class Antineoplastic Agent, Natural Source (Plant) Derivative; Antineoplastic Agent, Vinca Alkaloid

Vinorelbine (vi NOR el been)
Gene(s) of Interest
CYP3A4 *on page 189*
U.S. Brand Names Navelbine®
Synonyms Dihydroxydeoxynorvinkaleukoblastine; NVB
Pharmacologic Class Antineoplastic Agent, Natural Source (Plant) Derivative; Antineoplastic Agent, Vinca Alkaloid

- **Vioxx®** *see* Rofecoxib *on page 137*
- **Viracept®** *see* Nelfinavir *on page 118*
- **Vistaril®** *see* HydrOXYzine *on page 96*
- **Vivactil®** *see* Protriptyline *on page 133*
- **Vivelle®** *see* Estradiol *on page 80*
- **Vivelle-Dot®** *see* Estradiol *on page 80*
- **VLB** *see* VinBLAStine *on page 154*
- **VM-26** *see* Teniposide *on page 146*
- **Volmax®** *see* Albuterol *on page 46*
- **Voltaren®** *see* Diclofenac *on page 72*
- **Voltaren Ophthalmic®** *see* Diclofenac *on page 72*
- **Voltaren®-XR** *see* Diclofenac *on page 72*

Voriconazole (vor i KOE na zole)
Gene(s) of Interest
CYP2C9 *on page 183*
U.S. Brand Names VFEND®
Synonyms UK-109496
Pharmacologic Class Antifungal Agent, Oral; Antifungal Agent, Parenteral

- **VoSpire ER™** *see* Albuterol *on page 46*
- **VP-16** *see* Etoposide *on page 85*
- **VP-16-213** *see* Etoposide *on page 85*
- **Vumon** *see* Teniposide *on page 146*

Warfarin (WAR far in)
Gene(s) of Interest
CYP2C9 *on page 183*
(Continued)

Warfarin (Continued)
Protein C *on page 217*
Protein S *on page 218*
U.S. Brand Names Coumadin®
Canadian Brand Names Apo®-Warfarin; Gen-Warfarin; Taro-Warfarin
Pharmacologic Class Anticoagulant, Coumarin Derivative

- **Wellbutrin®** *see* BuPROPion *on page 58*
- **Wellbutrin SR®** *see* BuPROPion *on page 58*
- **Wesmycin®** *see* Tetracycline *on page 146*
- **Westcort®** *see* Hydrocortisone *on page 95*
- **Wigraine®** *see* Ergotamine *on page 79*
- **WR-139007** *see* Dacarbazine *on page 69*
- **Wytensin® [DSC]** *see* Guanabenz *on page 93*
- **Xalatan®** *see* Latanoprost *on page 102*
- **Xanax®** *see* Alprazolam *on page 47*
- **Xanax XR®** *see* Alprazolam *on page 47*
- **Xeloda®** *see* Capecitabine *on page 60*
- **Xopenex®** *see* Levalbuterol *on page 102*
- **Xylocaine®** *see* Lidocaine *on page 103*
- **Xylocaine® MPF** *see* Lidocaine *on page 103*
- **Xylocaine® Viscous** *see* Lidocaine *on page 103*
- **Yasmin®** *see* Ethinyl Estradiol and Drospirenone *on page 82*
- **Z4942** *see* Ifosfamide *on page 97*

Zafirlukast (za FIR loo kast)
Gene(s) of Interest
CYP2C9 *on page 183*
Leukotriene C4 Synthase *on page 206*
5-Lipoxygenase *on page 208*
U.S. Brand Names Accolate®
Synonyms ICI 204, 219
Pharmacologic Class Leukotriene Receptor Antagonist

- **Zagam®** *see* Sparfloxacin *on page 141*
- **Zanaflex®** *see* Tizanidine *on page 149*
- **Zantac®** *see* Ranitidine *on page 135*
- **Zantac® 75 [OTC]** *see* Ranitidine *on page 135*
- **Zarontin®** *see* Ethosuximide *on page 85*
- **Zaroxolyn®** *see* Metolazone *on page 111*
- **Z-Chlopenthixol** *see* Zuclopenthixol *on page 158*
- **ZD1694** *see* Raltitrexed *on page 135*
- **Zebeta®** *see* Bisoprolol *on page 56*
- **Zeldox** *see* Ziprasidone *on page 157*
- **Zestoretic®** *see* Lisinopril and Hydrochlorothiazide *on page 104*
- **Zestril®** *see* Lisinopril *on page 104*
- **Ziagen®** *see* Abacavir *on page 44*

ZOPICLONE

- **Zilactin-L® [OTC]** *see* Lidocaine *on page 103*
- **Zinecard®** *see* Dexrazoxane *on page 71*

Ziprasidone (zi PRAY si done)
Gene(s) of Interest
Alpha-1 Adrenergic Receptor *on page 161*
Cardiac Potassium Ion Channel *on page 177*
Cardiac Sodium Channel *on page 178*
D2 Receptor *on page 190*
D3 Receptor *on page 191*
5HT1A Receptor *on page 200*
5HT2A Receptor *on page 201*
5HT2C Receptor *on page 202*

U.S. Brand Names Geodon®

Synonyms Zeldox

Pharmacologic Class Antipsychotic Agent, Benzylisothiazolylpiperazine

- **Zithromax®** *see* Azithromycin *on page 54*
- **Zithromax® TRI-PAK™** *see* Azithromycin *on page 54*
- **Zithromax® Z-PAK®** *see* Azithromycin *on page 54*
- **Zocor®** *see* Simvastatin *on page 140*
- **Zoloft®** *see* Sertraline *on page 139*

Zolpidem (zole PI dem)
Gene(s) of Interest
CYP3A4 *on page 189*

U.S. Brand Names Ambien®

Pharmacologic Class Hypnotic, Nonbenzodiazepine

- **Zonalon®** *see* Doxepin *on page 76*
- **Zonegran®** *see* Zonisamide *on page 157*

Zonisamide (zoe NIS a mide)
Gene(s) of Interest
CYP3A4 *on page 189*

U.S. Brand Names Zonegran®

Pharmacologic Class Anticonvulsant, Miscellaneous

Zopiclone (ZOE pi clone)
Gene(s) of Interest
CYP2C9 *on page 183*
CYP3A4 *on page 189*

Canadian Brand Names Alti-Zopiclone; Apo®-Zopiclone; Gen-Zopiclone; Imovane®; Nu-Zopiclone; Rhovane®

Pharmacologic Class Hypnotic, Nonbenzodiazepine

- **ZORprin®** *see* Aspirin *on page 51*
- **Zovia™** *see* Ethinyl Estradiol and Ethynodiol Diacetate *on page 83*
- **Zovirax®** *see* Acyclovir *on page 45*

Zuclopenthixol (zoo kloe pen THIX ol)
Gene(s) of Interest
Alpha-1 Adrenergic Receptor *on page 161*
Cardiac Potassium Ion Channel *on page 177*
Cardiac Sodium Channel *on page 178*
D2 Receptor *on page 190*

Canadian Brand Names Clopixol®; Clopixol-Acuphase®; Clopixol® Depot

Synonyms Z-Chlopenthixol

Pharmacologic Class Antipsychotic Agent, Thioxanthene Derivative

- **Zyban®** *see* BuPROPion *on page 58*
- **Zydone®** *see* Hydrocodone and Acetaminophen *on page 94*
- **Zyloprim®** *see* Allopurinol *on page 47*
- **Zymar™** *see* Gatifloxacin *on page 91*
- **Zyprexa®** *see* Olanzapine *on page 121*
- **Zyprexa® Zydis®** *see* Olanzapine *on page 121*
- **Zyrtec®** *see* Cetirizine *on page 62*

ALPHABETICAL LISTING OF POTENTIAL POLYMORPHISMS

- **ABC20** see P-Glycoprotein on page 213
- **ABCB1** see P-Glycoprotein on page 213
- **ACE** see Angiotensin-Converting Enzyme on page 163
- **ADDA** see Alpha-Adducin on page 162
- **ADRB1** see Beta-1 Adrenergic Receptor on page 171
- **ADRB2** see Beta-2 Adrenergic Receptor on page 171
- **ADRB3** see Beta-3 Adrenergic Receptor on page 174
- **AGT** see Angiotensinogen on page 167
- **AG TR1** see Angiotensin II Type 1 Receptor on page 166

Aldosterone Synthase

Synonyms CYP11B2; P-450 C18 11-Beta Hydroxylase
Chromosome Location 8q21-22
Clinically-Important Polymorphisms Synonymous SNP in the 5'-flanking region (C-344T)
Discussion The conversion of 11-deoxycorticosterone to aldosterone requires three enzymatic reactions. Aldosterone synthase, a member of the cytochrome P450 enzyme family, mediates these reactions. The C-344T polymorphism, or a functional variant in linkage disequilibrium with it, is believed to contribute to the abnormal regulation of aldosterone secretion which may play a role in idiopathic low-renin hypertension (Rossi et al 2001). The CYP11B2 genotype may also influence the effect of risk factors for coronary events. Smoking and dyslipidemia have been shown to be more potent risk factors for nonfatal MI in males who carry the -344C allele (Hautanen et al 1999).

The -344C allele of CYP11B2 gene has been associated with a genetic predisposition to develop essential hypertension (Tsukada et al 2002). A relationship between the intima-media thickness of the large muscular femoral artery and the ACE gene has been noted to be apparent only in the presence of either the alpha-adducin 460W or the aldosterone synthase -344T allele (Balkestein et al 2002). The relationship between this genetic polymorphism and hypertension may be complex, as interactions between a number of genes, including angiotensin converting enzyme, alpha-adducin, and aldosterone synthase, appear to contribute to the prevalence and incidence of hypertension in Caucasians (Staessen et al 2001).

ACE inhibitors:
During ACE inhibitor therapy for a mean duration of 17 months in 107 patients with dilated cardiomyopathy, improvement in left ventricular ejection fraction was greater with the -344C allele compared to the TT genotype (Tiago et al 2002).

Angiotensin II type 1 receptor antagonists:
During treatment with irbesartan in patients with essential hypertension and left ventricular hypertrophy, systolic blood pressure reduction was greater with the -344TT genotype compared to -344TC and CC genotypes. There was no association between this genotype and diastolic blood pressure response (Kurland et al 2002). The C-344T polymorphism was not associated with regression of left ventricular mass during irbesartan treatment in this population (Kurland et al 2002).

May Alter Pharmacokinetics of Aldosterone synthase is not known to affect the metabolism of any drugs.

May Alter Pharmacodynamics of ACE inhibitors, angiotensin II type 1 receptor blockers, aldosterone antagonists

May Affect Disease Predisposition of Hypertension

Clinical Recommendations Data with the CYP11B2 gene to date are inconsistent. The CYP11B2 gene may interact with other genes in the renin-angiotensin system to influence response to renin-angiotensin system antagonists. The association between the CYP11B2 gene alone and response to ACE inhibitors or angiotensin II type 1 receptor blockers may be difficult to establish.

Counseling Points Since hypertension is a disease with polygenic etiology, carrier status of the aldosterone synthase variant allele does not necessarily predispose a person to developing hypertension or its sequelae.

References

Balkestein EJ, Wang JG, Struijker-Boudier HA, et al, "Carotid and Femoral Intima-media Thickness in Relation to Three Candidate Genes in a Caucasian Population," *J Hypertens*, 2002, 20(8):1551-61.

Hautanen A, Toivanen P, Manttari M, et al, "Joint Effects of an Aldosterone Synthase (CYP11B2) Gene Polymorphism and Classic Risk Factors on Risk of Myocardial Infarction," *Circulation*, 1999, 100(22):2213-8.

Kurland L, Melhus H, Karlsson J, et al, "Aldosterone Synthase (CYP11B2) -344 C/T Polymorphism Is Related to Antihypertensive Response: Result From the Swedish Irbesartan Left Ventricular Hypertrophy Investigation Versus Atenolol (SILVHIA) Trial," *Am J Hypertens*, 2002, 15(5):389-93.

Kurland L, Melhus H, Karlsson J, et al, "Polymorphisms in the Angiotensinogen and Angiotensin II Type 1 Receptor Gene Are Related to Change in Left Ventricular Mass During Antihypertensive Treatment: Results From the Swedish Irbesartan Left Ventricular Hypertrophy Investigation Versus Atenolol (SILVHIA) Trial," *J Hypertens*, 2002, 20(4):657-63.

Rossi E, Regolisti G, Perazzoli F, et al, "-344C/T Polymorphism of CYP11B2 Gene in Italian Patients With Idiopathic Low Renin Hypertension," *Am J Hypertens*, 2001, 14(9 Pt 1):934-41.

Staessen JA, Wang JG, Brand E, et al, "Effects of Three Candidate Genes on Prevalence and Incidence of Hypertension in a Caucasian Population," *J Hypertens*, 2001, 19(8):1349-58.

Tiago AD, Badenhorst D, Skudicky D, et al, "An Aldosterone Synthase Gene Variant Is Associated With Improvement in Left Ventricular Ejection Fraction in Dilated Cardiomyopathy," *Cardiovasc Res*, 2002, 54(3):584-9.

Tsukada K, Ishimitsu T, Teranishi M, et al, "Positive Association of CYP11B2 Gene Polymorphism With Genetic Predisposition to Essential Hypertension," *J Hum Hypertens*, 2002, 16(11):789-93.

♦ **ALOX5** *see* 5-Lipoxygenase *on page 208*

Alpha-1 Adrenergic Receptor

Chromosome Location 8p21-p11.2

Clinically-Important Polymorphisms ADRA1A; Arg347Cys

Discussion There are three pharmacologically defined α_1-adrenergic receptors with distinct sequences and tissue distribution. These include the α_{1A}, α_{1B}, and α_{1D} receptors. The distinct functional properties of these different α_1-adrenergic receptor subtypes have not been fully illuminated.

(Continued)

Alpha-1 Adrenergic Receptor *(Continued)*

α_1-adrenergic receptors are one of the key first messengers in the uncoupling protein pathway. They have an overlapping distribution on white and brown adipose tissue and within the hypothalamic paraventricular nucleus. Clozapine, via α_1-adrenergic antagonism, may disrupt peripheral, as well as central energy homeostasis and cause weight gain (Bymaster et al 1996).

Clozapine:
Individuals who are homozygous for the cysteine variant of the α_{1a}-adrenergic receptor were protected from clozapine-induced weight gain (Basile et al 2001).

May Alter Pharmacodynamics of Clozapine and other agents that affect the α_1-adrenergic receptor

References
Basile VS, Masellis M, McIntyre RS, et al, "Genetic Dissection of Atypical Antipsychotic-Induced Weight Gain: Novel Preliminary Data on the Pharmacogenetic Puzzle," *J Clin Psychiatry*, 2001, 62(Suppl 23):45-66 (review).

Bymaster FP, Hemrick-Luecke SK, Perry KW, et al, "Neurochemical Evidence for Antagonism by Olanzapine of Dopamine, Serotonin, Alpha$_1$-Adrenergic and Muscarinic Receptors *in vivo* in Rats," *Psychopharmacology (Berl)*, 1996, 124(1-2):87-94.

Alpha-Adducin

Synonyms ADDA

Chromosome Location 4p16.3

Clinically-Important Polymorphisms Nonsynonymous SNP at codon 460 *(G460W)*

Discussion Alpha-adducin is a cytoskeletal protein that is important in the assembly of the intracellular actin-spectrin network. It may also play a role in intracellular signaling and membrane ion transport. The alpha-adducin gene variant, *G460W*, has been associated with a salt-sensitive form of hypertension, renal sodium retention, and plasma renin activity (Manunta et al 1999, Cusi et al 1997). A relationship between the intima-media thickness of the large muscular femoral artery and the ACE gene has been noted to be apparent only in the presence of either the alpha-adducin *460W* allele or the aldosterone synthase *-344T* allele (Balkestein et al 2002).

Hydrochlorothiazide:
Significantly greater reductions in mean blood pressure were observed in hypertensive individuals with the *460W* allele during 2-month treatment with hydrochlorothiazide (Glorioso et al 1999). In a population-based-case-control study, treatment with a thiazide diuretic was associated with a significantly lower risk of the combined endpoint of myocardial infarction and stroke compared to other antihypertensive treatments among carriers of at least one *460W* allele (Psaty et al 2002).

May Alter Pharmacokinetics of Alpha-adducin is not known to affect the metabolism of any drugs.

May Alter Pharmacodynamics of Thiazide diuretics, loop diuretics

May Affect Disease Predisposition of Hypertension

Clinical Recommendations Genotyping for the *G460W* polymorphism may have a role in predicting the effects of diuretics on blood pressure and clinical outcomes in hypertensive patients.

Counseling Points Since hypertension is a disease with polygenic etiology, carrier status of the *460W* allele does not necessarily predispose a person to developing hypertension or its sequelae.

References
Balkestein EJ, Wang JG, Struijker-Boudier HA, et al, "Carotid and Femoral Intima-media Thickness in Relation to Three Candidate Genes in a Caucasian Population," *J Hypertens*, 2002, 20(8):1551-61.

Cusi D, Barlassina C, Azzani T, et al, "Polymorphisms of Alpha-Adducin and Salt Sensitivity in Patients With Essential Hypertension," *Lancet*, 1997, 349(9062):1353-7.

Glorioso N, Manunta P, Filigheddu F, et al, "The Role of Alpha-Adducin Polymorphism in Blood Pressure and Sodium Handling Regulation May Not Be Excluded by a Negative Association Study," *Hypertension*, 1999, 34(4 Pt 1):649-54.

Manunta P, Burnier M, D'Amico M, et al, "Adducin Polymorphism Affects Renal Proximal Tubule Reabsorption in Hypertension," *Hypertension*, 1999, 33(2):694-7.

Psaty BM, Smith NL, Heckbert SR, et al, "Diuretic Therapy, the Alpha-Adducin Gene Variant, and the Risk of Myocardial Infarction or Stroke in Persons With Treated Hypertension," *JAMA*, 2002, 287(13):1680-9.

Angiotensin-Converting Enzyme

Synonyms ACE

Chromosome Location 17q22-24

Clinically-Important Polymorphisms The ACE insertion/deletion *(I/ D)* polymorphism results in the presence or absence of a 287bp fragment in intron 16 of the ACE gene.

Discussion Angiotensin-converting enzyme mediates the conversion of angiotensin I to angiotensin II. The polymorphism of the human ACE gene contributes to circulating ACE activity. Genotype may influence the development of hypertension and cardiovascular disease. The *D* allele is associated with higher ACE levels as compared to the *I* allele (Kohno et al 1999, Ohmichi et al 1997, Danser et al 1995). Correlations between gene distribution and cardiovascular disease have been inconsistent. The ACE *DD* genotype has been associated with increased mortality and cardiac morbidity following coronary artery bypass grafting (Volzke et al 2002). The significance of this polymorphism may be difficult to distinguish, since blood pressure control is likely regulated by multiple factors. In addition, the influence of ACE genotype may be modified by environmental factors, including salt intake (van der Kleij et al 2002).

ACE inhibitors:
Although the data are inconsistent, the ACE *I/D* genotype has been correlated with the clinical effects of ACE inhibitors including blood pressure lowering (Ohmichi et al 1997, Stavroulakis et al 2000), reductions in left ventricular hypertrophy (Sasaki et al 1996, Kohno et al 1999), and improvements in endothelial function (Prasad et al 2000). The *II* genotype was associated with greater diastolic blood pressure reductions with ACE inhibitor therapy in Japanese hypertensives (Ohmichi et al 1997). In contrast, the *DD* genotype was associated with greater reductions in systolic and diastolic blood

(Continued)

Angiotensin-Converting Enzyme *(Continued)*

pressure with ACE inhibitor therapy in hypertensive European Caucasians (Stavroulakis et al 2000). Other studies found no association between the ACE *I/D* genotype and blood pressure response to renin-angiotensin system antagonists (Hingorani et al 1995, Kohno et al 1999, Sasaki et al 1996).

One study in Japanese hypertensive patients found that regression of cardiac mass after 1- and 2-years of treatment with an ACE inhibitor was greater with the *II* genotype, while another found that regression of cardiac mass regression after 1-year treatment with an ACE inhibitor was greater with the *DD* genotype (Kohno et al 1999, Sasaki et al 1996). The ACE gene was not associated with reduction in cardiac mass during 3-month treatment with irbesartan in another study (Kurland et al 2002).

Although the data are inconsistent, the *I/D* polymorphism has been associated with ACE inhibitor-induced cough. In a healthy volunteer study, cough threshold following 4 weeks of ACE inhibitor therapy was significantly reduced in volunteers with the *II* genotype (Takahashi et al 2001). However, a study in hypertensive subjects found no association between the ACE gene and the ACE inhibitor-induced cough (Zee et al 1998).

Angiotensin II type 1 receptor antagonists:

The *II* genotype was associated with greater diastolic blood pressure decline with 3-month treatment with irbesartan in 86 hypertensive European Caucasians compared to the *ID* and *DD* genotypes (Kurland et al 2001).

β-blockers:

In a retrospective study of heart failure patients, the ACE *D* allele was associated with greater transplant-free survival with β-blocker therapy compared to the *I* allele (McNamara 2001).

Statins:

In a study of individuals with coronary atherosclerosis who were treated with fluvastatin for 2.5 years, reductions in total and LDL cholesterol were greater in those with the *DD* genotype compared to those with the *ID* and *II* genotypes (Marian et al 2000).

In myocardial infarction survivors, the greatest reductions in fatal coronary heart disease or nonfatal myocardial infarction with pravastatin occurred in those with the Pl^{A2} allele of the glycoprotein IIIa subunit gene and either the ACE *ID* or *DD* genotype (Bray et al 2001).

Fibrates:

In a small clinical study, the ACE *DD* genotype was associated with greater increases in HDL cholesterol levels with gemfibrozil (Bosse et al 2002).

May Alter Pharmacokinetics of ACE is not known to alter the metabolism of any drugs.

May Alter Pharmacodynamics of ACE inhibitors, angiotensin II type 1 receptor blockers, β-blockers in heart failure, HMG CoA reductase inhibitors, fibrates

May Affect Disease Predisposition of In addition to cardiovascular disease, preliminary evidence suggests that the ACE-*DD*-genotype may be associated with other common adult diseases, including diabetes, psychiatric disease, depression, and some forms of cancer (Moskowitz et al 2002).

Laboratory Evaluation Clinical testing available

Clinical Recommendations Data with the ACE gene are inconsistent and often conflicting. The ACE gene may interact with other genes in the renin-angiotensin system to influence response to renin-angiotensin system antagonists. The association between the ACE gene alone and response to ACE inhibitors or angiotensin II type 1 receptor blockers may be difficult to establish.

Counseling Points Since hypertension is a disease with polygenic etiology, carrier status of the ACE variant allele does not necessarily predispose a person to developing hypertension or its sequelae.

References

Bosse Y, Pascot A, Dumont M, et al, "Influences of the PPAR Alpha-L162V Polymorphism on Plasma HDL(2)-Cholesterol Response of Abdominally Obese Men Treated With Gemfibrozil," *Genet Med*, 2002, 4(4):311-5.

Bray PF, Cannon CP, Goldschmidt-Clermont P, et al, "The Platelet Pl(A2) and Angiotensin-Converting Enzyme (ACE) D Allele Polymorphisms and the Risk of Recurrent Events After Acute Myocardial Infarction," *Am J Cardiol*, 2001, 88(4):347-52.

Danser AH, Schalekamp MA, Bax WA, et al, "Angiotensin-Converting Enzyme in the Human Heart. Effect of the Deletion/Insertion Polymorphism," *Circulation*, 1995, 92(6):1387-8.

Hingorani AD, Jia H, Stevens PA, et al, "Renin-Angiotensin System Gene Polymorphisms Influence Blood Pressure and the Response to Angiotensin-Converting Enzyme Inhibition," *J Hypertens*, 1995, 13(12 Pt 2):1602-9.

Kohno M, Yokokawa K, Minami M, et al, "Association Between Angiotensin-Converting Enzyme Gene Polymorphisms and Regression of Left Ventricular Hypertrophy in Patients Treated With Angiotensin-Converting Enzyme Inhibitors," *Am J Med*, 1999, 106(5):544-9.

Kurland LH, Melhus J, Karlsson T, et al, "Angiotensin-Converting Enzyme Gene Polymorphism Predicts Blood Pressure Response to Angiotensin II Receptor Type 1 Antagonist Treatment in Hypertensive Patients," *J Hypertens*, 2001, 19(10):1783-7.

Kurland LH, Melhus J, Karlsson T, et al, "Polymorphisms in the Angiotensinogen and Angiotensin II Type I Receptor Gene are Related to Change in Left Ventricular Mass During Antihypertensive Treatment: Results From the Swedish Irbesartan Left Ventricular Hypertrophy Investigation Versus Atenolol (SILVHIA) Trial," *J Hypertens*, 2002, 20(4):657-63.

Marian AJ, Safavi F, Ferlic L, et al, "Interactions Between Angiotensin-I Converting Enzyme Insertion/Deletion Polymorphism and Response of Plasma Lipids and Coronary Atherosclerosis to Treatment With Fluvastatin: The Lipoprotein and Coronary Atherosclerosis Study," *J Am Coll Cardiol*, 2000, 35(1):89-95.

McNamara DM, Holubkov R, Janosko K, et al, "Pharmacogenetic Interactions Between Beta-Blocker Therapy and the Angiotensin-Converting Enzyme Deletion Polymorphism in Patients With Congestive Heart Failure," *Circulation*, 2001, 103(12):1644-8.

Moskowitz DW, "Is Angiotensin I-Converting Enzyme a "Master" Disease Gene?" *Diabetes Technol Ther*, 2002, 4(5):683-711.

Ohmichi N, Iwai N, Uchida Y, et al, "Relationship Between the Response to the Angiotensin Converting Enzyme Inhibitor Imidapril and the Angiotensin Converting Enzyme Genotype," *Am J Hypertens*, 1997, 10(8):951-5.

Prasad A, Narayanan S, Husain S, et al, "Insertion-Deletion Polymorphism of the ACE Gene Modulates Reversibility of Endothelial Dysfunction With ACE Inhibition," *Circulation*, 2000, 102(1):35-41.

(Continued)

Angiotensin-Converting Enzyme *(Continued)*

Sasaki M, Oki T, Iuchi A, et al, "Relationship Between the Angiotensin Converting Enzyme Gene Polymorphism and the Effects of Enalapril on Left Ventricular Hypertrophy and Impaired Diastolic Filling in Essential Hypertension: M-mode and Pulsed Doppler Echocardiographic Studies," *J Hypertens*, 1996, 14(12):1403-8.

Stavroulakis GA, Makris TK, Krespi PG, et al, "Predicting Response to Chronic Antihypertensive Treatment With Fosinopril: The Role of Angiotensin-Converting Enzyme Gene Polymorphism," *Cardiovasc Drugs Ther*, 2000, 14(4):427-32.

Takahashi T, Yamaguchi E, Furuya K, et al, "The ACE Gene Polymorphism and Cough Threshold for Capsaicin After Cilazapril Usage," *Respir Med*, 2001, 95(2):130-5.

van der Kleij FG, de Jong PE, Henning RH, et al, "Enhanced Responses of Blood Pressure, Renal Function, and Aldosterone to Angiotensin I in the DD Genotype Are Blunted by Low Sodium Intake," *J Am Soc Nephrol*, 2002, 13(4):1025-33

Volzke H, Engel J, Kleine V, et al, "Angiotensin I-Converting Enzyme Insertion/Deletion Polymorphism and Cardiac Mortality and Morbidity After Coronary Artery Bypass Graft Surgery," *Chest*, 2002, 122(1):31-6

Zee RY, Rao VS, Paster RZ, et al, "Three Candidate Genes and Angiotensin-Converting Enzyme Inhibitor-Related Cough: A Pharmacogenetic Analysis," *Hypertension*, 1998, 31(4):925-8.

Angiotensin II Type 1 Receptor

Synonyms AG TR1; AT_1R

Chromosome Location 3q21-25

Clinically-Important Polymorphisms Synonymous SNP at nucleotide 1166 in the 3′ untranslated region *(A1166C)*

Discussion The angiotensin type 1 receptor mediates vasoconstriction, aldosterone secretion, and cardiac remodeling following stimulation by angiotensin II. The *1166C* allele has been shown to increase the arterial responsiveness to angiotensin II (VanGeel et al 2000). It has also been associated with aortic stiffness in hypertensive patients (Benetos et al 1996).

ACE inhibitors:

In hypertensive individuals, *1166C* allele carriers had threefold greater reductions in aortic stiffness with perindopril therapy compared to *1166AA* homozygotes (Benetos, Cambien et al 1996).

Angiotensin II type 1 receptor antagonists:

In healthy volunteers, a single dose of losartan resulted in a greater reduction in mean arterial pressure in *1166C* allele carriers compared to *1166AA* homozygotes (Miller et al 1999). However, in hypertensive patients treated with an ACE inhibitor, no association between the AT_1R gene and blood pressure reduction was found (Hingorani et al 1995).

During treatment with irbesartan in patients with essential hypertension and left ventricular hypertrophy, reductions in left ventricular mass were greater with the *1166AC* genotype compared to the *1166AA* genotype (Kurland et al 2002). However, the *1166AA* genotype did not remain an independent predictor of blood pressure response after regression analysis.

May Alter Pharmacokinetics of AT_1R is not known to alter the metabolism of any drugs.

May Alter Pharmacodynamics of ACE inhibitors, angiotensin II type 1 receptor blockers

May Affect Disease Predisposition of Hypertension, left ventricular hypertrophy, anxiety, depression, Alzheimer's disease

Clinical Recommendations Data with the AT_1R gene are inconsistent. The AT_1R gene may interact with other genes in the renin-angiotensin system to influence response to renin-angiotensin system antagonists. The association between the AT_1R gene alone and response to ACE inhibitors or angiotensin II type 1 receptor blockers may be difficult to establish.

Counseling Points Since hypertension is a disease with polygenic etiology, carrier status of the AT_1R variant allele does not necessarily predispose a person to developing hypertension.

References

Benetos A and Safar ME, "Aortic Collagen, Aortic Stiffness, and AT1 Receptors in Experimental and Human Hypertension," *Can J Physiol Pharmacol*, 1996, 74(7):862-6 (review).

Benetos A, Cambien F, Gautier S, et al, "Influence of the Angiotensin II Type 1 Receptor Gene Polymorphism on the Effects of Perindopril and Nitrendipine on Arterial Stiffness in Hypertensive Individuals," *Hypertension*, 1996, 28(6):1081-4.

Hingorani AD and Brown MJ, "A Simple Molecular Assay for the C1166 Variant of the Angiotensin II Type 1 Receptor Gene," *Biochem Biophys Res Commun*, 1995, 213(2):725-9.

Kurland L, Melhus H, Karlsson J, et al, "Aldosterone Synthase (CYP11B2) -344 C/T Polymorphism Is Related to Antihypertensive Response: Result From the Swedish Irbesartan Left Ventricular Hypertrophy Investigation Versus Atenolol (SILVHIA) Trial," *Am J Hypertens*, 2002, 15(5):389-93.

Miller JA, Thai K, and Scholey JW, "Angiotensin II Type 1 Receptor Gene Polymorphism Predicts Response to Losartan and Angiotensin II," *Kidney Int*, 1999, 56(6):2173-80.

van Geel PP, Pinto YM, Voors AA, et al, "Angiotensin II Type 1 Receptor A1166C Gene Polymorphism Is Associated With an Increased Response to Angiotensin II in Human Arteries," *Hypertension*, 2000, 35(3):717-21.

Angiotensinogen

Synonyms AGT

Chromosome Location 1q42-43

Clinically-Important Polymorphisms

Nonsynonymous SNP at codon 235 in exon 2 with a threonine instead of methionine *(M235T)*

Nonsynonymous SNP at codon 174 in exon 2 with methionine rather than threonine *(T174M)*

Discussion Angiotensinogen is the precursor to the formation of angiotensin I. Plasma angiotensinogen levels have been associated with the number of *235T* alleles (Winkelmann et al 1999). Since the systems regulating blood pressure involve multiple factors, the association of any single polymorphism with the development of hypertension may be difficult to establish. Studies evaluating the role of AGT polymorphisms have yielded inconsistent results. However, polymorphisms of this protein have been associated with differential responses to antihypertensive therapy. In one study, the *235T* allele was associated with the need for more multiple antihypertensive medications (Schunkert et al 1997).

ACE inhibitors:

The *235T* allele has been associated with enhanced blood pressure reduction during ACE inhibitor therapy compared to the *235M* genotype (Hingorani et al 1995).

(Continued)

Angiotensinogen *(Continued)*

Angiotensin II type 1 receptor antagonists:
During treatment with irbesartan in patients with essential hypertension and left ventricular hypertrophy, the *174TM* genotype and the *235T* allele were associated with the greatest reductions in left ventricular mass (Kurland et al 2002). The *174TM* genotype remained an independent predictor of drug response after stepwise multiple regression analysis.

May Alter Pharmacokinetics of The AGT gene is not known to alter the metabolism of any drugs.

May Alter Pharmacodynamics of ACE inhibitors, angiotensin II type 1 receptor blockers

May Affect Disease Predisposition of Hypertension, left ventricular hypertrophy

Clinical Recommendations Data suggest that the AGT gene may be an important predictor of response to renin-angiotensin system therapy in hypertension. The AGT gene may interact with other renin-angiotensin genes to determine responses to renin-angiotensin system antagonists.

Counseling Points Since hypertension is a disease with polygenic etiology, carrier status of the AGT variant allele does not necessarily predispose a person to developing hypertension.

References
Hingorani AD, Jia H, Stevens PA, et al, "Renin-Angiotensin System Gene Polymorphisms Influence Blood Pressure and the Response to Angiotensin-Converting Enzyme Inhibition," *J Hypertens*, 1995, 13(12 Pt 2):1602-9.

Kurland L, Melhus H, Karlsson J, et al, "Aldosterone Synthase (CYP11B2) -344 C/T Polymorphism Is Related to Antihypertensive Response: Result From the Swedish Irbesartan Left Ventricular Hypertrophy Investigation Versus Atenolol (SILVHIA) Trial," *Am J Hypertens*, 2002, 15(5):389-93.

Schunkert H, Hense HW, Gimenez-Roqueplo AP, et al, "The Angiotensinogen T235 Variant and the Use of Antihypertensive Drugs in a Population-Based Cohort," *Hypertension*, 1997, 29(2):628-33.

Winkelmann BR, Russ AP, Nauck M, et al, "Angiotensinogen M235T Polymorphism Is Associated With Plasma Angiotensinogen and Cardiovascular Disease," *Am Heart J*, 1999, 137(4 Pt 1):698-705.

♦ **APOE** *see* Apolipoprotein E *on page 168*

Apolipoprotein E

Synonyms APOE

Chromosome Location 19q13.2

Clinically-Important Polymorphisms Human APOE has three common alleles, *APOE2*, *APOE3*, and *APOE4*, resulting from nonsynonymous SNPs at codons 112 and 158.

Discussion Apolipoprotein E modulates cholesterol and phospholipid transport between cells of different types. Apolipoprotein is involved in lipid transport in both the plasma and within the brain. It mediates the binding of lipoproteins to members of the low density lipoprotein (LDL) receptor family. Genetic variation has been associated with plasma lipid profiles (including LDL, high density lipoprotein (HDL) and triglyceride concentrations). The APOE locus has been found to be a significant genetic determinant of cardiovascular disease. Some of the

APOLIPOPROTEIN E

variation in response to dietary modification has been reported to be associated with the *E4* allele. Additional variation in response to drug therapy are described under individual categories (below).

APOE and its receptors are expressed at high levels in the brain. The *APOE4* allele is associated with sporadic and late-onset familial Alzheimer disease. *APOE4* has been shown to correlate with the risk of developing Alzheimer's disease, age of onset, accumulation of plaques, and reduction of choline acetyltransferase activity in the hippocampus. *APOE4* allele copy number has an inverse relationship with residual brain choline acetyltransferase activity and nicotinic receptor binding sites in both the hippocampal formation and the temporal cortex of AD subjects. Individuals lacking the *APOE4* allele showed ChAT activities close or within age-matched normal control values. *APOE4* appears to play a crucial role in cholinergic transmission in Alzheimer's disease.

HMG CoA reductase inhibitors:

A relationship between the *APOE4* allele and response to statins has been described. In studies evaluating the effect of the *APOE* genotype on lipoprotein lipid changes during HMG CoA reductase therapy, the *E2* allele was associated with a more favorable drug response compared to other genotypes (Ordovas et al 1995, Nestel et al 1997). Other studies found no significant association between *APOE* genotype and lipoprotein response to HMG CoA reductase inhibitors (Sanllehy et al 1998).

In a large clinical trial of simvastatin therapy in myocardial infarction survivors, the greatest benefit from simvastatin therapy, in terms of mortality reduction, has been observed in patients with the *E4* allele (Gerdes et al 2000).

Cholinesterase inhibitors:

As a prognostic indicator, presence of the *APOE4* allele may signal the potential for a poor response to therapy with cholinesterase inhibitors. In a study of 40 patients with Alzheimer's disease, over 80% of *APOE4*-negative patients showed marked improvement in response to tacrine (ADAS scale). Deterioration of ADAS scores was noted in 60% of *APOE4* carriers (Poirier et al 1995). From the studies done to date analyzing genotype correlations to drug response, it is evident that there is an effect of *APOE4* (Poirier et al 1995, Farlow et al 1998, MacGowan et al 1998). The nature of this effect is well established for tacrine, with research showing that *E4* patients with AD respond poorer to this medication than those without an *E4* allele. Subsequent studies investigating galantamine, donepezil, and metrifonate have had mixed results depending on the agent studied, duration of treatment period, and primary outcome measure used (Wilcock et al 2000, Greenberg et al 2000, Farlow et al 1999). Further long-term studies utilizing the ADAS-Cog scale to assess patient response will determine which agents will be most beneficial to patients with or without an *E4* allele.

May Alter Pharmacokinetics of APOE is not known to alter the metabolism of any drugs.

(Continued)

Apolipoprotein E *(Continued)*

May Alter Pharmacodynamics of HMG-CoA reductase inhibitors, cholinesterase inhibitors

May Affect Disease Predisposition of Alzheimer's disease

Laboratory Evaluation Commercial testing available

Clinical Recommendations Data suggest that the *APOE* genotype may be useful in predicting clinical outcomes with HMG CoA reductase inhibitor therapy in patients with coronary heart disease. The *APOE* genotype may interact with the β-fibrinogen, stromelysin-1, ACE, and cholesterol ester transfer protein genes in predicting HMG CoA reductase inhibitor response. Data suggest that the *APOE* genotype may be related to response to the cholinesterase inhibitors. Some patients may have a better response to these medications based on their *APOE* genotype.

Counseling Points Carrier status for the *APOE4* allele has been associated with increased risk for developing coronary heart disease and Alzheimer's disease and for greater disease progression in individuals with coronary heart disease. Individuals who carry this allele should be encouraged to discuss the implications of their carrier status with their clinician or another healthcare professional.

References

Farlow MR, Cyrus PA, Nadel A, et al, "Metrifonate Treatment of AD: Influence of APOE Genotype," *Neurology*, 1999, 53(9):2010-6.

Farlow MR, Lahiri DK, Poirier J, et al, "Treatment Outcome of Tacrine Therapy Depends on Apolipoprotein Genotype and Gender of the Subjects With Alzheimer's Disease," *Neurology*, 1998, 50(3):669-77.

Gerdes LU, Gerdes C, Kervinen K, et al, "The Apolipoprotein Epsilon4 Allele Determines Prognosis and the Effect on Prognosis of Simvastatin in Survivors of Myocardial Infarction: A Substudy of the Scandinavian Simvastatin Survival Study," *Circulation*, 2000, 28;101(12):1366-71.

Greenberg SM, Tennis MK, Brown LB, et al, "Donepezil Therapy in Clinical Practice: A Randomized Crossover Study," *Arch Neurol*, 2000, 57(1):94-9.

MacGowan SH, Wilcock GK, and Scott M, "Effect of Gender and Apolipoprotein E Genotype on Response to Anticholinesterase in Alzheimer's Disease," *Int J Geriatr Psychiatry*, 1998, 13(9):625-30.

Nestel PJ, Simons L, Barter P, et al, "A Comparative Study of the Efficacy of Simvastatin and Gemfibrozil in Combined Hyperlipoproteinemia: Prediction of Response by Baseline Lipids, Apo E Genotype, Lipoprotein(a) and Insulin," *Atherosclerosis*, 1997, 21;129(2):231-9.

Ordovas JM, Lopez-Miranda J, Perez-Jimenez F, et al, "Effect of Apolipoprotein E and A-IV Phenotypes on the Low Density Lipoprotein Response to HMG CoA Reductase Inhibitor Therapy," *Atherosclerosis*, 1995, 113(2):157-66.

Poirier J, Delisle MC, Quirion R, et al, "Apolipoprotein E4 Allele as a Predictor of Cholinergic Deficits and Treatment Outcome in Alzheimer Disease," *Proc Natl Acad Sci U S A*, 1995, 92(26):12260-4.

Sanllehy C, Casals E, Rodriguez-Villar C, et al, "Lack of Interaction of Apolipoprotein E Phenotype With the Lipoprotein Response to Lovastatin and Gemfibrozil in Patients With Primary Hypercholesterolemia," *Metabolism*, 1998, 47(5):560-5.

Wilcock GK, Lilienfeld S, and Gaens E, "Efficacy and Safety of Galantamine in Patients With Mild to Moderate Alzheimer's Disease: Multicentre Randomised Controlled Trial. Galantamine International-1 Study Group," *BMJ*, 2000, 321(7274):1445-9.

- **AT$_1$R** *see* Angiotensin II Type 1 Receptor *on page 166*
- **B1AR** *see* Beta-1 Adrenergic Receptor *on page 171*
- **B2AR** *see* Beta-2 Adrenergic Receptor *on page 171*
- **B3AR** *see* Beta-3 Adrenergic Receptor *on page 174*

◆ **BDKRB2** *see* Bradykinin B2 Receptor *on page 175*

Beta-1 Adrenergic Receptor

Synonyms ADRB1; B1AR

Chromosome Location 10q24-26

Clinically-Important Polymorphisms Nonsynonymous SNPs at codon 49 in the amino terminus region (S49G) and codon 389 in the carboxy-terminus region (R389G)

Discussion In site-directed mutagenesis studies, the *S49G* polymorphism was associated with B1AR down-regulation and the *R389G* polymorphism was associated with basal- and agonist-mediated increases in adenylyl cyclase activities (Rathz et al 2002, Mason et al 1999). The *49S* allele has been associated with increased hospitalizations and poorer survival in heart failure patients (Borjesson et al 2000). The *389R/R* genotype has been associated with hypertension (Bengtsson et al 2001).

β-blockers:
  The *389R/R* and *49S/S* genotypes were associated with greater blood pressure response to metoprolol in hypertensive subjects (Zineh et al 2002).

May Alter Pharmacokinetics of The B1AR is not known to alter the metabolism of any drugs.

May Alter Pharmacodynamics of β-Blockers

May Affect Disease Predisposition of Hypertension

Clinical Recommendations The data suggest that the *B1AR* genotype may be an important determinant of blood pressure response to β-blocker therapy. Whether the B1AR gene interacts with intracellular signaling genes in determining β-blocker response remains to be determined.

Counseling Points Since hypertension is a disease with polygenic etiology, carrier status of the *389R/R* genotype does not necessarily predispose a person to developing hypertension or its sequelae. Heart failure patients with the *Ser49* allele should discuss the implications of carrier status with their clinician or another healthcare professional.

References

Bengtsson K, Melander O, Orho-Melander M, et al, "Polymorphism in the Beta(1)-Adrenergic Receptor Gene and Hypertension," *Circulation*, 2001, 104(2):187-90.

Borjesson M, Magnusson Y, Hjalmarson A, et al, "A Novel Polymorphism in the Gene Coding for the Beta(1)-Adrenergic Receptor Associated With Survival in Patients With Heart Failure," *Eur Heart J*, 2000, 21(22):1853-8.

Mason DA, Moore JD, Green SA, et al, "A Gain-of-Function Polymorphism in a G-Protein Coupling Domain of the Human Beta$_1$-Adrenergic Receptor," *J Biol Chem*, 1999, 274(18):12670-4.

Rathz DA, Brown KM, Kramer LA, et al, "Amino Acid 49 Polymorphisms of the Human Beta$_1$-Adrenergic Receptor Affect Agonist-Promoted Trafficking," *J Cardiovasc Pharmacol*, 2002, 39(2):155-60.

Zineh I, Puckett SP, McGorray DF, et al, "Beta$_1$-Adrenergic Receptor Polymorphisms Predict Antihypertensive Response to Beta-Blockers," *Circulation*, 2002, 106(19):Suppl 11-574 (abstract).

Beta-2 Adrenergic Receptor

Synonyms ADRB2; B2AR

Chromosome Location 5q31-32

(Continued)

Beta-2 Adrenergic Receptor *(Continued)*
Clinically-Important Polymorphisms

Receptor coding region: R16G, Q27E, and T164I

Multiple SNPs have also been identified in the promoter region (including at amino acid position R-19C)

Discussion The β_2-adrenergic receptor is a membrane bound, G-protein linked receptor. This receptor subtype plays a role in smooth muscle contraction and lipolysis. It is involved in the regulation of vascular tone, bronchial constriction, and uterine contraction. Variant forms of the β_2-adrenergic receptor gene display functional differences which may be clinically important. Frequently encountered SNPs include those at position 16 and 27 coding region and at codon-19 in the promoter region. A less common SNP occurs at codon 164. The codon 16, 27, and -19 SNPs appear to be in linkage disequilibrium.

Receptor polymorphisms influence receptor function *in vitro*, although evidence regarding exact relationships is conflicting. A common polymorphism resulting in a change from arginine to glycine at amino acid 16 (R16G) enhances agonist-promoted downregulation of receptor expression *in vitro* (Green et al 1994).

The *Q27E* genotype has been associated with fat mass, body mass index, and obesity in females. Lipolysis and fat oxidation promoted by acute submaximal exercise has been observed to be blunted in females with the *27QQ* genotype (Macho-Azcarate et al 2002).

The *T164I* polymorphism is found in approximately 4% of humans. It has been associated with decreased receptor signaling and, blunted cardiac response in transgenic mice. In addition, this polymorphism has been associated with decreases in exercise capacity and decreased survival in patients with congestive heart failure (Liggett et al 1998, Wagoner et al 2000).

Polymorphism of the β_2-adrenergic receptor may be related to variation in airway hyper-reactivity as well as responsiveness to β_2-agonist drugs. Although early studies suggested a relationship between *B2AR* genotype and airway hyper-responsiveness and asthma severity, the correlations have been inconsistent, and in some cases contradictory. A dynamic model of receptor kinetics, which attempts to account for downregulation from endogenous catecholamines in the *16G* genotype prior to exposure to pharmacologic agents, has been proposed (Liggett et al 2000). Under this model, tachyphylaxis to the effects of a β_2-agonist would be more apparent in patients with the *16R* genotype.

Since multiple polymorphisms may occur in both the sequences which encode the receptor as well as its regulatory sequences, the evaluation of haplotypes may yield more appropriate correlations to phenotype and drug response. Combinations of alleles may be more important in determining the relationship to phenotype than individual SNPs, and may explain why earlier investigations have yielded contrasting results.

β_2-adrenergic agonists:

The relationship of receptor polymorphisms to β-adrenergic receptor agonists appears to be complicated by discrepancies between observations made *in vitro* versus *in vivo* clinical trials. The *16G* genotype demonstrates enhanced down-regulation after exposure to stimulation *in vitro* (Green et al 1994). However, *in vivo* responses generally indicate that the *16G* genotype may be less likely to demonstrate tachyphylaxis. A potential explanation may be that the receptor populations in *16G* individuals have been previously down-regulated by exposure to endogenous catecholamines (Liggett et al 2000).

A small number of frequently occurring, functionally-relevant haplotype pairs have been confirmed (Drysdale et al 2000). Future studies will be required to clarify the pharmacodynamic effects of haplotypes both *in vitro* and *in vivo*.

Acute administration to children with the *16R* genotype has been shown to produce a higher number of positive responses to bronchodilator therapy (Martinez et al 1997). However, diminished responses to β-agonist therapy has been shown to occur following regular use of β_2-agonists in patients with the *16R* genotype (Israel et al 2000). Lower morning peak expiratory flow rates have been demonstrated in patients who are homozygous for the *16R* genotype following regular albuterol use (Israel et al 2001). Significant changes in the dose-response curves for terbutaline with respect to inotropic and chronotropic responses have also been associated with the *16R* genotype (Brodde et al 2001).

Although acute responses and extent of tachyphylaxis differ in patients with the *16G* genotype, use of a long-acting β_2-agonist (formoterol) maintained asthma control in a group of 24 patients with this genotype (Lipworth et al 2000).

May Alter Pharmacodynamics of β_2-adrenergic agonists

May Affect Disease Predisposition of Asthma, obesity, congestive heart failure

References

Brodde OE, Buscher R, Tellkamp R, et al, "Blunted Cardiac Responses to Receptor Activation in Subjects With Thr164Ile Beta(2)-Adrenoceptors," *Circulation*, 2001, 103(8):1048-50.

Drysdale CM, McGraw DW, Stack CB, et al, "Complex Promoter and Coding Region Beta-2 Adrenergic Receptor Haplotypes Alter Receptor Expression and Predict *in vivo* Responsiveness," *Proc Natl Acad Sci U S A*, 2000, 97(19):10483-8.

Green S, Turki J, Innis M, et al, "Amino-Terminal Polymorphisms of the Human Beta-2 Adrenergic Receptor Impart Distinct Agonist-Promoted Regulatory Properties," *Biochemistry*, 1994, 33(32):9414-9.

Israel E, Drazen JM, Liggett SB, et al, "Effect of Polymorphism of the Beta-2 Adrenergic Receptor on Response to Regular Use of Albuterol in Asthma," *Int Arch Allergy Immunol*, 2001, 124(1-3):183-6.

Israel E, Drazen JM, Liggett SB, et al, "The Effect of Polymorphisms of the Beta-2 Adrenergic Receptor on the Response to Regular Use of Albuterol in Asthma," *Am J Respir Crit Care Med*, 2000, 162(1):75-80.

Liggett SB, "Pharmacogenetics of Beta-1 and Beta-2 Adrenergic Receptors," *Pharmacology*, 2000, 61(3):167-73 (review).

Liggett SB, "Polymorphisms of the Beta$_2$-Adrenergic Receptor," *N Engl J Med*, 2002, 346(7):536-8

(Continued)

Beta-2 Adrenergic Receptor *(Continued)*

Liggett SB, Wagoner LE, Craft LL, et al, "The Ile164 Beta₂-Adrenergic Receptor Polymorphism Adversely Affects the Outcome of Congestive Heart Failure," *J Clin Invest*, 1998, 102(8):1534-9.

Lipworth BJ, Dempsey OJ, Aziz I, et al, "Effects of Adding a Leukotriene Antagonist or a Long-Acting Beta(2)-Agonist in Asthmatic Patients With the Glycine-16 Beta(2)-Adrenoceptor Genotype," *Am J Med*, 2000, 109(2):114-21.

Macho-Azcarate T, Marti A, Gonzalez A, et al, "Gln27Glu Polymorphism in the Beta₂-Adrenergic Receptor Gene and Lipid Metabolism During Exercise in Obese Women," *Int J Obes Relat Metab Disord*, 2002, 26(11):1434-41.

Martinez FD, Graves PE, Baldini M, et al, "Association Between Genetic Polymorphisms of the Beta-2 Adrenergic Receptor and Response to Albuterol in Children With and Without a History of Wheezing," *J Clin Invest*, 1997, 100(12):3184-8.

Taylor DR and Kennedy MA, "Beta-Adrenergic Receptor Polymorphisms and Drug Responses in Asthma," *Pharmacogenomics*, 2002, 3(2):173-84 (review).

Taylor DR and Kennedy MA, "Genetic Variation of the Beta(2)-Adrenoceptor: Its Functional and Clinical Importance in Bronchial Asthma," *Am J Pharmacogenomics*, 2001, 1(3):165-74 (review).

Wagoner LE, Craft LL, Singh B, et al, "Polymorphisms of the Beta(2)-Adrenergic Receptor Determine Exercise Capacity in Patients With Heart Failure," *Circ Res*, 2000, 86(8):834-40.

Beta-3 Adrenergic Receptor

Synonyms ADRB3; B3AR

Chromosome Location 8p12-11.2

Clinically-Important Polymorphisms T64R

Discussion A polymorphism in the β₃-adrenergic receptor gene (*T64R*) has been associated with insulin resistance (Widen et al 1995), the time of onset of type 2 diabetes mellitus (Walston et al 1995), and an increased capacity for obese individuals to gain weight (Clement et al 1995).

Clozapine:

The *T64R* polymorphism was associated with a higher mean change in weight during treatment with clozapine (Basile et al 2001).

May Alter Pharmacodynamics of Clozapine

References

Basile VS, Masellis M, McIntyre RS, et al, "Genetic Dissection of Atypical Antipsychotic-Induced Weight Gain: Novel Preliminary Data on the Pharmacogenetic Puzzle," *J Clin Psychiatry*, 2001, 62(Suppl 23):45-66 (review).

Clement K, Vaisse C, Manning BS, et al, "Genetic Variation in the Beta 3-adrenergic Receptor and an Increased Capacity to Gain Weight in Patients With Morbid Obesity," *N Engl J Med*, 1995, 333(6):352-4.

Walston J, Silver K, Bogardus C, et al, "Time of Onset of Noninsulin-Dependent Diabetes Mellitus and Genetic Variation in the Beta₃-Adrenergic-Receptor Gene," *N Engl J Med*, 1995, 333(6):343-7.

Widen E, Lehto M, Kanninen T, et al, "Association of a Polymorphism in the Beta₃-Adrenergic Receptor Gene With Features of the Insulin Resistance Syndrome in Finns," *N Engl J Med*, 1995, 333(6):348-51.

Beta-Fibrinogen

Synonyms FGB

Chromosome Location 4q28

Clinically-Important Polymorphisms Synonymous SNP in the promoter region *G-455A*

Discussion Elevated fibrinogen levels have been linked to an increased risk for thrombosis (myocardial infarction, deep venous thrombosis, stroke). However, it is not clear whether fibrinogen is a cause of thrombosis or simply a marker for other risk factors. The *G-455A* polymorphism in the gene that encodes for the β-chain is associated with elevated fibrinogen levels. The *-455AA* genotype was associated with higher plasma fibrinogen levels and greater progression of atherosclerotic disease than other β-fibrinogen genotypes (de Maat et al 1998).

HMG CoA reductase inhibitors:
Treatment with pravastatin in patients with coronary heart disease offset the greater progression of coronary atherosclerosis observed with the *455AA* genotype in the placebo group (de Maat et al 1998).

May Alter Pharmacokinetics of β-fibrinogen is not known to alter the metabolism of any drugs.

May Alter Pharmacodynamics of HMG CoA reductase inhibitors

May Affect Disease Predisposition of Thrombosis, deep venous thrombosis

Clinical Recommendations Data suggest that the β-fibrinogen genotype may be useful in predicting clinical outcomes with HMG CoA reductase inhibitor therapy in patients with coronary heart disease. The β-fibrinogen genotype may interact with the apolipoprotein E, stromelysin-1, ACE, and cholesterol ester transfer protein genes in predicting HMG CoA reductase inhibitor response.

Counseling Points Carrier status for the *-455AA* genotype has been associated with greater disease progression in individuals with coronary heart disease. Individuals with coronary heart disease who carry this allele should be encouraged to discuss the implications of their carrier status with their clinician or another healthcare professional.

References
de Maat MP, Kastelein JJ, Jukema JW, et al, "-455G/A Polymorphism of the Beta-Fibrinogen Gene Is Associated With the Progression of Coronary Atherosclerosis in Symptomatic Men: Proposed Role For an Acute-Phase Reaction Pattern of Fibrinogen. REGRESS Group," *Arterioscler Thromb Vasc Biol*, 1998, 18(2):265-71 (review).

♦ **BKB2R** *see* Bradykinin B2 Receptor *on page 175*

Bradykinin B2 Receptor

Synonyms BDKRB2; BKB2R

Chromosome Location 14q32.1-32.2

Clinically-Important Polymorphisms Synonymous SNP in promoter region *(C-58T)*

Discussion With respect to the regulation of vascular tone, the BKB2R and angiotensin II type 1 receptor are antagonistic. Stimulation of bradykinin receptors leads to vasodilatation and enhanced sodium excretion. In addition to their effects on the formation of angiotensin II, ACE inhibitors increase bradykinin concentrations. Increased bradykinin concentrations may play a role in the development of ACE inhibitor-induced cough.

(Continued)

Bradykinin B2 Receptor *(Continued)*

ACE inhibitors:
Although data are inconsistent, the BKB2R has been associated with the ACE inhibitor-induced cough. Among hypertensives treated with an ACE inhibitor, the frequency of the *-58T* allele was significantly higher in those who developed a cough compared to cough-free individuals (Mukae et al 2000). Other investigators reported no association between the BKB2R gene and a cough during ACE inhibitor therapy (Zee et al 1998).

May Alter Pharmacokinetics of Bradykinin B_2 receptor is not known to alter the metabolism of any drugs.

May Alter Pharmacodynamics of ACE inhibitors

Clinical Recommendations Because of the benefits of ACE inhibitor therapy, the inconsistencies in the data, and the fact that some study subjects with the *-58T* allele did not develop a cough with ACE inhibitors, the association between the BKB2R gene and an ACE inhibitor-induced cough is unlikely to influence prescribing practices.

References
Mukae S, Aoki S, Itoh S, et al, "Bradykinin B(2) Receptor Gene Polymorphism Is Associated With Angiotensin-Converting Enzyme Inhibitor-Related Cough," *Hypertension*, 2000, 36(1):127-31.

Zee RY, Rao VS, Paster RZ, et al, "Three Candidate Genes and Angiotensin-Converting Enzyme Inhibitor-Related Cough: A Pharmacogenetic Analysis," *Hypertension*, 1998, 31(4):925-8.

♦ **BRCA-1** *see BRCA Genes on page 176*
♦ **BRCA-2** *see BRCA Genes on page 176*

BRCA Genes

Synonyms BRCA-1; BRCA-2

Chromosome Location 17q21; 13q12.3

Clinically-Important Polymorphisms Three "founder" BRCA mutations include the 185delAG mutation, the 5382insC mutation, and the 6174 delT mutation. A large number of other mutations have also been described.

Discussion BRCA-1 and BRCA-2 are believed to be tumor suppression genes. They are located on the long arms of chromosomes 17 and 13, respectively. Both are large genes, distributed over approximately 100,000 base pairs of genomic DNA, and each encodes a large, negatively-charged protein. Inactivating mutations identified to date are distributed throughout both genes, with an increased frequency of two distinct BRCA-1 mutations and one BRCA-2 mutation in individuals of Ashkenazi Jewish descent.

Women carriers of germline BRCA-1 mutations have a lifetime risk of breast cancer exceeding 80% and of ovarian cancer approaching 60%. BRCA-2 mutations are associated with a similar increase in breast cancer, although the risk of ovarian cancer is elevated, it is not as high as the BRCA-1 mutants. Approximately 0.5% of women carry one of these mutations; however, the frequency may be as high as 2% in certain ethnic groups. In the case of BRCA-1 carriers, the risk of developing breast cancer prior to menopause is particularly increased.

Their risk of contralateral breast cancer is also significantly higher as compared to the general population (4.2% to 53% vs 2%), and the grade of contralateral tumors is more aggressive. The hereditary breast cancer associated with BRCA-2 appears to be more heterogeneous than the BRCA-1 phenotype. It should be noted that 20% to 30% of BRCA carriers never develop breast or ovarian cancer, therefore, other factors must modify or offset this risk.

In general, women have a 10% lifetime risk of developing breast cancer and a 2% to 3% chance of ovarian cancer. Women with the BRCA1/BRCA2 mutations have an 80% chance of breast cancer and 60% chance of ovarian cancer. Patients and their families with these mutations are frequently referred for genetic testing counseling.

Oral contraceptives:
Among carriers of BRCA-1, women who use oral contraceptives for 5 years or more have a 33% increase in the risk of early onset breast cancer as compared to BRCA1 carriers who never used this form of contraception (Narod et al 2002).

May Alter Pharmacodynamics of Oral contraceptives

May Affect Disease Predisposition of Breast cancer, ovarian cancer

Laboratory Evaluation Commercial testing available

Clinical Recommendations Category 2 ASCO genetic test; consult ASCO Guidelines

References
Narod SA, Dube MP, Klijn J, et al, "Oral Contraceptives and the Risk of Breast Cancer in BRCA1 and BRCA2 Mutation Carriers," *J Natl Cancer Inst*, 2002, 94(23):1773-9.

Cardiac Potassium Ion Channel

Synonyms k-channel

Chromosome Location 11-KVLQT1; 7-HERG; 21-KCNE1, KCNE2

Clinically-Important Polymorphisms
Missense mutations in the KCNE2 leading to Q9E and M54T form of the MinK-related peptide-1
Nonsynonymous SNP in the KCNE2 gene leading to the T8A form of the MinK-related peptide-1
R583C in the C-terminal of the KVLQT1 protein
R784W in the C-terminal of the HERG protein

Discussion KCNE1 and KvLQT1 encode subunits of the IKs channel, while KCNE2 and HERG encode subunits of the IKr channel. Variations in these genes have been identified as a cause of the most common form of congenital long QT syndrome. It has been proposed that predisposition to arrhythmias with QT-prolonging agents may be related to the presence of mutations in the genes which encode potassium channel proteins. Some cases of drug-induced QT prolongation have been related to genetic causes.

QT-prolonging agents:
Phenotypic expression of a heterozygous mutation has been described in a patient who developed drug-induced cardiac arrest with cisapride, clarithromycin, and quinidine (Abbott et al 1999)
(Continued)

Cardiac Potassium Ion Channel (Continued)

and a prolonged QT interval with procainamide and sulfamethoxazole (Sesti et al 2000).

May Alter Pharmacokinetics of The cardiac potassium channel is not known to affect the metabolism of any drugs.

May Alter Pharmacodynamics of QT-prolonging agents, Class I and III antiarrhythmics, selected fluoroquinolones, some antipsychotics, TCAs

May Affect Disease Predisposition of Arrhythmia

Clinical Recommendations It remains to be seen whether molecular screening for mutations of candidate genes may allow identification of individuals at risk of drug-induced arrhythmias.

Counseling Points Genetic variants in the cardiac potassium channel may influence a patient's risk for congenital long QT syndrome. Patients who have a genetic variant in this location should discuss the implications of the variant on their risk for arrhythmia with their clinician or another healthcare professional.

References

Abbott GW, Sesti F, Splawski I, et al, "MiRP1 Forms IKr Potassium Channels With HERG and Is Associated With Cardiac Arrhythmia," *Cell*, 1999, 97(2):175-87.

Bianchi L, Priori SG, Napolitano C, et al, "Mechanisms of I(Ks) Suppression in LQT1 Mutants," *Am J Physiol Heart Circ Physiol*, 2000, 279(6):H3003-11

Napolitano C, Schwartz PJ, Brown AM, et al, "Evidence for a Cardiac Ion Channel Mutation Underlying Drug-Induced QT Prolongation and Life-Threatening Arrhythmias," *J Cardiovasc Electrophysiol*, 2000, 11(6):691-6.

Sesti F, Abbott GW, Wei J, et al, "A Common Polymorphism Associated With Antibiotic-Induced Cardiac Arrhythmia," *Proc Natl Acad Sci U S A*, 2000, 97(19):10613-8.

Cardiac Sodium Channel

Synonyms SCN5A

Chromosome Location 3p21

Clinically-Important Polymorphisms G615E, L618F, F1250L in the intracellular domain of the alpha subunit region; L1825P in the C-terminus region

Discussion Subclinical mutations in SCN5A increase activity of the sodium channel and have been associated with congenital long QT syndromes and may increase the risk for drug-induced arrhythmias (Sesti et al 2000).

QT-prolonging agents:

A novel missense mutation (L1825P) was identified in an elderly Japanese woman who developed torsade de pointes during treatment with cisapride (Makita et al 2002). The G615E, L618F, and F1250L mutations of the SNC5A gene were identified in patients who developed torsade de pointes during treatment with quinidine and sotalol (Sesti et al 2000).

May Alter Pharmacokinetics of The SNC5A gene is not known to affect the metabolism of any drugs.

May Alter Pharmacodynamics of QT-prolonging agents, Class I and III antiarrhythmics, selected fluoroquinolones, some antipsychotics, TCAs

May Affect Disease Predisposition of Arrhythmia

Clinical Recommendations It remains to be seen whether molecular screening for mutations of candidate genes may allow identification of individuals at risk of drug-induced arrhythmias.

Counseling Points Genetic variants in the cardiac sodium channel may influence a patient's risk for congenital long QT syndrome. Patients who have a genetic variant in this location should discuss the implications of the variant on their risk for arrhythmia with their clinician or another healthcare professional.

References

Makita NM, Horie T, Nakamura T, et al, "Drug-Induced Long QT Syndrome Associated With a Subclinical SCN5A Mutation," *Circulation*, 2002, 106(10):1269-74.

Sesti F, Abbott GW, Wei J, et al, "A Common Polymorphism Associated With Antibiotic-Induced Cardiac Arrhythmia," *Proc Natl Acad Sci U S A*, 2000, 97(19):10613-8.

♦ **CETP** *see Cholesteryl Ester Transfer Protein on page 179*

Cholesteryl Ester Transfer Protein

Synonyms CETP

Chromosome Location 16q21

Clinically-Important Polymorphisms Presence *(B1)* or absence *(B2)* of a restriction site for the TaqI enzyme in intron 1 *(B1/B2)*.

Discussion The CETP is involved in the metabolism of high-density lipoprotein (HDL). The *B1B1* genotype has been associated with higher CETP concentrations, increased triglycerides and reduced high-density lipoprotein (HDL)-levels, and increased progression of coronary atherosclerosis (Kuivenhoven et al 1998).

HMG CoA reductase inhibitors:

Among men with atherosclerosis, treatment with pravastatin slowed atherosclerosis progression in *B1B1* carriers, but not in those with the *B2B2* genotype. There was no association between the *B1/B2* genotype and changes in lipoprotein lipid levels with pravastatin (Kuivenhoven et al 1998).

There was no association between the *B1/B2* genotype and the ability of pravastatin to reduce the risk of coronary events in a large study of men with hypercholesterolemia and no history and myocardial infarction.

Fibrates:

Among men with coronary heart disease, the *B1B1* genotype was associated with greater reductions in triglyceride levels with gemfibrozil compared to the *B1B2* and *B2B2* genotypes (Brousseau et al 2002).

May Alter Pharmacokinetics of CETP is not known to alter the metabolism of any drugs.

May Alter Pharmacodynamics of HMG CoA reductase inhibitors, fibrates

May Affect Disease Predisposition of Atherosclerosis

Clinical Recommendations It is unclear whether the *CETP* gene will be useful in predicting response to HMG CoA-reductase inhibitors. The *CETP* genotype may interact with the apolipoprotein E, fibrinogen, stromelysin-1, and ACE genes in predicting HMG CoA-reductase inhibitor response.

(Continued)

Cholesteryl Ester Transfer Protein *(Continued)*

Counseling Points Carrier status for the *B1B1* genotype has been associated with greater disease progression in individuals with coronary heart disease. Individuals with coronary heart disease who carry this allele should be encouraged to discuss the implications of their carrier status with their clinician or another healthcare professional.

References

Brousseau ME, O'Connor JJ Jr, Ordovas JM, et al, "Cholesteryl Ester Transfer Protein Taql B2B2 Genotype Is Associated With Higher HDL Cholesterol Levels and Lower Risk of Coronary Heart Disease End Points in Men With HDL Deficiency: Veterans Affairs HDL Cholesterol Intervention Trial," *Arterioscler Thromb Vasc Biol*, 2002, 22(7):1148-54.

Kuivenhoven JA, Jukema JW, Zwinderman AH, et al, "The Role of a Common Variant of the Cholesteryl Ester Transfer Protein Gene in the Progression of Coronary Atherosclerosis. The Regression Growth Evaluation Statin Study Group," *N Engl J Med*, 1998, 338(2):86-93.

COMT

Synonyms COMT-L; val-COMT

Chromosome Location 22q11

Clinically-Important Polymorphisms Val(158)Met (also known as Val(108)Met when in soluble form)

Discussion Catechol-O-methyltransferase catalyzes a methyl group transfer from S-adenosylmethionine to catecholamines, including the neurotransmitters dopamine, epinephrine, and norepinephrine. Catechol-O-methyltransferase mediates metabolism of catecholamines, and is an important regulator of both dopaminergic and noradrenergic neurotransmission. This is also one of the major degradative pathways of drugs used in the treatment of hypertension, asthma, and Parkinson disease.

COMT is found in two forms in tissues, a soluble form (S-COMT) and a membrane-bound form (MB-COMT). A methionine substitution for valine at codon 158 results in a gene product which is three to four times less active than the high-activity allele. The genes exhibit codominant expression, with heterozygotes demonstrating intermediate activity. Polymorphism of the COMT gene is common in the human population, with up to 25% of Caucasians being homozygous for the low-activity allele (COMT-L). This genotype appears to be less common in Asians than in Caucasians.

The *val-158-met* genotype has been linked to the expression of a variety of complex disease states, and may be a contributing factor in their development. The role of a single polymorphism in these diseases is likely to be limited, given the complex pathogenesis of these disorders. Associations include Parkinson's disease (Goudreau et al 2002), schizophrenia (Bilder et al 2002, Harrison et al 2003), Alzheimer's disease (Qu et al 2001), atherosclerosis (Mehrabian et al 2002), ADHD (Kirley et al 2002, Qian et al 2003), panic disorder (Woo et al 2002), and breast cancer incidence in a limited population (Kocabas et al 2002).

CYP1A2

Opiates:
Individuals who are homozygous for the *met-158* gene demonstrated diminished μ-opioid responses, correlating with higher sensory and affective ratings of pain. In contrast, individuals who were homozygous for the *val-158* allele withstood significantly greater saline doses than other volunteers and rated the resulting pain as less bothersome. Some of the variability in pain tolerance and opiate requirements may be linked to these observations.

May Alter Pharmacodynamics of Opiates/narcotic analgesics

May Affect Disease Predisposition of Alzheimer's disease, anxiety disorder, atherosclerosis, attention deficit disorder, breast cancer, panic disorder, Parkinson's disease, schizophrenia

References

Bilder RM, Volavka J, Czobor P, et al, "Neurocognitive Correlates of the COMT Val(158)Met Polymorphism in Chronic Schizophrenia," *Biol Psychiatry*, 2002, 52(7):701-7.

Enoch MA, Schuckit MA, Johnson BA, et al, "Genetics of Alcoholism Using Intermediate Phenotypes," *Alcohol Clin Exp Res*, 2003, 27(2):169-76.

Goudreau JL, Maraganore DM, Farrer MJ, et al, "Case-Control Study of Dopamine Transporter-1, Monoamine Oxidase-B, and Catechol-O-methyl Transferase Polymorphisms in Parkinson's Disease," *Mov Disord*, 2002, 17(6):1305-11.

Harrison PJ and Owen MJ, "Genes for Schizophrenia? Recent Findings and Their Pathophysiological Implications," *Lancet*, 2003, 361(9355):417-9 (review).

Kirley A, Hawi Z, Daly G, et al, "Dopaminergic System Genes in ADHD: Toward a Biological Hypothesis," *Neuropsychopharmacology*, 2002, 27(4):607-19.

Kocabas NA, Sardas S, Cholerton S, et al, "Cytochrome P450 CYP1B1 and Catechol O-methyltransferase (COMT) Genetic Polymorphisms and Breast Cancer Susceptibility in a Turkish Population," *Arch Toxicol*, 2002, 76(11):643-9.

Qian Q, Wang Y, Zhou R, et al, "Family-Based and Case-Control Association Studies of Catechol-O-methyltransferase in Attention Deficit Hyperactivity Disorder Suggest Genetic Sexual Dimorphism," *Am J Med Genet*, 2003, 118B(1):103-9.

Qu T, Manev R, and Manev H, "5-Lipoxygenase (5-LOX) Promoter Polymorphism in Patients With Early-Onset and Late-Onset Alzheimer's Disease," *J Neuropsychiatry Clin Neurosci*, 2001, 13(2):304-5.

Zubieta JK, Heitzeg MM, Smith YR, et al, "COMT val158met Genotype Affects μ-Opioid Neurotransmitter Responses to a Pain Stressor," *Science*, 2003, 299(5610):1240-3.

♦ **COMT-L** *see* COMT *on page 180*

CYP1A2

Related Information

Cytochrome P450 Enzymes: Substrates, Inhibitors, and Inducers *on page 23*

Synonyms Cytochrome P450 Isoenzyme 1A2

Chromosome Location 15q22-qter

Clinically-Important Polymorphisms

C-A in first intron at position 734 (*C-C* genotype) has low potential for induction.

G-A in 5' flanking region at -2964 associated with a significant decrease in CYP1A2 activity (identified in Japanese smokers).

Discussion CYP1A2 is an important drug-metabolizing enzyme. Decreases in activity may lead to significant changes in serum concentrations of individual drugs, which may lead to toxicity. Only a small number of substrates have been specifically studied; however, these results may generalize to other drugs which share this pathway, (Continued)

CYP1A2 *(Continued)*

particularly when this pathway serves as the primary route of drug metabolism.

Clozapine:

Polymorphisms of 1A2 have been linked to clinically-relevant pharmacokinetic data with the antipsychotics. The levels of 1A2 have been found to be elevated in clozapine nonresponders (Bender and Eap 1998). Recently a C to A transversion in the first intron of CYP1A2 was found. This SNP is associated with variation in 1A2 inducibility due to cigarette smoke. The *A/A* genotype is more inducible than the *C/A* or *C/C* genotype (Sachse et al 1999). This may have clinical implications for patients with schizophrenia who smoke. A G to A transversion in the 5' flanking region of 1A2 at position -2964 has also been associated with decreased 1A2 activity in Japanese subjects (Nakajima et al 1999). Other authors have examined these polymorphisms in relation to clozapine pharmacokinetics and unable to find a relationship (Masellis et al 1998).

The role of the *C-A* polymorphism of CYP1A2 in interindividual variations in clozapine-induced weight gain was evaluated. Patients with the *C/C* genotype exhibited higher mean weight gain, but no strong association was observed (Basile et al 2001).

Haloperidol:

No relationship between polymorphism and haloperidol or reduced haloperidol concentrations have been identified.

Polymorphisms of 1A2 have also been associated with tardive dyskinesia. AIMS scores in subjects with a *C/C* genotype was 2.7- to 3.4-fold higher than those with a *C/A* or *A/A* genotype (Basile et al 2000). In smokers, the AIMS scores were 5.4-fold to 4.7-fold greater with a *C/C* genotype compared to the other groups.

Olanzapine:

Other authors found no relationship between 1A2 and 2D6 phenotypes and olanzapine pharmacokinetics (Hagg et al 2001).

Trazodone:

No association between phenotype and steady-state concentrations of trazodone and mCPP in both smokers and nonsmokers.

May Alter Pharmacokinetics of Caffeine, clomipramine, clozapine, cyclobenzaprine, doxepin, fluvoxamine, mirtazapine, pimozide, propranolol, ropinirole, tacrine, thiothixene, trifluoperazine, verapamil, other CYP1A substrates

Counseling Points CYP1A2 is involved in the metabolism of many psychiatric medications. Polymorphisms within 1A2 may result in lower plasma concentrations of these medications which may predispose patients to disease relapse. Patients who smoke may be at a higher risk for these changes in metabolism.

References

Basile VS, Masellis M, McIntyre RS, et al, "Genetic Dissection of Atypical Antipsychotic-Induced Weight Gain: Novel Preliminary Data on the Pharmacogenetic Puzzle," *J Clin Psychiatry*, 2001, 62(Suppl 23):45-66 (review).

Basile VS, Ozdemir V, Masellis M, et al, "A Functional Polymorphism of the Cytochrome P450 1A2 (CYP1A2) Gene: Association With Tardive Dyskinesia in Schizophrenia," *Mol Psychiatry*, 2000, 5(4):410-7.

Bender S and Eap CB, "Very High Cytochrome P4501A2 Activity and Nonresponse to Clozapine," *Arch Gen Psychiatry*, 1998, 55(11):1048-50.

Hagg S, Spigest O, Lakso HA, et al, "Olanzapine Disposition in Humans Is Unrelated to CYP1A2 and CYP2D6 Phenotypes," 2001, *Eur J Clin Pharmacol*, 57(6-7):493-7.

Masellis M, Basile VS, Macciardi FM, et al, "Genetic Prediction of Antipsychotic Response Following Switch From Typical Antipsychotics to Clozapine," *XXIst Collegium Internationale Neuro Psychopharmacologicum (CINP) Congress*, Glasgow, Scotland, 1998.

Nakajima M, Yokoi T, Mizutani M, et al, "Genetic Polymorphism of the 5'-Flanking Region of the Human CYP1A2 Gene: Effect on the CYP1A2 Inducibility in Humans," *J Biochem (Tokyo)*, 1999, 125(4):803-8.

Sachse C, Brockmoller J, Bauer S, et al, "Functional Significance of a C-->A Polymorphism in Intron 1 of the Cytochrome P450 CYP1A2 Gene Tested With Caffeine," *Br J Clin Pharmacol*, 1999, 47(4):445-9.

CYP2C9

Related Information
Cytochrome P450 Enzymes: Substrates, Inhibitors, and Inducers *on page 23*

Synonyms Cytochrome P450 Isoenzyme 2C9

Chromosome Location 10q24

Clinically-Important Polymorphisms The three common allelic variants identified for the CYP2C9 gene are CYP2C9*1 (wild-type), CYP2C9*2 and CYP2C9*3. The *2 and *3 alleles are associated with reduced activity.

Discussion CYP2C9 is an important drug-metabolizing enzyme. Decreases in activity may lead to significant changes in serum concentrations of individual drugs, which may lead to toxicity. Only a small number of substrates have been specifically studied; however, these results may generalize to other drugs which share this pathway, particularly when this pathway serves as the primary route of drug metabolism.

Warfarin:
The S-isomer of warfarin, which has 5-fold greater anticoagulant activity than the R-isomer, is metabolized by the CYP2C9 enzyme (Hirsh et al 2001). Several investigators have reported significantly lower warfarin clearance rates, lower warfarin dose requirements, more difficulty with warfarin initiation, and greater bleeding risk among CYP2C9*2 and CYP2C9*3 allele carriers compared to CYP2D9*1 homozygotes (Aithal et al 1999, Steward et al 1997, Higashi et al 2002).

Angiotensin II type 1 receptor blockers:
Losartan is metabolized to E-3174 by CYP2C9. In healthy volunteers, plasma concentrations of E-3174 were significantly lower in those with the CYP2C9*1/*3 and *2/*3 genotypes compared to those with the CYP2C9*1/*1 and *1/*2 genotypes (Yasar et al 2002).

In hypertensive subjects, treatment with irbesartan resulted in significantly greater reductions in diastolic blood pressure with the
(Continued)

CYP2C9 *(Continued)*

CYP2C9*1/CYP2C9*2 genotype compared to the CYP2C9*1/CYP2C9*1 genotype (Hallberg et al 2002).

Phenytoin:

The mean dose of phenytoin required to achieve therapeutic serum concentrations has been correlated to CYP2C9 genotype. Individuals carrying at least one variant CYP2C9 allele required a mean phenytoin dose, which was approximately 37% lower than the mean dose required in individuals with the wild-type allele. A maintenance dose <200 mg/day was required in 47% of variant carriers, while 58% of normals required a dose >300 mg/day (van der Weide et al 2001).

Case reports of toxicity have been attributed to the CYP2C9 genotype, including a patient who was homozygous for the CYP2C9*3 allele (Brandolese et al 2001). In addition, rare alleles may be responsible for idiosyncratic toxicity, as noted in a female African-American who presented with phenytoin toxicity and was later determined to carry a null allele of the CYP2C9 isoenzyme (Kidd et al 2001).

In a regression analysis which included CYP2C9, 2C19 and MDR1, the number of variant CYP2C9 alleles was a major determinant, and the number of MDR1*T alleles further contributed to the prediction of phenytoin plasma levels. CYP2C19*2 did not appear to contribute to individual variability. The regression equation explained 15.4% of the variability of phenytoin data (Kerb et al 2001).

Glyburide and glimepiride:

Significant pharmacokinetic differences have been noted to be associated with CYP2C9 genotype. In subjects determined to be homozygous for the CYP2C9*3 allele, the median AUC of glyburide was 280% while that of glimepiride was 267% as compared to subjects with the CYP2C9*1/*1 genotype. However, responses to glyburide and glimepiride, as determined from blood glucose values, were not significantly affected by the CYP2C9 genotype (Niemi et al 2002).

May Alter Pharmacokinetics of Fluoxetine, fosphenytoin, ketamine, mephenytoin, phenytoin, selegiline, sertraline, and other CYP2C9 substrates; see above.

Counseling Points Some patients with polymorphism of CYP2C9 may require less drug to reach steady-state concentrations.

References

Aithal GP, Day CP, Kesteven PJ, et al, "Association of Polymorphisms in the Cytochrome P450 CYP2C9 With Warfarin Dose Requirement and Risk of Bleeding Complications," 1999, 353(9154):717-9.

Brandolese R, Scordo MG, Spina E, et al, "Severe Phenytoin Intoxication in a Subject Homozygous for CYP2C9*3," *Clin Pharmacol Ther*, 2001, 70(4):391-4.

Hallberg P, Karlsson J, Kurland L, et al, "The CYP2C9 Genotype Predicts the Blood Pressure Response to Irbesartan: Results From the Swedish Irbesartan Left Ventricular Hypertrophy Investigation vs Atenolol (SILVHIA) Trial," *J Hypertens*, 2002, 20(10):2089-93.

Higashi MK, Veenstra DL, Kondo LM, et al, "Association Between CYP2C9 Genetic Variants and Anticoagulation-Related Outcomes During Warfarin Therapy," *JAMA*, 2002, 287(13):1690-8.

Hirsh J, Dalen J, Anderson DR, et al, "Oral Anticoagulants: Mechanism of Action, Clinical Effectiveness, and Optimal Therapeutic Range," *Chest*, 2001, 119(1 Suppl):8S-21S (review).

Kerb R, Aynacioglu AS, Brockmoller J, et al, "The Predictive Value of MDR1, CYP2C9, and CYP2C19 Polymorphisms for Phenytoin Plasma Levels," *Pharmacogenomics J*, 2001, 1(3):204-10.

Kidd RS, Curry TB, Gallagher S, et al, "Identification of a Null Allele of CYP2C9 in an African-American Exhibiting Toxicity to Phenytoin," *Pharmacogenetics*, 2001, 11(9):803-8.

Lee CR, Goldstein JA, and Pieper JA, "Cytochrome P450 2C9 Polymorphisms: A Comprehensive Review of the *in vitro* and Human Data," *Pharmacogenetics*, 2002, 12(3):251-63 (review).

Niemi M, Cascorbi I, Timm R, et al, "Glyburide and Glimepiride Pharmacokinetics in Subjects With Different CYP2C9 Genotypes," *Clin Pharmacol Ther*, 2002, 72(3):326-32.

Steward DJ, Haining RL, Henne KR, et al, "Genetic Association Between Sensitivity to Warfarin and Expression of CYP2C9*3," *Pharmacogenetics*, 1997, 7(5):361-7.

van der Weide J, Steijns LS, van Weelden MJ, et al, "The Effect of Genetic Polymorphism of Cytochrome P450 CYP2C9 on Phenytoin Dose Requirement," *Pharmacogenetics*, 2001, 11(4):287-91.

Yasar U, Forslund-Bergengren C, Tybring G, et al, "Pharmacokinetics of Losartan and Its Metabolite E-3174 in Relation to the CYP2C9 Genotype," *Clin Pharmacol Ther*, 2002, 71(1):89-98.

CYP2C19

Related Information

Cytochrome P450 Enzymes: Substrates, Inhibitors, and Inducers *on page 23*

Synonyms Cytochrome P450 Isoenzyme 2C19

Chromosome Location 10q24.1-q24.3

Clinically-Important Polymorphisms *2 through *8: inactive (in up to 20% of Asians [*2 and *3], 3% of Caucasians, 19% of African Americans, 8% of Africans, up to 71% of Pacific islanders)

Discussion CYP2C19 is an important drug-metabolizing enzyme. Decreases in activity may lead to significant changes in serum concentrations of individual drugs, which may lead to toxicity. Only a small number of substrates have been specifically studied; however, these results may generalize to other drugs which share this pathway, particularly when this pathway serves as the primary route of drug metabolism.

Proton pump inhibitor:

Metabolism of proton pump inhibitors may influence their kinetics and efficacy. In a clinical evaluation, gastroesophageal reflux disease cure with lansoprazole was correlated to both the grade of disease prior to treatment and CYP2C19 genotype status. The cure rate in the homozygous extensive metabolizer phenotype was 46%, while the cure rate in patients with the poor metabolizer phenotype was 85% (Furuta et al 2002).

Cure rates for *H. pylori* infection by dual therapy (rabeprazole/amoxicillin) were dependent on CYP2C19 genotype. Dual therapy was apparently effective for heterozygous extensive metabolizer and poor metabolizer genotypes. However, efficacy could be improved

(Continued)

CYP2C19 *(Continued)*

for patients with homozygous extensive metabolizer genotypes through the use of high-dose dual therapy. The authors proposed that genotyping could be a useful tool to aid in the optimal dual treatment with these agents (Furuta et al 2001).

The development of low vitamin B_{12} serum concentrations in association with long-term omeprazole may be dependent on CYP2C19 genotype. Patients with mutations in the CYP2C19 genes were noted to have lower serum concentrations as compared to individuals with the wild-type genotype. These differences were only apparent after long-term treatment (Sagar et al 1999).

Phenytoin:

In a regression analysis which included CYP2C9, 2C19, and MDR1, the number of mutant CYP2C9 alleles was a major determinant, and the number of MDR1*T alleles further contributed to the prediction of phenytoin plasma levels. CYP2C19*2 did not appear to contribute to individual variability. The regression equation explained 15.4% of the variability of phenytoin data (Kerb et al 2001).

May Alter Pharmacokinetics of Proton pump inhibitors, citalopram, clomipramine, diazepam, escitalopram, fosphenytoin, imipramine, mephenytoin, mephobarbital, methsuximide, moclobemide, phenobarbital, phenytoin, propranolol, sertraline, trimipramine, other CYP2C19 substrates

Laboratory Evaluation Commercial testing available

References

Furuta T, Shirai N, Takashima M, et al, "Effects of Genotypic Differences in CYP2C19 Status on Cure Rates for *Helicobacter pylori* Infection by Dual Therapy With Rabeprazole Plus Amoxicillin," *Pharmacogenetics*, 2001, 11(4):341-8.

Furuta T, Shirai N, Watanabe F, et al, "Effect of Cytochrome P4502C19 Genotypic Differences on Cure Rates for Gastroesophageal Reflux Disease by Lansoprazole," *Clin Pharmacol Ther*, 2002, 72(4):453-60.

Kerb R, Aynacioglu AS, Brockmoller J, et al, "The Predictive Value of MDR1, CYP2C9, and CYP2C19 Polymorphisms for Phenytoin Plasma Levels," *Pharmacogenomics J*, 2001, 1(3):204-10.

Sagar M, Janczewska I, Ljungdahl A, et al, "Effect of CYP2C19 Polymorphism on Serum Levels of Vitamin B12 in Patients on Long-Term Omeprazole Treatment," *Aliment Pharmacol Ther*, 1999, 13(4):453-8.

CYP2D6

Related Information

Cytochrome P450 Enzymes: Substrates, Inhibitors, and Inducers *on page 23*

Synonyms Cytochrome P450 Isoenzyme 2D6

Chromosome Location 22q13.1

Clinically-Important Polymorphisms CYP2D6*2 (increased activity), CYP2D6*3 (diminished/absent), CYP2D6*4 (diminished/absent), CYP2D6*5 (diminished/absent), CYP2D6*10 (diminished activity), CYP2D6*17 (diminished activity)

Discussion CYP2D6 is an important drug-metabolizing enzyme. Decreases in activity may lead to significant changes in serum concentrations of individual drugs, which may lead to toxicity. Only a small number of substrates have been specifically studied; however, these results may generalize to other drugs which share this pathway, particularly when this pathway serves as the primary route of drug metabolism.

Significant variation in CYP2D6 activity has been associated with key polymorphisms, and these variations occur with different frequencies among populations. In Americans and Europeans, between 1% and 5% of individuals carry two or more copies of the variant CYP2D6*2 allele which confers the ultrarapid metabolizer phenotype for CYP2D6 substrates (Agundez et al 1995, Dahl et al 1995).

Several genotypes are associated with diminished or absent CYP2D6 activity. The variant CYP2D6*10 allele, with a frequency of about 50% in Asians (Ingelman-Sundberg et al 1999), and the variant CYP2D6*17 allele, with a frequency of about 34% in black Africans (Masimirembwa et al 1996), are associated with reduced CYP2D6 activity. CYP2D6 alleles associated with an absence of CYP2D6 activity include CYP2D6*3, CYP2D6*4, and CYP2D6*5. Two alleles associated with an absence of activity are found in approximately 7% of Caucasians, but fewer than 3% of black Africans and 1% of Asians. Low activity may lead to a reduced formation of an active metabolite (and a loss of drug effect), or reduced capacity for metabolism/detoxification may lead to toxicity from normal dosages of a drug metabolized by this pathway.

β-blockers:
In Chinese subjects, the CYP2D6*10A allele was associated with higher metoprolol plasma concentrations and lower urinary metoprolol metabolite levels compared to the CYP2D6*1 allele (Huang et al 1999).

Clozapine:
CYP2D6 has been implicated in the metabolism of clozapine, but no relationship has been found (Arranz et al 1995).

Haloperidol:
CYP2D6 has been shown to have a relationship with the development of tardive dyskinesia (Ellingrod et al 2002), although other investigators have not found a relationship between 2D6 poor metabolizers and the occurrence of tardive dyskinesia (Arthur et al 1995, Armstrong et al 1997, Andreasen et al 1997, Ohmori et al 1999). Patients heterozygous for the CYP2D6*3 or *4 alleles who smoke cigarettes may have the highest risk for the development of abnormal movements and tardive dyskinesia compared to those homozygous for the *1 allele or nonsmokers (20% vs 78%) (Ellingrod et al 2002). These subjects may shunt antipsychotic metabolism through other pathways induced by cigarette smoke. This induction may result in formation of neurotoxic metabolites leading to increased AIMS scores and a higher incidence of tardive dyskinesia, compared to subjects without these alleles.

(Continued)

CYP2D6 (Continued)

SSRIs:
Case reports of toxicity have been attributed to CYP2D6 mutations. Case reports of diminished response were retrospectively attributed to a duplication of the gene encoding 2D6. Most SSRIs are inhibitors of CYP2D6 and may cause toxic concentrations of tricyclic antidepressants when used in combination.

Olanzapine:
No relationship between 1A2 and 2D6 phenotypes and olanzapine pharmacokinetics has been found (Hagg et al 2001).

A relationship between polymorphism of 2D6 and weight gain from olanzapine has been found. Subjects with a heterozygous *1/*3, *4 2D6 genotype experienced a statistically significantly larger percentage change in BMI than the homozygous*1/*1 group (128% vs 112%) (Ellingrod et al 2002). Thus, polymorphisms of CYP isoenzymes may be the trigger needed for excessive weight gain and other morbidity associated with olanzapine and other AAPs.

Tricyclic antidepressants:
In poor metabolizers, the mean half-life of desipramine was 125 hours, while the mean half-life in extensive metabolizers was 22 hours.

Codeine:
Conversion to morphine is mediated by CYP2D6. Deficient activity of this isoenzyme may be associated with decreased effectiveness of codeine.

Serotonin 5HT$_{1D}$ agonists:
Genotypic variation may influence the efficacy of serotonin agonists in the treatment of chemotherapy-induced nausea and vomiting. Variation in 2D6 metabolism has been correlated to a lack of response to tropisetron and ondansetron (50). In a population of 270 patients categorized by extent of CYP2D6-mediated metabolism, 7.8% were categorized as poor metabolizers and 1.5% were "ultraextensive" metabolizers. The ultraextensive phenotype experienced significantly more episodes of vomiting than extensive metabolizers, while poor metabolizers did not experience episodes of vomiting.

May Alter Pharmacokinetics of CYP2D6 substrates
Carvedilol, flecainide, metoprolol, mexiletine, propafenone, propranolol, timolol, desipramine, tricyclic antidepressants

May Alter Pharmacodynamics of Haloperidol, SSRIs, olanzapine, codeine

Laboratory Evaluation Commercial testing available

References
Agundez JA, Ledesma MC, Ladero JM, et al, "Prevalence of CYP2D6 Gene Duplication and Its Repercussion on the Oxidative Phenotype in a White Population," *Clin Pharmacol Ther*, 1995, 57(3):265-9.

Andreasen OA, MacDwan T, Gulbandsen et al, "Nonfunctional CYP2D6 Alleles and Risk for Neuroleptic-Induced Movement Disorders in Schizophrenic Patients," *Psychopharmacol (Berl)*, 1997, 131:174-9.

Armstrong M, Daly AK, Blennerhassett R, et al, "Antipsychotic Drug-Induced Movement Disorders in Schizophrenics in Relation to CYP2D6 Genotype," *Br J Psychiatry*, 1997, 170:23-6.

Arranz MJ, Dawson E, Shaikh S, et al, "Cytochrome P4502D6 Genotype Does Not Determine Response to Clozapine," *Br J Clin Pharmacol*, 1995, 39(4):417-20.

Arthur H, Dahl ML, Siwers B, et al, "Polymorphic Drug Metabolism in Schizophrenic Patients With Tardive Dyskinesia," *J Clin Psychopharmacol*, 1995, 15(3):211-6.

Dahl ML, Johansson I, Bertilsson L, et al, "Ultrarapid Hydroxylation of Debrisoquine in a Swedish Population. Analysis of the Molecular Genetic Basis," *J Pharmacol Exp Ther*, 1995, 274(1):516-20.

Ellingrod VL, Miller D, Schultz SK, et al, "CYP2D6 Polymorphisms and Atypical Antipsychotic Weight Gain," *Psychiatr Genet*, 2002, 12(1):55-8.

Ellingrod VL, Schultz SK, and Arndt S, "Abnormal Movements and Tardive Dyskinesia in Smokers and Nonsmokers With Schizophrenia Genotyped for Cytochrome P450 2D6," *Pharmacotherapy*, 2002, 22(11):1416-9.

Hagg S, Spigest O, Lakso HA, et al, "Olanzapine Disposition in Humans in Unrelated to CYP1A2 and CYP2D6 Phenotypes," *Eur J Clin Pharmacol*, 2001, 57(6-7):493-7.

Huang J, Chuang SK, Cheng CL, et al, "Pharmacokinetics of Metoprolol Enantiomers in Chinese Subjects of Major CYP2D6 Genotypes," *Clin Pharmacol Ther*, 1999, 65(4):402-7.

Ingelman-Sundberg M, Oscarson M, and McLellan RA, "Polymorphic Human Cytochrome P450 Enzymes: An Opportunity for Individualized Drug Treatment," *Trends Pharmacol Sci*, 1999, 20(8):342-9 (review).

Masimirembwa C, Persson I, Bertilsson L, et al, "A Novel Mutant Variant of the CYP2D6 Gene (CYP2D6*17) Common in a Black African Population: Association With Diminished Debrisoquine Hydroxylase Activity," *Br J Clin Pharmacol*, 1996, 42(6):713-9.

Ohmori O, Kojima H, Shinkai T, et al, "Genetic Association Analysis Between CYP2D6*2 Allele and Tardive Dyskinesia in Schizophrenic Patients," *Psychiatry Res*, 1999, 87(2-3):239-44.

CYP3A4

Related Information
Cytochrome P450 Enzymes: Substrates, Inhibitors, and Inducers *on page 23*

Chromosome Location 7q21.1

Clinically-Important Polymorphisms
A number of polymorphisms have been identified. CYP3A4*1 represents the wild type. CYP3A4*3 has been referred to as CYP3A4-V (variant).

A number of other SNPs which produce coding changes have been identified. *In vitro*, CYP3A4*17 demonstrates a lower turnover for probe substrates, while CYP3A4*18 demonstrates a higher turnover rate. Other SNPs which produce coding changes include CYP3A4*3, CYP3A4*15, and CYP3A4*19. A large number of other variants have been described, including CYP3A4*1B, CYP3A4*2, CYP3A4*4, CYP3A4*5, CYP3A4*6, CYP3A4*8, CYP3A4*11, CYP3A4*12, and CYP3A4*13.

Racial variability in the frequency of individual SNPs has been identified. In one series, CYP3A*15 was identified only in Black populations with an allelic frequency of 4%. CYP3A4*17 and CYP3A4*3 were identified in Caucasians with allelic frequencies 2% and 4%, respectively. CYP3A4*18 and CYP3A4*19 were only observed in Asians at allelic frequencies of 2% (Dai et al 2001).

Discussion
The expression of CYP3A4 varies 40-fold in individual human livers, and metabolism of CYP3A4 substrates varies at least 10-fold *in vivo*. The CYP3A family is encoded by 4 separate genes and
(Continued)

CYP3A4 *(Continued)*

2 pseudogenes. Many studies have not been able to establish a predictive value to a known genotype. Conclusive correlations between individual polymorphisms have not been limited to date.

Although the genetic component of the interindividual variability of CYP3A4 enzyme activity seems to be high, a key role for the variant alleles has not been able to be identified in patients low CYP3A4 activity. Unknown mutations that affect CYP3A4 or other functionally-related genes may be associated with low CYP3A4 activity (Garcia-Martin et al 2002).

Cyclophosphamide:
Cyclophosphamide requires activation by CYP3A3/4 to its active form. A variant allele has been described which occurs in 45% of African Americans and only 9% of Caucasians. This variant has been associated with a decrease in the activation of cyclophosphamide, potentially resulting in diminished efficacy. In addition, variability in metabolism of substrates may lead to enhanced toxicity. Decreased survival has been associated with the variant allele (Petros 2002).

May Alter Pharmacokinetics of Cyclophosphamide, other CYP3A4 substrates

May Alter Pharmacodynamics of Cyclophosphamide, other CYP3A4 substrates

Laboratory Evaluation Commercial testing available

References
Dai D, Tang J, Rose R, et al, "Identification of Variants of CYP3A4 and Characterization of Their Abilities to Metabolize Testosterone and Chlorpyrifos," *J Pharmacol Exp Ther*, 2001, 299(3):825-31.

Garcia-Martin E, Martinez C, Pizarro RM, et al, "CYP3A4 Variant Alleles in White Individuals With Low CYP3A4 Enzyme Activity," *Clin Pharmacol Ther*, 2002, 71(3):196-204.

Petros WP, *Proc AACR*, 2002, 42:1435.

- **CYP11B2** *see* Aldosterone Synthase *on page 160*
- **Cytochrome P450 Isoenzyme 1A2** *see* CYP1A2 *on page 181*
- **Cytochrome P450 Isoenzyme 2C9** *see* CYP2C9 *on page 183*
- **Cytochrome P450 Isoenzyme 2C19** *see* CYP2C19 *on page 185*
- **Cytochrome P450 Isoenzyme 2D6** *see* CYP2D6 *on page 186*
- **D_2** *see* D2 Receptor *on page 190*
- **D_{2L}** *see* D2 Receptor *on page 190*

D2 Receptor
Synonyms D_2; D_{2L}; D_{2S}; DRD2

Chromosome Location 11q23

Clinically-Important Polymorphisms -141 C insertion/deletion

Discussion Dopamine-2 receptors are of paramount importance in mental health, especially in regard to antipsychotics. Estimates of clinical potency of antipsychotic agents correlates with their potency *in vitro* to inhibit binding of ligands to D_2 dopamine receptors. Almost all antipsychotics have high affinity for D_2 receptors. Atypical antipsychotics also have affinity for the D_2 receptors, but some (clozapine, quetiapine) have lower affinities than others. It appears that blockade of dopamine at the D_2 receptor is required for a drug to possess antipsychotic activity.

Clozapine:
No significant association with response

Tardive dyskinesia:
Increased frequency of the *A2* allele in patients with tardive dyskinesia (Chen et al 1997)

May Alter Pharmacodynamics of Antipsychotic agents and potentially other D2 receptor antagonists

May Affect Disease Predisposition of Alzheimer's disease, anxiety disorder, affective disorder, schizophrenia, alcoholism, substance abuse, Parkinson's disease

References
Chen CH, Wei FU, Koong FJ, et al, "Association of the Taq-I A Polymorphism of Dopamine D2 Receptor Gene and Tardive Dyskinesia in Schizophrenia," *Biol Psychiatry*, 1997, 41(7):827-9.

♦ **D_{2S}** *see* D2 Receptor *on page 190*
♦ **D_3** *see* D3 Receptor *on page 191*

D3 Receptor

Synonyms D_3; DRD3

Chromosome Location 3q13.3

Clinically-Important Polymorphisms Serine to Glycine (Ser9Gly), a novel polymorphism in the promoter region of the gene (*-205 A/G*) (Ishiguro et al 2000), polymorphism associated with the development of tardive dyskinesias. It is also predictive of the occurrence of tardive dyskinesia.

Discussion There are two major categories of dopamine receptors, namely the D_1-like and D_2-like. The D_1-like receptors include D_1 and D_5 receptors. The D_2-like receptors include two isoforms of the D_2 receptor, the D_3 receptor, and the D_4 receptor. The D_1 and D_5 receptors activate adenylyl cyclase. The D_2 receptors possess several actions, including the inhibition of adenylyl cyclase activity, suppression of calcium currents, and activation of potassium currents. The effector system to which the D_3 and D_4 receptors couple has not been defined with certainty.

Polymorphism of the D_3 receptor has been related to the development of tardive dyskinesia. Excess of the *Gly/Gly* genotype has been found in patients with tardive dyskinesia (Steen et al 1997, Segman et al 1999, Basile et al 1999, and Lovlie et al 2000), although this was not replicated by Rietschel et al (2000).

Clozapine:
No significant association with response (Shaikh et al 1996, Malhotra et al 1998).

Olanzapine:
A cohort of 50 individuals of Basque origin who received olanzapine for at least 3 months were assessed using the PANSS scale. The
(Continued)

D3 Receptor *(Continued)*

average improvement in positive symptoms was higher in those individuals with the *Gly9* and *-205-G* alleles (Staddon et al 2002).

May Alter Pharmacodynamics of Aripiprazole, haloperidol, olanzapine, ziprasidone, risperidone, and potentially other antipsychotics

May Affect Disease Predisposition of Alzheimer's disease, anxiety disorder, affective disorder, schizophrenia, alcoholism, substance abuse, Parkinson's disease

References

Basile VS, Masellis M, Badri F, et al, "Association of the Mscl Polymorphism of the Dopamine D3 Receptor Gene With Tardive Dyskinesia in Schizophrenia," *Neuropsychopharmacology*, 1999, 21(1):17-27.

Ishiguro H, Okuyama Y, Toru M, et al, "Mutation and Association Analysis of the 5' Region of the Dopamine D3 Receptor Gene in Schizophrenia Patients: Identification of the Ala38Thr Polymorphism and Suggested Association Between DRD3 Haplotypes and Schizophrenia," *Mol Psychiatry*, 2000, 5(4):433-8.

Lovlie R, Daly AK, Blennerhassett R, et al, "Homozygosity for Gly-9 Variant of the Dopamine D3 Receptor and Risk for Tardive Dyskinesia in Schizophrenic Patients," *Int J Neuropsychopharmacol*, 2000, 3(1):61-6.

Malhotra AK, Goldman D, Buchanan RW, et al, "The Dopamine D3 Receptor (DRD3) Ser9Gly Polymorphism and Schizophrenia: A Haplotypes Relative Risk Study and Association With Clozapine Response," *Mol Psychiatry*, 1998, 3(1):72-5.

Rietschel M, Krauss H, Muller DJ, et al, "Dopamine D3 Receptor Variant and Tardive Dyskinesia," *Eur Arch Psychiatry Clin Neurosci*, 2000, 250(1):31-5.

Segman R, Neeman T, Heresco-Levy U, et al, "Genotypic Association Between the Dopamine D3 Receptor Gene and Tardive Dyskinesia in Chronic Schizophrenia," *Mol Psychiatry*, 1999, 4(3):247-53.

Shaikh S, Collier DA, Sham P, et al, "Allelic Association Between a Ser-9-Gly Polymorphism of the D3 Receptor Gene and Schizophrenia," *Hum Genet*, 1996, 97(6):714-9.

Staddon S, Arranz MJ, Mancama D, et al, "Clinical Applications of Pharmacogenetics in Psychiatry," *Psychopharmacology (Berl)*, 2002, 162(1):18-23 (review).

Steen VM, Lovlie R, MacEwan T, et al, "Dopamine D3 Receptor Gene Variant and Susceptibility to Tardive Dyskinesia in Schizophrenic Patients," *Mol Psychiatry*, 1997, 2(2):139-45.

♦ **D$_4$** see D4 Receptor *on page 192*

D4 Receptor

Synonyms D$_4$; DRD4

Chromosome Location 11p15.5

Clinically-Important Polymorphisms Exon III 48bp vntr; Exon I 12 bp repeat, Exon I 13 bp deletion; Gly11Arg

Discussion There are two major categories of dopamine receptors, namely the D$_1$-like and D$_2$-like. The D$_1$-like receptors include D$_1$ and D$_5$ receptors. The D$_2$-like receptors include two isoforms of the D$_2$ receptor, the D$_3$ receptor, and the D$_4$ receptor. The D$_1$ and D$_5$ receptors activate adenylyl cyclase. The D$_2$ receptors possess several actions, including the inhibition of adenylyl cyclase activity, suppression of calcium currents, and activation of potassium currents. The effector system to which the D$_3$ and D$_4$ receptors couple has not been defined with certainty.

Clozapine:
   No significant association established between polymorphisms of the D_4 receptor and therapeutic effect (Rao et al 1994, Shaikh et al 1995, Rietschel et al 1996, Kohn et al 1997).

May Alter Pharmacodynamics of Haloperidol, risperidone, and potentially other antipsychotic agents

May Affect Disease Predisposition of Alzheimer's disease, anxiety disorder, affective disorder, schizophrenia, alcoholism, substance abuse, Parkinson's disease

References

Kohn Y, Ebstein RP, Heresco-Levy U, et al, "Dopamine D4 Receptor Gene Polymorphisms: Relation to Ethnicity, No Association With Schizophrenia and Response to Clozapine in Israeli Subjects," *Eur J Neuropsychopharmacol*, 1997, 7(1):39-43.

Rao PA, Picckar D, Gejman PV, et al, "Allelic Variation in the D3 Dopamine Receptor (DRD4) Gene Does Not Predict Response to Clozapine," *Arch Gen Psychiatry*, 1994, 51(11):912-7.

Rietschel M, Naber D, Oberlander H, et al, "Efficacy and Side Effects of Clozapine: Testing for Association With Allelic Variation in the Dopamine D4 Receptor Gene," *Neuropsychopharmacology*, 1996, 15(5):491-6.

Shaikh S, Collier DA, Sham P, et al, "Analysis of Clozapine Response and Polymorphism of the Dopamine D4 Receptor Gene (DRD4) in Schizophrenic Patients," *Am J Med Genet*, 1995, 60(6):541-5.

♦ **Diaphorase-4** see NAD(P)H Quinone Oxidoreductase *on page 212*

Dihydropyrimidine Dehydrogenase

Synonyms DPD; DPYD

Chromosome Location 1p22

Discussion A deficiency in dihydropyrimidine dehydrogenase (DPD) is inherited as an autosomal recessive trait. It has been estimated that up to 3% of the Caucasian population are deficient in DPD activity. Enzyme deficiencies are related in up to 17 different reported mutations which are associated with an 8- to 21-fold variability in enzymatic activity. Of note, cimetidine (and possibly all H-2s) have been identified as inhibitors of DPD.

Fluorouracil:
   Approximately 80% of a dose of fluorouracil is metabolized by DPD. Deficiency has been correlated to a prolongation of fluorouracil's half-life and increased neurological and hematological toxicity (Collie-Duguid et al 2000).

May Alter Pharmacokinetics of Fluorouracil, capecitabine

References

Collie-Duguid ES, Etienne MC, Milano G, et al, "Known Variant DPYD Alleles Do Not Explain DPD Deficiency in Cancer Patients," *Pharmacogenetics*, 2000, 10(3):217-23.

♦ **DPD** see Dihydropyrimidine Dehydrogenase *on page 193*

♦ **DPYD** see Dihydropyrimidine Dehydrogenase *on page 193*

♦ **DRD2** see D2 Receptor *on page 190*

♦ **DRD3** see D3 Receptor *on page 191*

♦ **DRD4** see D4 Receptor *on page 192*

♦ **DT-Diaphorase** see NAD(P)H Quinone Oxidoreductase *on page 212*

♦ **EC 1.6.99.2** see NAD(P)H Quinone Oxidoreductase *on page 212*

EPITHELIAL SODIUM CHANNEL BETA-SUBUNIT

♦ **ENaC-Beta** *see* Epithelial Sodium Channel Beta-Subunit *on page 194*

Epithelial Sodium Channel Beta-Subunit

Synonyms ENaC-Beta
Chromosome Location 16p12
Clinically-Important Polymorphisms Nonsynonymous SNP in exon 12 (*T594M*)

Discussion The ENaC is an important regulator of epithelial cell sodium exchange. Sodium reabsorption through ENaC within the distal nephron regulates sodium balance, and contributes to regulation of circulating blood volume and blood pressure. Expression of ENaC is regulated by aldosterone. Rare genetic disorders of sodium channel activity (Liddle's syndrome and pseudohypoaldosteronism type 1) have been described. Liddle's syndrome is an autosomal dominant trait resulting in pseudoaldosteronism and salt-sensitive hypertension. Systemic pseudohypoaldosteronism type I is an autosomal recessive disorder that arises from loss of function mutations. These result in a severe salt-wasting syndrome in neonates, which is resistant to mineralocorticoid supplementation. In addition to genetic syndromes, additional polymorphisms of the epithelial cell sodium channel have been described. The *T594M* polymorphism occurs in approximately 5% of persons of African descent and has been associated with hypertension (Baker et al 1998).

Amiloride:
  Monotherapy with amiloride 10 mg twice a day was shown to control blood pressure as effectively as two antihypertensive medications in hypertensive individuals of African descent with the *T594M* polymorphism (Baker et al 2002).

May Alter Pharmacokinetics of The ENaC gene is not known to affect the metabolism of any drugs.
May Alter Pharmacodynamics of Amiloride
May Affect Disease Predisposition of Hypertension
Clinical Recommendations Genotyping for the *T594M* polymorphism may have a role in the management of individuals of African descent with drug-resistant hypertension.
Counseling Points Carrier status of the *T594M* polymorphism may influence sodium sensitivity and risk for hypertension. Individuals should discuss the implications of having this variant with their clinician or another healthcare professional.

References
Baker EH, Dong YB, Sagnella GA, et al, "Association of Hypertension With T594M Mutation in Beta Subunit of Epithelial Sodium Channels in Black People Resident in London," *Lancet*, 1998, 351(9113):1388-92.
Baker EH, Duggal A, Dong Y, et al, "Amiloride, A Specific Drug for Hypertension in Black People With T594M Variant?" *Hypertension*, 2002, 40(1):13-7.

♦ **F5** *see* Factor V *on page 194*

Factor V
Synonyms F5
Chromosome Location 1q23

GLUCOSE-6-PHOSPHATE DEHYDROGENASE

Clinically-Important Polymorphisms Factor V Leiden results from a nonsynonymous SNP at nucleotide 1691 (G/A) resulting in the *506Q* polymorphism.

Discussion The *506Q* mutation in the factor V gene (factor V Leiden) is an established risk factor for venous thrombosis. This mutation confers resistance to activated protein C.

Oral contraceptives:

The factor V Leiden mutation occurs in about 5% of the Caucasian population and has been correlated with an increased risk of venous thrombosis, and may predispose to thrombosis in patients receiving estrogens, including oral contraceptives (Vandenbroucke et al 1994). Differences in the potential for venous thrombosis have been observed in some, but not all studies evaluating second and third generation oral contraceptives. Estrogen-induced changes in factor V attenuated by a second-generation progestin, but not by a third generation progestin, have been proposed as a basis for greater risk of thrombosis associated with third generation agents (Kemmeren et al 2002).

May Alter Pharmacokinetics of The factor V Leiden gene is not known to alter the pharmacokinetics of any drugs

May Alter Pharmacodynamics of Oral contraceptives, estrogen

May Affect Disease Predisposition of Thrombosis, deep venous thrombosis

Laboratory Evaluation Screening for the *506Q* polymorphism should be considered in potential oral contraceptive users with a positive family history of thrombosis.

Clinical Recommendations Individuals with the *506Q* allele who used oral contraceptive are at markedly increased risk for venous thromboembolism. Clinicians should consider alternative contraceptive methods in *506Q* carriers, especially if other genetic mutations in the coagulation cascade are also present.

References

Kemmeren JM, Algra A, Meijers JC, et al, "Effect of Second- and Third-Generation Oral Contraceptives on Fibrinolysis in the Absence or Presence of the Factor V Leiden Mutation," *Blood Coagul Fibrinolysis*, 2002, 13(5):373-81.

Vandenbroucke JP, Koster T, Briet E, et al, "Increased Risk of Venous Thrombosis in Oral-Contraceptive Users Who Are Carriers of Factor V Leiden Mutation," *Lancet*, 1994, 344(8935):1453-7.

- ♦ **Fc Gamma RIIa** *see* Platelet Fc Gamma Receptor *on page 216*
- ♦ **FCG R2A** *see* Platelet Fc Gamma Receptor *on page 216*
- ♦ **FGB** *see* Beta-Fibrinogen *on page 174*
- ♦ **G6PD** *see* Glucose-6-Phosphate Dehydrogenase *on page 195*
- ♦ **GB3** *see* G-Protein Beta-3 Subunit *on page 197*

Glucose-6-Phosphate Dehydrogenase

Synonyms G6PD

Chromosome Location Xq28

Clinically-Important Polymorphisms Over 300 variants have been described that result in deficient enzymatic activity.
(Continued)

Glucose-6-Phosphate Dehydrogenase
(Continued)

Discussion Glucose-6-phosphate dehydrogenase is an enzyme that catalyzes the oxidation of glucose-6-phosphate to 6-phosphogluconate, reducing NADP to NADPH. NADPH is involved in protecting erythrocytes from oxidative stress. Over 300 variants of the G6PD enzyme have been reported, resulting in a wide range of potential enzymatic activity and symptoms. Glucose-6-phosphate dehydrogenase deficiency is inherited as an X-linked genetic trait.

Over 200 million people are estimated to have a genetic deficiency of the G6PD enzyme. Individuals from the Mediterranean basin, Southeast Asia, Africa, and India have a higher prevalence of this trait. Variants in the extent of G6PD-deficiency have been noted. The reduction in enzyme activity is more pronounced in older red blood cells, resulting in hemolysis when the red cell is no longer able to maintain its integrity. Severity of the deficiency determines the point at which red cells are lysed. Severe deficiency leads to a dramatic reduction in RBC lifespan, and a chronic hemolytic anemia. Females may experience difficulty carrying a pregnancy to term.

In patients with less severe deficiency, exposure to certain chemicals or infections may trigger hemolysis. Some foods, including fava beans, have been associated with hemolytic reactions. Exposure to specific drugs and/or drug classes may lead to acute hemolysis. This has been described for primaquine, chloramphenicol, acetanilide, phenacetin, vitamin K, sulfonamides, and nitrofurans. Case reports have identified other drugs (ie, acetaminophen), which may not be directly related to hemolysis.

May Alter Pharmacodynamics of Quinine derivatives, sulfonamides, chloramphenicol, nitrofuran-containing drugs

Laboratory Evaluation Commercial testing for G6PD is available.

Glycoprotein IIIa Receptor

Synonyms GPIIIa

Chromosome Location 17q21.32

Clinically-Important Polymorphisms Nonsynonymous SNP resulting in substitution of Leu(Pl^{A1}) or Pro(Pl^{A2}) at codon 33 in exon 2

Discussion Fibrinogen binds to glycoprotein IIb/IIIa receptors expressed on the platelet surface to cross link adjacent platelets as the final common pathway of platelet aggregation. Although data are inconsistent, the GPIIIa *P1$^{A1/A2}$* polymorphism has been associated with platelet aggregation and the effects of aspirin on platelet aggregation in *in vitro* studies.

Antiplatelet therapy:

The GPIIIa *Pl^{A2}* allele was associated with greater restenosis and risk for subacute coronary thrombosis during combination therapy with aspirin and ticlopidine in patients who had undergone coronary artery stent implantation (Kastrati et al 2000, Walter et al 1997).

HMG CoA reductase inhibitors:
    In myocardial infarction survivors, the greatest reductions in fatal coronary heart disease or nonfatal myocardial infarction with pravastatin occurred in those with the Pl^{A2} allele and either the ACE *ID* or ACE *DD* genotype (Bray et al 2001).

May Alter Pharmacokinetics of GPIIIa is not known to alter the metabolism of any drugs.

May Alter Pharmacodynamics of Aspirin, ticlopidine, clopidogrel, glycoprotein IIb/IIIa antagonists, dipyridamole, HMG CoA reductase inhibitors

May Affect Disease Predisposition of Coronary thrombosis

Clinical Recommendations The data suggest that the GPIIIa may be a predictor of the effectiveness of antiplatelet therapy in preventing subacute thrombosis following coronary artery stent implantation.

References
    Bray PF, Cannon CP, Goldschmidt-Clermont P, et al, "The Platelet PI(A2) and Angiotensin-Converting Enzyme (ACE) D Allele Polymorphisms and the Risk of Recurrent Events After Acute Myocardial Infarction," *Am J Cardiol*, 2001, 88(4):347-52.

    Kastrati A, Koch W, Gawaz M, et al, "PlA Polymorphism of Glycoprotein IIIa and Risk of Adverse Events After Coronary Stent Placement," *J Am Coll Cardiol*, 2000, 36(1):84-9.

    Walter DH, Schachinger V, Elsner M, et al, "Platelet Glycoprotein IIIa Polymorphisms and Risk of Coronary Stent Thrombosis," *Lancet*, 1997, 350(9086):1217-9.

- **GNAS1** see Gs Protein Alpha-Subunit *on page 198*
- **GNB3** see G-Protein Beta-3 Subunit *on page 197*
- **GP170** see P-Glycoprotein *on page 213*
- **GPIIIa** see Glycoprotein IIIa Receptor *on page 196*

G-Protein Beta-3 Subunit
Synonyms GB3; GNB3
Chromosome Location 12p13
Clinically-Important Polymorphisms Synonymous SNP in exon 10 (*C825T*)

Discussion The *825T* allele has been associated with enhanced intracellular signal transduction and sodium hydrogen exchange *in vitro*, and reduced plasma renin activity in hypertensive patients (Siffert et al 1995, Schunkert et al 1998). The *T* allele has also been linked to risk for hypertension in some populations.

Antidepressants:
    An association between the *TT* homozygosity and response to antidepressant treatment after 4 weeks was identified (Zill et al 2000).

Hydrochlorothiazide:
    Compared to the *825CC* genotype, the *825TT* genotype was associated with significantly greater blood pressure response to 4-week treatment with hydrochlorothiazide in hypertensive patients (Turner et al 2001). After linear regression, the overall contribution of the *C825T* polymorphism to drug response was approximately 5%.

May Alter Pharmacodynamics of Thiazide diuretics, loop diuretics, antidepressants (tricyclics and SSRIs), and potentially other CYP2D6 substrates

May Affect Disease Predisposition of Hypertension, depression
(Continued)

G-Protein Beta-3 Subunit *(Continued)*

Clinical Recommendations Future studies may show that the GNB3 gene interacts with other genes, such as the alpha-adducin gene, to determine response to diuretics in hypertension. The GNB3 gene alone appears to contribute minimally to thiazide diuretic response.

Counseling Points Since hypertension is a disease with polygenic etiology, carrier status of the *GNB3* variant allele does not necessarily predispose a person to developing hypertension or its sequelae.

References

Kirchheiner J, Brosen K, Dahl ML, et al, "CYP2D6 and CYP2C19 Genotype-Based Dose Recommendations for Antidepressants: A First Step Towards Subpopulation-Specific Dosages," *Acta Psychiatr Scand*, 2001, 104(3):173-92.

Morita S, Shimoda K, Someya T, et al, "Steady-State Plasma Levels of Nortriptyline and Its Hydroxylated Metabolites in Japanese Patients: Impact of CYP2D6 Genotype on the Hydroxylation of Nortriptyline," *Clin Psychopharmacol*, 2000, 20(2):141-9.

Schunkert H, Hense HW, Doring A, et al, "Association Between a Polymorphism in the G Protein Beta3 Subunit Gene and Lower Renin and Elevated Diastolic Blood Pressure Levels," *Hypertension*, 1998, 32(3):510-3.

Siffert W, Rosskopf D, Moritz A, et al, "Enhanced G Protein Activation in Immortalized Lymphoblasts From Patients With Essential Hypertension," *J Clin Invest*, 1995, 96(2):759-66.

Turner ST, Schwartz GL, Chapman AB, et al, "C825T Polymorphism of the G Protein Beta(3)-Subunit and Antihypertensive Response to a Thiazide Diuretic," *Hypertension*, 2001, 37(2 Part 2):739-43.

Zill P, Baghai TC, Zwanzger P, et al, "Evidence for an Association Between a G-Protein Beta3-Gene Variant With Depression and Response to Antidepressant Treatment," *Neuroreport*, 2000, 11(9):1893-7.

Gs Protein Alpha-Subunit

Synonyms GNAS1

Chromosome Location 20q13

Clinically-Important Polymorphisms Synonymous SNP at codon 131 creating a restriction site for the *Fok*I restriction enzyme; T/C point mutation in exon 5; ATT → ATC at codon 131

Discussion Gs is a ubiquitous protein that couples receptors to adenylyl cyclase, which is required to generate intracellular cAMP following receptor stimulation. Mutations of Gs(alpha) are present in endocrine tumors, fibrous dysplasia of bone, and McCune-Albright syndrome.

Reports of altered levels of the stimulatory G-proteins in depression have been presented. Investigations into whether a polymorphism in the stimulatory alpha subunit of G-proteins may be associated with major depression or response to antidepressant medications has been reported (Zill et al 2002).

The Gs-proteins mediate activation of adenylyl cyclase by the β-adrenoceptor. Alteration of the GNAS1 has been associated with essential hypertension. A polymorphism has been identified which may be recognized by the presence (+) or absence (-) of a restriction site for the enzyme *Fok*I.

Antidepressants:

No evidence of an association between the alpha subunit of G-protein and major depression and response to antidepressant medication was reported (Zill et al 2002).

β-blockers:

In a retrospective study, the frequency of the *FokI+* allele was higher in hypertensive individuals who had a good response (>15 mm Hg decline in mean arterial pressure) to β-blocker therapy compared to those with a poor response (<11 mm Hg decline in mean arterial pressure) (Jia et al 1999). The *GNAS1* genotype was the only independent predictor of BP response identified in a multiple linear regression analysis.

May Alter Pharmacokinetics of The GNAS1 gene is not known to alter the metabolism of any drugs.

May Alter Pharmacodynamics of β-adrenergic receptor antagonists, antidepressants (cyclic and SSRIs)

May Affect Disease Predisposition of Depression, endocrine neoplasia

Clinical Recommendations The role of the GNAS1 in predicting β-blocker response must be confirmed in a prospectively designed study before its clinical utility will be realized.

Counseling Points Since hypertension is a disease with polygenic etiology, carrier status of the *GNAS1* variant allele does not necessarily predispose a person to developing hypertension or its sequelae.

References

Jia H, Hingorani AD, Sharma P, et al, "Association of the G(s)alpha Gene With Essential Hypertension and Response to Beta-Blockade," *Hypertension*, 1999, 34(1):8-14.

Zill P, Baghai TC, Zwanzger P, et al, "Association Analysis of a Polymorphism in the G-Protein Stimulatory Alpha Subunit in Patients With Major Depression," *Am J Med Genet*, 2002, 114(5):530-2.

Histamine 1 and 2 Receptors

Synonyms HR1; HR2

Chromosome Location 3p25; 5q35.3

Clinically-Important Polymorphisms -1018G/A, -1068A/G, Asp349Glu, Leu449Ser, Lys19Asn, Phe358D

Discussion Histaminic activity is believed to be involved in schizophrenia. Within the brain, histaminic receptors project from the tuberomammillary nucleus of the posterior hypothalamus, with both H1 and H2 receptors being present in the caudate, putamen, neocortex, and hippocampus. There are at least four types of histamine receptors (H1, H2, H3, and H4). The H1 receptor has a role in sleep, wakefulness, feeding, and drinking, while the H2 receptor is primarily involved in gastrointestinal functions.

Clozapine:

No relationship between clozapine response and these polymorphisms have been found. Additionally, no relationship between these polymorphisms and weight gain from clozapine have been found (Basile et al 2001).

May Alter Pharmacodynamics of Clozapine, olanzapine, and other H1 and H2 receptor antagonists

May Affect Disease Predisposition of Schizophrenia, obesity

References

Basile VS, Masellis M, McIntyre RS, et al, "Genetic Dissection of Atypical Antipsychotic-
(Continued)

Histamine 1 and 2 Receptors *(Continued)*

Induced Weight Gain: Novel Preliminary Data on the Pharmacogenetic Puzzle," *J Clin Psychiatry*, 2001, 62(Suppl 23):45-66 (review).

Mancama D, Arranz MJ, Munro J, et al, "The Histamine-1 and Histamine-2 Receptor Genes - Candidates for Schizophrenia and Clozapine Drug Response," *GeneScreen*, 2000, 1:29-34.

- **HLA** *see* Human Leukocyte Antigen *on page 206*

HLA-A1

Synonyms MMC-IA

Chromosome Location 6p21.3

Discussion

Clozapine:

Clozapine responders vs nonresponders 76% predictive value (a combination of 6 polymorphisms were included in the analysis) (Arranz et al 2000).

The ability to predict response may be linked, at least in part, to a genetic polymorphism of HLA-A1, an allele that has a higher distribution in the Scandinavian population than the incidence noted in granulocytopenic patients (Lahdelma et al 2001).

May Alter Pharmacodynamics of Clozapine

May Affect Disease Predisposition of Schizophrenia, clozapine-induced agranulocytosis

References

Arranz MJ, Munro J, Birkett J, et al, "Pharmacogenetic Prediction of Clozapine Response," *Lancet*, 2000, 355(921):1615-6.

Lahdelma L, Ahokas A, Andersson LC, et al, "Mitchell B. Balter Award. Human Leukocyte Antigen-A1 Predicts a Good Therapeutic Response to Clozapine With a Low Risk of Agranulocytosis in Patients With Schizophrenia," *J Clin Psychopharmacol*, 2001, 21(1):4-7.

- **HR1** *see* Histamine 1 and 2 Receptors *on page 199*
- **HR2** *see* Histamine 1 and 2 Receptors *on page 199*

5HT1A Receptor

Discussion Serotonin receptor subtypes are grouped into several classes. The 5HT1 class are G protein receptors and include multiple isoforms within the class. The 5HT1 receptor subset includes at least five receptor subtypes (5HT1A, 1B, 1D, 1E, 1F) and is linked to inhibition of adenylyl cyclase activity or to regulation of potassium or calcium channels. The 5HT1A receptors are most abundant in the dorsal raphe nucleus. They are also found in the hippocampus and amygdala. Activities associated with these receptor locations include temperature regulation, mood changes, and anxiety, respectively. The 5HT1A receptors are located both presynaptically (somatodendritic autoreceptor) and postsynaptically.

Clozapine:

No significant association with weight gain (Basile et al 2001) in the C antinucleotide repeat polymorphism.

May Alter Pharmacodynamics of Aripiprazole, ziprasidone, SSRIs

May Affect Disease Predisposition of Anxiety disorder, affective disorder

References

Basile VS, Masellis M, McIntyre RS, et al, "Genetic Dissection of Atypical Antipsychotic-Induced Weight Gain: Novel Preliminary Data on the Pharmacogenetic Puzzle," *J Clin Psychiatry*, 2001, 62(Suppl 23):45-66 (review).

5HT2A Receptor

Synonyms HTR2

Chromosome Location 13q14-q21

Clinically-Important Polymorphisms T102C, Thr25Asn, His452Tyr, T516C, and -G1438A

Discussion Serotonin receptor subtypes are grouped into several classes. The 5HT2 class are G protein receptors and include multiple isoforms within the class. The 5HT2 receptor subset includes at least three receptor subtypes (5HT2A, 2B, 2C) and is linked to activation of phospholipase C. Areas of high concentration of 5HT2A receptors include the neocortex, olfactory tubercle, and several nuclei arising from the brainstem.

Clozapine:

The *C/C* genotype has been associated with a lack of response to clozapine (Arranz et al 1995) and in 1998 these same authors (Arranz et al 1998) found that homozygosity for the *-1438G* allele was also higher among nonresponders than responders (58% vs 32%, p=0.001). The *His452Tyr* polymorphism has also been associated with clozapine response (Arranz et al 1996, Badri et al 1996) with the presence of the *Tyr452* variant being tied to a poorer response (Arranz et al 1998).

Multiple authors have been unable to replicate these findings (Malhotra et al 1996, Arranz et al 1998, Masellis et al 1998, Ishigaki et al 1996, Jonsson et al 1996, Sasaki et al 1996).

Olanzapine:

Negative symptom response has been associated with the *102T/T* genotype and *-1438A/A* genotype (Ellingrod et al 2002).

Tardive dyskinesia:

Two studies have found a relationship between SNPs of the 5HT2A receptor and tardive dyskinesia (Segman et al 2001, Tan et al 2001), although subsequent studies were unable to replicate these results (Basile et al 2000). In comparing patients with tardive dyskinesia to normal controls, there was a significant excess of the *102C* and *-1438G* alleles in patients with tardive dyskinesia. The *102C/C* and *-1438G/G* genotypes were also significantly associated with higher abnormal involuntary movement scale (AIMS) trunk dyskinesia scores.

May Alter Pharmacodynamics of Atypical antipsychotics (except quetiapine)

May Affect Disease Predisposition of Schizophrenia

References

Arranz MJ, Collier DA, Munro J, et al, "Analysis of the Structural Polymorphisms in the 5HT2A Receptor and Clinical Response to Clozapine," *Neurosci Lett*, 1996, 217(2-3):177-8.

Arranz MJ, Dawson E, Shaikh S, et al, "Cytochrome P4502D6 Genotype Does Not Determine Response to Clozapine," *Br J Clin Pharmacol*, 1995, 39(4):417-20.

(Continued)

5HT2A Receptor *(Continued)*

Arranz MJ, Munro J, Owen MJ, et al, "Evidence for Association Between Polymorphisms in the Promoter and Coding Regions of the 5HT2A Receptor Gene and Response to Clozapine," *Mol Psychiatry*, 1998, 3(1):61-6.

Badri F, Masellis M, Petronis A, et al, "Dopamine and Serotonin System Genes May Predict Clinical Response to Clozapine," *Am J Hum Genet*, 1996, 59:A247.

Basile VS, Ozdemir V, Masellis M, et al, "Lack of Association Between Serotonin-2A Receptor Gene (HTR2A) Polymorphisms and Tardive Dyskinesia in Schizophrenia," *Mol Psychiatry*, 2001, 6(2):230-4.

Ellingrod VL, Perry PJ, Lund BL, et al, "5HT2A and 5HT2C Receptor Polymorphisms and Predicting Clinical Response to Olanzapine in Schizophrenia," *J Clin Psychopharmacol*, 2002, 22(6):622-4.

Ishigaki T, Xie DW, Liu JC, et al, "Intact 5HT2A Receptor Exons and the Adjoining Intron Regions in Schizophrenia," *Neuropsychopharmacology*, 1996, 14(5):339-47.

Jonsson E, Nothen MM, Bunzel R, et al, "5HT2a Receptor T102C Polymorphism and Schizophrenia," *Lancet*, 1996, 347(9018):1831.

Malhotra AK, Goldman D, Buchanan R, et al, "5HT2a Receptor T102C Polymorphism and Schizophrenia," *Lancet*, 1996, 347(9018):1830-1.

Masellis M, Basile VS, Meltzer HY, et al, "Serotonin Subtype 2 Receptor Genes and Clinical Response to Clozapine in Schizophrenia Patients," *Neuropsychopharmacology*, 1998, 19(2):123-32.

Sasaki T, Hattori M, Fukuda R, et al, "5HT2a Receptor T102C Polymorphism and Schizophrenia," *Lancet*, 1996, 347(9018):1832.

Segman RH, Heresco-Levy U, Finkel B, et al, "Association Between the Serotonin 2A Receptor Gene and Tardive Dyskinesia in Chronic Schizophrenia," 2001, *Mol Psychiatry*, 6(2):225-9.

Tan EC, Chong SA, Mahendran R, et al, "Susceptibility to Neuroleptic-Induced Tardive Dyskinesia and the T102C Polymorphism in the Serotonin Type 2A Receptor," *Biol Psychiatry*, 2001, 50(2):144-7.

5HT2C Receptor

Synonyms HTR2C

Chromosome Location Xq24

Clinically-Important Polymorphisms Cys23Ser, -759C/T

Discussion Serotonin receptor subtypes are grouped into several classes. The 5HT2 class are G protein receptors and include multiple isoforms within the class. The 5HT2 receptor subset includes at least three receptor subtypes (5HT2A, 2B, 2C) and is linked to activation of phospholipase C. 5HT2C receptors are abundant in the choroid plexus and its pharmacology is similar to the 5HT2A receptor.

This receptor has been associated with weight gain. Significantly less weight gain was noted in patients with the *-759T* variant allele than in those without this allele. This was noted in first-episode patients with schizophrenia (Reynolds et al 2002).

Clozapine:

The *Ser* allele has been associated with a positive change in GAS scores (Sodhi et al 1995). Other authors were unable to confirm these results (Rietschel et al 1997, Masellis et al 1998, Malhotra et al 1996). There was a trend for patients carrying only the serine variant to have higher mean weight gain following treatment with clozapine (Basile et al 2001). Patients with the *-759T* variant allele showed significantly less weight gain than those without this allele. The effect was strongest in male patients and not apparent in female patients (Reynolds et al 2003). At least three authors have found a relationship between weight gain from clozapine and presence of the *-759C* allele (Basile et al 2003, Reynolds et al 2003), while one research group was unable to find an association (Tsai et al 2003).

Olanzapine:
Presence of a *-759C* allele has been associated with weight gain of greater than 10% over baseline in 6 weeks (Ellingrod et al submitted).

Tardive dyskinesia:
The frequency of the 5HT2C *Ser* allele has been found to be significantly higher in patients with tardive dyskinesia, versus those without tardive dyskinesia and normal controls (27.2% vs 14.6%, 14.2%, respectively). The 5HT2C *Ser* and DRD3 *Gly* alleles contributed to 4.2% and 4.7% of the variance seen in orofacial dyskinesia scores (Segman et al 2000).

May Alter Pharmacodynamics of Atypical antipsychotics (except quetiapine)

May Affect Disease Predisposition of Schizophrenia

References

Basile VS, Masellis M, DeLuca V, et al, "-759C/T Genetic Variation of the 5HT2C Receptor and Clozapine Induced Weight Gain," *Lancet*, 2003, 360:1790-1.

Basile VS, Masellis M, McIntyre RS, et al, "Genetic Dissection of Atypical Antipsychotic-Induced Weight Gain: Novel Preliminary Data on the Pharmacogenetic Puzzle," *J Clin Psychiatry*, 2001, 62(Suppl 23):45-66 (review).

Ellingrod VL, Perry PJ, Ringold JC, et al, (submitted), "Weight Gain Associated With the -759 C/T Polymorphism of the 5HT2C Receptor and Olanzapine," *Am J Med Genetics*.

Malhotra AK, Goldman D, Ozaki N, et al, "Clozapine Response and the 5HT2C Cys23Ser Polymorphism," *Neuroreport*, 1996, 7(13):2100-2.

Masellis M, Basile VS, Meltzer HY, et al, "Serotonin Subtype 2 Receptor Genes and Clinical Response to Clozapine in Schizophrenia Patients," *Neuropsychopharmacology*, 1998, 19(2):123-32.

Reynolds GP, Zhang ZJ, and Zhang XB, "Association of Antipsychotic Drug-Induced Weight Gain With 5-HT2C Receptor Gene Polymorphism," *Lancet*, 2002, 359(9323):2086-7.

Reynolds GP, Zhang Z, and Zhang X, "Polymorphism of the Promoter Region of the Serotonin 5-HT(2c) Receptor Gene and Clozapine-Induced Weight Gain," *Am J Psychiatry*, 2003, 160(4):677-9.

Rietschel M, Naber D, Fimmers R, et al, "Efficacy and Side Effects of Clozapine Not Associated With Variation in the 5-HT2c Receptor," *Neuroreport*, 1997, 8(8):1999-2003.

Segman RH, Heresco-Levy U, Finkel B, et al, "Association Between the Serotonin 2C Receptor Gene and Tardive Dyskinesia in Chronic Schizophrenia: Additive Contribution of the 5-HT2Cser and DRD3gly to Susceptibility," *Psychopharmacology (Berl)*, 2000, 152(4):408-13.

Sodhi MS, Arranz MJ, Curtis D, et al, "Association Between Clozapine Response and Allelic Variation in the 5-HT2C Receptor Gene," *Neuroreport*, 1995, 7(1):169-72.

Tsai SJ, Hong CJ, Yu YW, et al, "-759C/T Genetic Variation of the 5HT2C Receptor and Clozapine Induced Weight Gain," *Lancet*, 2002, 360(9347):1790.

5HT6 Receptor

Synonyms HTR6

Chromosome Location 1p36-p35

Clinically-Important Polymorphisms The *T267C* polymorphism was evaluated, and a larger change in BPRS score was associated
(Continued)

5HT6 Receptor *(Continued)*

with the *T/T* genotype (Yu et al 1999). This has not been replicated (Masellis et al 2000).

Discussion The 5HT6 receptor is a G protein receptor and is linked to activation of adenylyl cyclase. Clozapine has a high affinity for 5HT6 receptors.

May Alter Pharmacodynamics of Clozapine, olanzapine

References
Masellis M, Basile VS, Meltzer HY, et al, "Lack of Association Between the T.C267 Serotonin 5HT6 Receptor Gene (HTR6) Polymorphism and Prediction of Response to Clozapine in Schizophrenia," *Schizophr Res*, 2001, 47(1):49-58.
Yu YW, Tsai SJ, Lin CH, et al, "Serotonin-6 Receptor Variant (C267T) and Clinical Response to Clozapine," *Neuroreport*, 1999, 10(6):1231-3.

- **HTR2** *see* 5HT2A Receptor *on page 201*
- **HTR2C** *see* 5HT2C Receptor *on page 202*
- **HTR6** *see* 5HT6 Receptor *on page 203*
- **HTT** *see* 5HT Transporter *on page 204*
- **5HTT** *see* 5HT Transporter *on page 204*
- **5HTTLPR** *see* 5HT Transporter *on page 204*

5HT Transporter

Synonyms HTT; 5HTT; 5HTTLPR; SERT; SLC6A4

Chromosome Location 17q11.1-q12

Clinically-Important Polymorphisms A 45 bp insertion results in a long variant (l) of this gene. The short variant has been associated with a reduced transcriptional efficiency of the 5HTT gene promoter. The "s" variant has also been linked to a greater risk of "switching" in bipolar patients. Additionally an intronic variable number of tandem repeats (VNTR) polymorphism has been found in intron 2. This polymorphism has three alleles (*Stin2.9*, *Stin2.10*, and *Stin2.12*).

Discussion The serotonin transporter is selective for serotonin and is in part responsible for the termination of its action at the postsynaptic receptors.

The selective serotonin re-uptake inhibitors (SSRIs) bind to the serotonin transporter (5HTT) and inhibit its capacity to transport serotonin (5HT). A functional polymorphism in the promoter region of 5HTT (5HTTLPR) has been identified. Two variants, an insertion (long allele) and a deletion (short allele) have been identified. The long allele is associated with higher expression of brain 5HTT. In addition, an association between this polymorphism and the development of mental disorders has been reported by some investigators. These findings have not been replicated in all studies. Gene polymorphisms have been associated with greater response to SSRIs. Further investigation is warranted to evaluate the relationships between genotype, susceptibility to mental disorders, and response to antidepressants (Weizman et al 2000).

The 5HTT gene (SLC6A4) has 2 known polymorphisms. Variants have been correlated to the pathogenesis of antidepressant-induced mania in bipolar disorder. If replicated, polymorphism in the 5HTT gene may be useful as a predictor of mania/hypomania in bipolar patients (Mundo et al 2001).

SSRIs:

The long form of this gene has been associated with a greater response to fluvoxamine, paroxetine, and fluvoxamine in unipolar and bipolar depression (Smeraldi et al 1998, Zanardi et al 2000, Pollock et al 2000, Kim et al 2000). Response to SSRIs for major depressive disorder, has been reported to be associated with genotype, however the associations have been inconsistent. In some studies, the presence of the *l* allele has been linked to enhanced response (Smeraldi et al 1998, Zanardi et al 2000, Pollock et al 2000), while in other reports the *s/s* genotype was reported to have an improved response (Kim et al 2000). Additionally, no relationship between nortriptyline and 5HTTLPR genotype has been found (Pollock et al 2000).

In obsessive compulsive disorder, a negative response to medication has been associated with the *l* variant (McDougle et al 1998). Additionally, no relationship between 5HTTLPR genotype and response to SSRIs or clomipramine was found in OCD by other authors (Billet et al 1997).

Clozapine:

No relationship between clozapine response and these polymorphisms have been found (Arranz et al 2000).

Tardive dyskinesia:

No relationship has been found between this polymorphism of 5HTTLPR, AIMS score, or the diagnosis of tardive dyskinesia (Chong et al 2000).

May Alter Pharmacodynamics of SSRIs
May Affect Disease Predisposition of Depression
References

Arranz MJ, Bolonna AA, Munro J, et al, "The Serotonin Transporter and Clozapine Response," *Mol Psychiatry*, 2000, 5(2):124-5.

Billett EA, Richter MA, King N, et al, "Obsessive-Compulsive Disorder, Response to Serotonin Reuptake Inhibitors and Serotonin Transporter Gene," *Mol Psychiatry*, 1997, 2(5):403-6.

Chong SA, Tan EC, Tan CH, et al, "Tardive Dyskinesia Is Not Associated With the Serotonin Gene Polymorphism (5-HTTLPR) in Chinese," *Am J Med Genet*, 2000, 96(6):712-5.

Kim DK, Lim SW, Lee S, et al, "Serotonin Transporter Gene Polymorphism and Antidepressant Response," *Neuroreport*, 2000, 11(1):215-9.

McDougle CJ, Epperson CN, Price LH, et al, "Evidence for Linkage Disequilibrium Between Serotonin Transporter Gene (SLC6A4) and Obsessive Compulsive Disorder," *Mol Psychiatry*, 1998, 3(3):270-3.

Mundo E, Walker M, Cate T, et al, "The Role of Serotonin Transporter Protein Gene in Antidepressant-Induced Mania in Bipolar Disorder: Preliminary Findings," *Arch Gen Psychiatry*, 2001, 58(6):539-44.

Pollock BG, Ferrell RE, Mulsant BH, et al, "Allelic Variation in the Serotonin Transporter Promoter Affects Onset of Paroxetine Treatment Response in Late Life Depression," *Neuropsychopharmacology*, 2000, 23(5):587-90.

Smeraldi E, Zanardi R, Benedetti F, et al, "Polymorphism Within the Promoter of the Serotonin Transporter Gene and Antidepressant Efficacy of Fluvoxamine," *Mol Psychiatry*, 1998, 3(6):508-11.

(Continued)

5HT Transporter (Continued)

Weizman A and Weizman R, "Serotonin Transporter Polymorphism and Response to SSRIs in Major Depression and Relevance to Anxiety Disorders and Substance Abuse," *Pharmacogenomics*, 2000, 1(3):335-41.

Zanardi R, Benedetti F, DiBella D, et al, "Efficacy of Paroxetine in Depression Is Influenced by a Functional Polymorphism Within the Promoter of the Serotonin Transporter Gene," *J Clin Psychopharmacol*, 2000, 20(1):105-7.

Human Leukocyte Antigen

Synonyms HLA

Chromosome Location 6p21.3

Clinically-Important Polymorphisms HLA-B*5701, HLA-DR7, HLA-DQ3 haplotype

Discussion

Abacavir:

Life-threatening hypersensitivity reactions to abacavir are known to occur in about 5% of all patients. The gene for HLA is polymorphic and believed to contribute to the interpatient variability in antigen interaction with T cells. Researchers have noted a strong association between the HLA gene and hypersensitivity reactions to abacavir. In a study of 200 patients, the HLA-B*5701, HLA-DR7, HLA-DQ3 haplotype was present in 13 (72%) of the 18 patients with abacavir hypersensitivity, and none of the 167 patients who tolerated abacavir. It is unclear whether this gene participates in triggering the hypersensitivity or is closely linked to a gene that mediates this reaction. The presence of HLA-B5701, HLA-DR7, and HLA-DQ3 had a positive predictive value for hypersensitivity of 100%, and a negative predictive value of 97%. The researchers concluded that withholding abacavir in patients with HLA-B5701, HLA-DR7, and HLA-DQ3 would substantially reduce the prevalence of hypersensitivity (estimating a reduction from 9% to 2.5% in this study population), without denying the use of the agent inappropriately. It remains to be seen whether genetic screening for these markers, or perhaps additional genes, will become a standard for patients who may be candidates for this therapy. However, this study indicates the potential for these procedures to improve the safety of drug therapy (Mallal et al 2002).

May Alter Pharmacodynamics of Abacavir

References

Mallal S, Nolan D, Witt C, et al, "Association Between Presence of HLA-B*5701, HLA-DR7, and HLA-DQ3 and Hypersensitivity to HIV-1 Reverse-Transcriptase Inhibitor Abacavir," *Lancet*, 2002, 359(9308):727-32.

♦ **k-channel** *see* Cardiac Potassium Ion Channel *on page 177*
♦ **LDLR** *see* Low-Density Lipoprotein Receptor *on page 209*

Leukotriene C4 Synthase

Synonyms LTC(4) Synthase

Chromosome Location 5q35

Clinically-Important Polymorphisms A-444C in the promoter region

Discussion Leukotrienes are important mediators of inflammation, and have been implicated in the pathogenesis of allergic disorders, asthma and other inflammatory diseases. Leukotrienes have been implicated as a contributing factor in a number of disease states, including Alzheimer's disease (Manev et al 2000).

The synthesis of leukotrienes may be influenced by polymorphisms of the promoter regions for leukotriene C(4) synthase. Leukotriene C(4) synthase is the initial enzyme in the pathway which produces leukotrienes from arachidonic acid. Although leukotrienes synthesized by LTC(4) play a role in the pathogenesis of asthma, the pathogenesis of this disorder, as well as other inflammatory diseases, is complex. The association between individual polymorphisms and the asthmatic phenotype has not been adequately defined.

Aspirin (sensitivity and asthma):

Approximately 10% of patients with asthma have a form in which symptoms are exacerbated by aspirin (as well as most other nonsteroidal anti-inflammatory agents). This syndrome is characterized by significant basal overproduction of cysteinyl leukotrienes (cysLT). This has been correlated to elevated expression of leukotriene C(4) synthase. The exacerbation of symptoms by aspirin-like drugs is related to inhibition of cyclooxygenase, the second pathway for arachidonic acid conversion, and results in overproduction of cysteinyl leukotrienes.

Several investigations have attempted to evaluate the relationship between polymorphisms and aspirin-sensitive asthma. The frequency of the (-444) allele appears to correlate with upregulation of the cys-leukotriene pathway. However, associations with the development of aspirin-induced asthma have been inconsistent. For example, this polymorphism was associated with a relative risk of 3.89 for the aspirin-intolerant phenotype in Polish patients. A subsequent study in the United States demonstrated that the C-444 allele was not statistically different among patients between aspirin-intolerant asthmatics, aspirin-tolerant asthmatics, and unaffected control subjects. In addition, functional studies have been unable to demonstrate significant upregulatory or downregulatory effects in the transcription of the leukotriene C4 synthetase gene related to the -444 allele (Van Sambeek et al 2000). Basal levels of specific leukotrienes (LTE4) and the increment of urinary LTE4 on venous aspirin challenge did not differ between wild-type homozygotes and carriers of the C-allele (Kawagishi et al 2002).

May Alter Pharmacodynamics of Aspirin (exacerbation of asthma), nonsteroidal anti-inflammatory agents (exacerbation of asthma), leukotriene receptor antagonists

May Affect Disease Predisposition of Asthma

Clinical Recommendations While a polymorphism in leukotriene C4 synthetase may contribute to the development of aspirin-intolerant asthma, it does not appear to be a single factor in regulating this response. It has been suggested that this gene may be in linkage disequilibrium with another mutation which may be more directly related to the phenomenon.
(Continued)

Leukotriene C4 Synthase *(Continued)*

References

Coffey M and Peters-Golden M, "Extending the Understanding of Leukotrienes in Asthma," *Curr Opin Allergy Clin Immunol*, 2003, 3(1):57-63.

Fowler SJ, Hall IP, Wilson AM, et al, "5-Lipoxygenase Polymorphism and *in vivo* Response to Leukotriene Receptor Antagonists," *Eur J Clin Pharmacol*, 2002, 58(3):187-90.

Kawagishi Y, Mita H, Taniguchi M, et al, "Leukotriene C4 Synthase Promoter Polymorphism in Japanese Patients With Aspirin-Induced Asthma," *J Allergy Clin Immunol*, 2002, 109(6):936-42.

Manev H, "5-Lipoxygenase Gene Polymorphism and Onset of Alzheimer's Disease," *Med Hypotheses*, 2000, 54(1):75-6.

Nanavaty U, Goldstein AD, and Levine SJ, "Polymorphisms in Candidate Asthma Genes," *Am J Med Sci*, 2001, 321(1):11-6.

Palmer LJ, Silverman ES, Weiss ST, et al, "Pharmacogenetics of Asthma," *Am J Respir Crit Care Med*, 2002, 165(7):861-6 (review).

Sanak M, Pierzchalska M, Bazan-Socha S, et al, "Enhanced Expression of the Leukotriene C(4) Synthase Due to Overactive Transcription of an Allelic Variant Associated With Aspirin-Intolerant Asthma," *Am J Respir Cell Mol Biol*, 2000, 23(3):290-6.

5-Lipoxygenase

Synonyms ALOX5; 5-LO; 5-LOX

Chromosome Location 10q11.2

Clinically-Important Polymorphisms

Three to six tandem repeats of GGGCGG in promoter region of the 5-lipoxygenase gene contribute to the clinical response to leukotriene receptor antagonists.

Mutant forms of the transcription factor binding region may be significantly less effective than the activity driven by the wild type transcription factor binding region.

Discussion Five lipoxygenase (5-LO) is a critical enzyme in the synthesis of leukotrienes from arachidonic acid. Leukotrienes mediate a number of smooth muscle effects, including bronchoconstriction. Increased expression of 5-lipoxygenase in pulmonary artery endothelial cells has been observed in pulmonary hypertension and has been associated with allergenic stimuli. *In situ* leukotriene blockade has been noted to decrease gene expression of 5-LO and its activator protein (FLAP) (Chu et al 2000). Mutations of the 5-LOX gene promoter have been reported to occur with a frequency as high as 25%. These mutations decrease expression of the 5-LOX gene.

A phenotype favoring allergic responses appears to be induced by leukotrienes. Although leukotrienes synthesized by 5-LO play a role in the pathogenesis of asthma, the association between genetic polymorphisms and the asthmatic phenotype has not been adequately defined.

Leukotriene receptor antagonists:

In 52 patients (40 homozygous wild type, 12 heterozygous), the influence of 5-lipoxygenase promoter region polymorphisms and response to leukotriene receptor antagonists were evaluated. An analysis of genotype and response to lipoxygenase inhibitors failed to demonstrate a significant difference between homozygous wild types and heterozygotes in terms of bronchodilator response or bronchial hyper-responsiveness with leukotriene receptor antagonists (Fowler et al 2002, Sampson et al 2000, Drazen et al 1999).

In an investigation of a possible correlation between polymorphisms of the core promoter region of the 5-lipoxygenase gene and clinical response to leukotriene receptor antagonists, no difference between homozygous wild types and heterozygotes could be identified in terms of bronchodilator response or bronchial hyper-responsiveness to adenosine monophosphate (Fowler et al 2002).

May Affect Disease Predisposition of Asthma

References
- Chu SJ, Tang LO, Watney E, et al, "*In situ* Amplification of 5-Lipoxygenase and 5-Lipoxygenase-Activating Protein in Allergic Airway Inflammation and Inhibition by Leukotriene Blockade," *J Immunol*, 2000, 165(8):4640-8.
- Drazen JM, Yandava CN, Dube L, et al, "Pharmacogenetic Association Between ALOX5 Promoter Genotype and the Response to Antiasthma Treatment," *Nat Genet*, 1999, 22(2):168-70.
- Fowler SJ, Hall IP, Wilson AM, et al, "5-Lipoxygenase Polymorphism and *in vivo* Response to Leukotriene Receptor Antagonists," *Eur J Clin Pharmacol*, 2002, 58(3):187-90.
- Sampson AP, Siddiqui S, Buchanan D, et al, "Variant LTC(4) Synthase Allele Modifies Cysteinyl Leukotriene Synthesis in Eosinophils and Predicts Clinical Response to Zafirlukast," *Thorax*, 2000, 55(Suppl 2):S28-31.

♦ **5-LO** *see* 5-Lipoxygenase *on page 208*

Low-Density Lipoprotein Receptor

Synonyms LDLR

Chromosome Location 19p13.3

Clinically-Important Polymorphisms AvaII (exon 13), HincII (exon 12), PvuII (intron 15) restriction fragment length polymorphisms

Discussion The LDLR is responsible for the hepatic uptake of low density lipoproteins from the plasma. Many mutations have been reported, and have been associated with forms of familial hypercholesterolemia. Familial hypercholesterolemia is an autosomal dominant disorder characterized by elevated low-density lipoproteins, as well as premature coronary artery disease.

HMG CoA reductase inhibitors:
The AvaII and PvuII polymorphisms were associated with the cholesterol-lowering response to fluvastatin in patients with primary hypercholesterolemia, with less reduction in total cholesterol, LDL cholesterol, and apolipoprotein B levels after 16 weeks among A+A+ (AvaII) and P+P+ (PvuII) homozygotes (Salazar et al 2000).

May Alter Pharmacokinetics of LDLR is not known to alter the metabolism of any drugs.

May Alter Pharmacodynamics of HMG CoA reductase inhibitors

May Affect Disease Predisposition of Hypercholesterolemia

Clinical Recommendations The association between the LDLR gene and clinical outcomes during HMG CoA reductase therapy should be determined before genotyping for this polymorphism is considered clinically useful.

Counseling Points Carrier status for a variant LDLR allele may increase the risk for hypercholesterolemia. Individuals should discuss
(Continued)

Low-Density Lipoprotein Receptor (Continued)

the implications of carrier status with their clinician or another healthcare professional. In addition, carriers of the variant allele should be encouraged to follow recommended guidelines for cholesterol screening.

References
Salazar LA, Hirata MH, Forti N, et al, "Pvu II Intron 15 Polymorphism at the LDL Receptor Gene Is Associated With Differences in Serum Lipid Concentrations in Subjects With Low and High Risk for Coronary Artery Disease From Brazil," *Clin Chim Acta*, 2000, 293(1-2):75-88.

- **5-LOX** see 5-Lipoxygenase on page 208
- **LTC(4) Synthase** see Leukotriene C4 Synthase on page 206
- **Matrix Metalloproteinase 3** see Stromelysin-1 on page 219
- **MDR-1** see P-Glycoprotein on page 213

Methylenetetrahydrofolate Reductase

Synonyms MHFR; MTHFR
Chromosome Location 1p36.3
Clinically-Important Polymorphisms C677T

Discussion Methylenetetrahydrofolate reductase regulates the intracellular folate pool which is used in the synthesis of DNA and protein. A homozygous variant, *C677T*, occurs in up to 10% of Caucasians. Homozygotes for this variant exhibit diminished activity (only 35% of normal enzyme capacity) and accumulate 5,10-methylenetetrahydrofolate, or CH2THF (Schwahn et al 2001).

Fluorouracil:
Severe myelosuppression was reported in breast cancer patients with the *C677T* polymorphism after receiving CMF (cyclophosphamide, methotrexate, and 5FU). An excess of CH2THF may increase the ability of 5FU to inhibit thymydilate synthetase, resulting in increased myelosuppression.

Raletrexid:
In a phase 1 trial with the thymydilate synthetase inhibitor, raletrexid, individuals with polymorphism of this enzyme had no toxicities associated with raletrexid (Schwahn et al 2001).

May Alter Pharmacodynamics of Fluorouracil, capecitabine

Clinical Recommendations Pending additional clinical investigation, analysis of MHFR polymorphisms are not recommended for routine clinical use.

References
Schwahn B and Rozen R, "Polymorphisms in the Methylenetetrahydrofolate Reductase Gene: Clinical Consequences," *Am J Pharmacogenomics*, 2001, 1(3):189-201 (review).

- **MHFR** see Methylenetetrahydrofolate Reductase on page 210
- **MMC-IA** see HLA-A1 on page 200
- **MMP3** see Stromelysin-1 on page 219
- **MTHFR** see Methylenetetrahydrofolate Reductase on page 210
- **Multidrug Resistance Gene** see P-Glycoprotein on page 213

N-Acetyltransferase 2 Enzyme

Synonyms NAT2

Chromosome Location 8p22

Clinically-Important Polymorphisms At least 11 single nucleotide polymorphisms contributing to the slow, rapid, and intermediate acetylator phenotypes

Discussion Acetylator phenotype may influence the activation and/or metabolism of a variety of compounds. For a number of medications metabolized by NAT2, the development of specific adverse events has been correlated to acetylator phenotype (see below).

Isoniazid:

Isoniazid (INH) is metabolized by hepatic N-acetylation to yield a variety of metabolites. These compounds include acetylhydrazine, which has been characterized as a potent hepatotoxin. INH can cause clinically-significant and even fatal hepatic injury in 1% of patients and elevated liver enzymes in 10% to 20% of patients. The frequency of hepatic injury has been correlated to acetylator phenotype.

Procainamide:

Slow acetylators are at risk of developing antinuclear antibodies and lupus-like syndrome during hydralazine or procainamide therapy (Woosley et al 1978).

Fast acetylators have increased conversion of procainamide to N-acetylprocainamide, its active metabolites possessing potent class III antiarrhythmic effects. In fast acetylators, a normal procainamide dose can lead to supratherapeutic levels of N-acetylprocainamide (NAPA), prolongation of the QT interval, and an increased risk for ventricular arrhythmias.

Hydralazine:

Slow acetylators are at risk of developing antinuclear antibodies and lupus-like syndrome during hydralazine therapy (Mansilla-Tinoco et al 1982).

Sulfonamides:

Adverse effects to sulfamethoxazole-trimethoprim, such as rash, granulocytopenia, or liver impairment, were noted to be considerably higher in children with mutations of the NAT2 encoding gene. It has been suggested that the NAT2 genotype may provides the basis for the detection of hypersensitivity to TMP-SMX (Zielinska et al 1998). No association was evident between the slow acetylator phenotype and leprosy treatment outcome, although the mean percentage of sulfamethazine acetylated in patients with the slow acetylator phenotype was significantly higher than that observed for the same phenotype in controls.

May Alter Pharmacokinetics of Hydralazine, isoniazid, procainamide, sulfonamides

References

Mansilla-Tinoco R, Harland SJ, Ryan PJ, et al, "Hydralazine, Antinuclear Antibodies, and the Lupus Syndrome," *Br Med J (Clin Res Ed)*, 1982, 284(6320):936-9.

(Continued)

N-Acetyltransferase 2 Enzyme *(Continued)*

Woosley RL, Drayer DE, Reidenberg MM, et al, "Effect of Acetylator Phenotype on the Rate at Which Procainamide Induces Antinuclear Antibodies and the Lupus Syndrome," *N Engl J Med*, 1978, 298(21):1157-9.

Zielinska E, Niewiarowski W, Bodalski J, et al, "Genotyping of the Arylamine N-acetyltransferase Polymorphism in the Prediction of Idiosyncratic Reactions to Trimethoprim-Sulfamethoxazole in Infants," *Pharm World Sci*, 1998, 20(3):123-30

NAD(P)H Quinone Oxidoreductase

Synonyms Diaphorase-4; DT-Diaphorase; EC 1.6.99.2; NQO1; Quinone Oxidoreductase

Chromosome Location 16q22.1

Clinically-Important Polymorphisms Three alleles of the human reduced nicotinamide adenine dinucleotide phosphate:quinone oxidoreductase-1 (NQO1) gene are known: Wild-type, *609C>T* variant, and *465C>T* variant; these are designed as NQO1*1 and NQO1*2, and NQO1*3

Discussion Mammalian NAD(P)H:quinone oxidoreductase (NQO1) catalyzes the two-electron reduction of quinones and plays one of the main roles in the bioactivation of quinoidal drugs. NQO1 has often been suggested to be involved in cancer prevention by means of detoxification of electrophilic quinones. Underactive variants of NQO1 seem to increase the risk of AML. NQO1 has been associated with the development of ALL (along with many other genetic factors), and the prognosis of patients with CYPIA1 and NQO1 variants has been noted to be worse than that of patients who lack these variants (Krajinovic et al 2001). NQO1 C609T has also been reported to be associated with lung cancer, colorectal cancer, and urological malignancies.

Mitomycin-C:
Studies have suggested that patients homozygous for a C to T transition at position 609 of the cDNA sequence of NQO1 may be resistant to mitomycin C. Resistance appears to result from a diminished activation of mitomycin C. In addition, gene expression has been shown to correlate with chemosensitivity (Pan et al 1995). However, several enzyme systems, including DTD, P450 reductase, GSH and GST may act in concert to determine chemosensitivity. This may include additive or antagonistic effects, depending on intracellular concentrations. An isolated mutation in NQO1 may not result in predictable effect on MMC activity (Phillips et al 2001).

May Alter Pharmacodynamics of Mitomycin C

May Affect Disease Predisposition of Secondary AML carcinogenesis

References

Krajinovic M, Labuda D, and Sinnett D, "Childhood Acute Lymphoblastic Leukemia: Genetic Determinants of Susceptibility and Disease Outcome," *Rev Environ Health*, 2001, 16(4):263-79 (review).

Pan SS, Forrest GL, Akman SA, et al, "NAD(P)H:Quinone Oxidoreductase Expression and Mitomycin C Resistance Developed by Human Colon Cancer HCT 116 Cells," *Cancer Res*, 1995, 55(2):330-5.

Phillips RM, Burger AM, Fiebig HH, et al, "Genotyping of NAD(P)H:Quinone Oxidoreductase (NQO1) in a Panel of Human Tumor Xenografts: Relationship Between Genotype

Status, NQO1 Activity, and the Response of Xenografts to Mitomycin C Chemotherapy *in vivo*(1)," *Biochem Pharmacol*, 2001, 62(10):1371-7.

- **NAT2** see N-Acetyltransferase 2 Enzyme *on page 211*
- **NQO1** see NAD(P)H Quinone Oxidoreductase *on page 212*
- **P-450 C18 11-Beta Hydroxylase** see Aldosterone Synthase *on page 160*

P-Glycoprotein

Synonyms ABC20; ABCB1; GP170; MDR-1; Multidrug Resistance Gene; PGP; PGY1

Chromosome Location 7q21.1

Clinically-Important Polymorphisms

MDR1*2: Synonymous *C3435T* polymorphism in exon 26; nonsynonymous SNP (*G2677T*) in exon 21; synonymous SNP (*C1236T*) in exon 12. These SNPs appear to be in linkage disequilibrium.

MDR1*2 has been identified in 62% of European Americans and 13% of African Americans.

Discussion Concentration of P-glycoprotein in intestinal epithelial cells and in a subset of lymphoid cells is substantially lower in people with the *T/T* genotype than those with the *C/C* genotype. A higher frequency of the *C/C* genotype has been reported in West Africans and African Americans (142 of 172 [83%] and 25 of 41 [61%], respectively), than in white people (139 of 537 [26%]) (p=<0.0001) (Schaeffeler et al 2001).

Digoxin:

In *in vitro* studies, the *3435T* allele was associated with twofold lower *MDR1* gene expression and reduced PGP activity compared to *3435C* allele (Hoffmeyer et al 2000). In healthy volunteers, plasma digoxin levels were 4 times higher in those with the *3435TT* genotype than *CC* homozygotes after a single, oral digoxin dose (Hoffmeyer et al 2000). However, these findings have not been consistently replicated.

The area under the plasma concentration-time curve from time zero to 4 hours [AUC(0-4)] and C_{max} values of digoxin were higher in subjects with the *3435TT* genotype than in those with the *3435CC*. Significant differences for AUC(0-4) and C_{max} were substantiated by haplotype analysis. Haplotype 12 (*2677G/3435T*), which had a frequency of 13.3% in a randomly drawn Caucasian sample (n=687), was associated with higher AUC(0-4) values than were found in noncarriers. Haplotype 11 (*2677G/3435C*) had lower AUC(0-4) values compared with those of noncarriers. Analysis of *MDR1* haplotypes is superior to unphased SNP analysis to predict *MDR1* (Johne et al 2002).

The bioavailability of digoxin in *G/G2677C/C3435*, *G/T2677C/T3435*, and *T/T2677T/T3435* subjects were 67.6% +/- 4.3%, 80.9% +/- 8.9%, and 87.1% +/- 8.4%, respectively, and the difference between *G/G2677C/C3435* and *T/T2677T/T3435* subjects was statistically significant (p=<.05). The *MDR1* variants were also associated with differences in disposition kinetics of digoxin, with the renal clearance being almost 32% lower in *T/T2677T/T3435*

(Continued)

P-Glycoprotein *(Continued)*

subjects (1.9 ± 0.1 mL/min/kg) than *G/G2677C/C3435* subjects (2.8 ± 0.3 mL/min/kg), and *G/T2677C/T3435* subjects having an intermediate value (2.1 ± 0.6 mL/min/kg).

Coadministration of clarithromycin did not consistently affect digoxin clearance or renal clearance. However, a significant increase in digoxin bioavailability was observed in *G/G2677C/C3435* subjects (67.6% ± 4.3% versus 85.4% ± 6.1%; p <.05) but not in the other 2 genotype groups (Kurata et al 2002).

Fexofenadine:

*MDR1*1* and *MDR1*2* variants were associated with differences in fexofenadine levels, consistent with the *in vitro* data, with the area under the plasma level-time curve being almost 40% greater in the **1/*1* genotype compared with the **2/*2* and the **1/*2* heterozygotes having an intermediate value, suggesting enhanced *in vivo* P-glycoprotein activity among subjects with the *MDR1*2* allele (Kim et al 2001).

Antiretroviral agents:

The influence of genotype on the efficacy of antiretroviral therapy was evaluated in 123 patients. Median drug concentrations in patients with the *MDR1 3435 TT*, *CT*, and *CC* genotypes were at the 30th, 50th, and 75th percentiles, respectively. Patients with the *MDR1 TT* genotype had a greater rise in CD4-cell count at 6 months after treatment than the *CT* or *CC* genotype, and the best recovery of naive CD4-cells. Therefore, the *MDR1* genotype appears to predict immune recovery after the initiation of antiretroviral treatment (Fellay et al 2002).

Defective PGP expression in HIV-1 infection has been noted to increase with the progression of HIV-1 infection. Larger studies of patients with HIV-1 infection are needed to determine the effects of opportunistic infection and antiretroviral therapy on the expression of PGP. Potentially, the expression of PGP may serve as another surrogate marker for the progression of HIV-1 infection (Andreana et al 1996).

Cyclosporine:

Although PGP is suspected to influence cyclosporine concentrations, some data suggests that the *MDR-1 C3435T* mutation (in addition to the CYP3A4-V variant) is not a major determinant of cyclosporine A efficacy in renal transplant recipients (von Ahsen et al 2001). No relationship between the pharmacokinetics of cyclosporine and *C3435T* genotype have been found (Min et al 2002).

Corticosteroids:

Glucocorticoids are known Pgp substrates. Inflammatory bowel disease (IBD), which is poorly responsive to medical therapy, has been noted to correlate to MDR expression. This may be related to the role of Pgp in determining the response of IBD patients to glucocorticoid therapy (Farrell et al 2000).

Paclitaxel:

Resistance to paclitaxel has been attributed to overexpression of P-glycoprotein (PGP) (Kao et al 2000).

Tacrolimus:

In a small series, a mutation at position 2677 in exon 21 of Pgp, as well as high tacrolimus concentrations and hepatic dysfunction were demonstrated as positive predictors of tacrolimus-induced neurotoxicity (Yamauchi et al 2002).

Nortriptyline (Orthostasis):

The multidrug resistance gene *MDR1* encodes a P-glycoprotein that regulates passage of many substances across the blood-brain barrier. A significant association was noted between nortriptyline-induced postural hypotension and *3435C>T*. Homozygosity for *3435T* may be a risk factor for nortriptyline-induced postural hypotension (Roberts et al 2002).

Phenytoin:

Although some of the interindividual differences in phenytoin metabolism can be attributed to polymorphisms in CYP2C9, a large component of individual variability remains still unexplained. A portion of this variability may be attributed to variable uptake by P-glycoprotein. Phenytoin plasma levels correlate with the *MDR-1 C3435T* polymorphism associated with intestinal PGP activity. The *MDR1*CC* genotype was found to be more common in individuals with low phenytoin levels.

In a regression analysis which included CYP2C9, 2C19, and MDR1, the number of mutant CYP2C9 alleles was a major determinant, and the number of *MDR1*T* alleles further contributed to the prediction of phenytoin plasma levels. CYP2C19*2 did not appear to contribute to individual variability. The regression equation explained 15.4% of the variability of phenytoin data (Kerb et al 2001).

May Alter Pharmacokinetics of Protease inhibitors, corticosteroids, cyclosporine, digoxin, fexofenadine, paclitaxel, tacrolimus, nortriptyline, phenytoin

References

Andreana A, Aggarwal S, Gollapudi S, et al, "Abnormal Expression of a 170-Kilodalton P-Glycoprotein Encoded by MDR1 Gene, a Metabolically Active Efflux Pump, in CD4+ and CD8+ T Cells From Patients With Human Immunodeficiency Virus Type 1 Infection," *AIDS Res Hum Retroviruses*, 1996, 12(15):1457-62.

Farrell RJ, Murphy A, Long A, et al, "High Multidrug Resistance (P-Glycoprotein 170) Expression in Inflammatory Bowel Disease Patients Who Fail Medical Therapy," *Gastroenterology*, 2000, 118(2):279-88.

Fellay J, Marzolini C, Meaden ER, et al, "Response to Antiretroviral Treatment in HIV-1-Infected Individuals With Allelic Variants of the Multidrug Resistance Transporter 1: A Pharmacogenetics Study," *Lancet*, 2002, 359(9300):30-6.

Hoffmeyer S, Burk O, von Richter O, et al, "Functional Polymorphisms of the Human Multidrug-Resistance Gene: Multiple Sequence Variations and Correlation of One Allele With P-Glycoprotein Expression and Activity *in vivo*," *Proc Natl Acad Sci U S A*, 2000, 97(7):3473-8.

Johne A, Kopke K, Gerloff T, et al, "Modulation of Steady-State Kinetics of Digoxin by Haplotypes of the P-Glycoprotein MDR1 Gene," *Clin Pharmacol Ther*, 2002, 72(5):584-94.

(Continued)

P-Glycoprotein *(Continued)*

Kao CH, Hsieh JF, Tsai SC, et al, "Quickly Predicting Chemotherapy Response to Paclitaxel-Based Therapy in Non-small Cell Lung Cancer by Early Technetium-99m Methoxyisobutylisonitrile Chest Single-Photon-Emission Computed Tomography," *Clin Cancer Res*, 2000, 6(3):820-4.

Kerb R, Aynacioglu AS, Brockmoller J, et al, "The Predictive Value of MDR1, CYP2C9, and CYP2C19 Polymorphisms for Phenytoin Plasma Levels," *Pharmacogenomics J*, 2001, 1(3):204-10.

Kim RB, Leake BF, Choo EF, et al, "Identification of Functionally Variant MDR1 Alleles Among European Americans and African Americans," *Clin Pharmacol Ther*, 2001, 70(2):189-99.

Kurata Y, Ieiri I, Kimura M, et al, "Role of Human MDR1 Gene Polymorphism in Bioavailability and Interaction of Digoxin, a Substrate of P-Glycoprotein," *Clin Pharmacol Ther*, 2002, 72(2):209-19

Min DI and Ellingrod VL, "C3435T Mutation in Exon 26 of the Human MDR1 Gene and Cyclosporine Pharmacokinetics in Healthy Subjects," *Ther Drug Monit*, 2002, 24(3):400-4.

Roberts RL, Joyce PR, Mulder RT, et al, "A Common P-Glycoprotein Polymorphism Is Associated With Nortriptyline-Induced Postural Hypotension in Patients Treated for Major Depression," *Pharmacogenomics J*, 2002, 2(3):191-6.

Schaeffeler E, Eichelbaum M, Brinkmann U, et al, "Frequency of C3435T Polymorphism of MDR1 Gene in African People," *Lancet*, 2001, 358(9279):383-4.

von Ahsen N, Richter M, Grupp C, et al, "No Influence of the MDR-1 C3435T Polymorphism or a CYP3A4 Promoter Polymorphism (CYP3A4-V Allele) on Dose-Adjusted Cyclosporin A Trough Concentrations or Rejection Incidence in Stable Renal Transplant Recipients," *Clin Chem*, 2001, 47(6):1048-52.

Yamauchi A, Ieiri I, Kataoka Y, et al, "Neurotoxicity Induced by Tacrolimus After Liver Transplantation: Relation to Genetic Polymorphisms of the ABCB1 (MDR1) Gene," *Transplantation*, 2002, 74(4):571-2.

- **PGP** *see P-Glycoprotein on page 213*
- **PGY1** *see P-Glycoprotein on page 213*

Platelet Fc Gamma Receptor

Synonyms Fc Gamma RIIa; FCG R2A

Chromosome Location 1q23

Clinically-Important Polymorphisms Nonsynonymous SNP in the extracellular domain of the receptor *(R131H)*

Discussion The platelet Fc gamma receptor is widely expressed on hematopoietic cells. There are two known alleles (*131R* and *131H*). These differ in their ability to bind to specific proteins. Clearance of autoantibody-sensitized platelets through Fc gamma receptors on phagocytic cells is one of the main mechanisms of thrombocytopenia in idiopathic thrombocytopenic purpura (ITP).

Heparin-induced thrombocytopenia (HIT) is a severe complication of heparin treatment. HIT antibodies activate platelets via the platelet Fc gamma receptor. The impact of this polymorphism on the clinical presentation and course of HIT is under investigation. It has been speculated that reduced clearance of immune complexes in patients with the *131R* allele may result in prolonged activation of endothelial cells and platelets, which may lead to thrombotic complications.

Heparin:

The *R131H* polymorphism has been associated with an increased risk of type II heparin-induced thrombocytopenia (HIT) (Carlsson et al 1998). In a study comparing healthy individuals, patients with a history of HIT, and patients with a history of thrombocytopenia from other causes, the frequency of the *131R/R* genotype was greater among those with a history of HIT than among the other two groups. In a subgroup of HIT patients studied prospectively, the *131R/R* genotype was more common among those who developed thromboembolic complications (Carlsson et al 1998).

May Alter Pharmacokinetics of Platelet Fc gamma receptor gene is not known to alter the metabolism of any drugs.

May Alter Pharmacodynamics of Heparin

Clinical Recommendations Data suggest that the Fc gamma receptor gene may be useful in identifying patients at high risk for developing HIT in whom alternative anticoagulant therapy should be initiated.

References

Carlsson LE, Santoso S, Baurichter G, et al, "Heparin-Induced Thrombocytopenia: New Insights Into the Impact of the FcgammaRIIa-R-H131 Polymorphism," *Blood*, 1998, 92(5):1526-31.

♦ **PROC** *see* Protein C *on page 217*

Protein C

Synonyms PROC

Chromosome Location 2q13-14

Clinically-Important Polymorphisms Numerous functional defects have been described which result in defective interaction with one or more substrate molecules, including thrombomodulin, phospholipids, factor Va, and factor VIIIa (type II deficiencies). In addition, decreased synthesis of normally functioning protein C has been described (type I).

SNPs at nucleotides -1654 (C/T), -1641 (A/G), and -1476 (A/T) have been identified in the protein C gene promoter region.

Discussion Protein C deficiency predisposes an individual to venous thrombosis and embolic events. First described in 1981, protein C is required to inactivate factor Va and factor VIIIa. Initially thrombomodulin is activated by thrombin. Protein C then combines with thrombomodulin resulting in the activation of Protein C. Activated protein C may combine with an additional molecule, protein S, on the platelet surface, where it inactivates factor Va and factor VIIIa.

Protein C deficiency is classified as a deficiency of functional protein (type I deficiency), or a functional defect in the synthesized protein in spite of normal circulating concentrations (type II deficiency). Approximately 0.2% of the general population are estimated to have a deficiency of protein C.

The combination of the *-C1654T* and *-A1641G* polymorphisms has been associated with protein C concentrations and risk of venous thromboembolism (Aiach et al 1999).

Warfarin:
  Skin necrosis is a rare, but potentially severe, complication of warfarin therapy. The risk of this reaction is increased in patients with deficiency in protein C and/or S.

(Continued)

Protein C *(Continued)*

May Alter Pharmacodynamics of Warfarin

Laboratory Evaluation Future studies may support genotyping for the protein C polymorphisms in potential warfarin users with a family history of thrombosis.

Clinical Recommendations Warfarin should be avoided or started in low doses with concurrent heparin therapy and gradually dose increases over several weeks in patients with a genetic predisposition for protein C deficiency.

References

Aiach M, Nicaud V, Alhenc-Gelas M, et al, "Complex Association of Protein C Gene Promoter Polymorphism With Circulating Protein C Levels and Thrombotic Risk," *Arterioscler Thromb Vasc Biol*, 1999, 19(6):1573-6.

Protein S

Chromosome Location 3p11-11.2

Clinically-Important Polymorphisms Numerous abnormalities have been reported, including deficiency in circulating concentrations (type I), unbound form of the protein (type III), and functional defects despite adequate circulating concentrations of protein (type II).

Discussion Protein S is a cofactor for the inactivation of factor Va and factor VIIIa. It acts in conjunction with protein C, which is the protein which is responsible for this inactivation (also see Protein C listing). Activated protein C combines with protein S on platelet surfaces to degrade factor Va and factor VIIIa. Protein S circulates in bound and unbound (free) forms.

Protein S deficiency may be classified according to the nature of the deficiency. Type I protein S deficiency results from inadequate synthesis of protein S, leading to low circulating levels of fully-functional protein. Type II deficiency is defined by functional defects in protein S molecules, which circulate in normal amounts. An unusual deficiency, type III, is related to altered protein binding of protein S, resulting in low concentrations of unbound protein S, although total concentrations are normal. In Caucasians, the incidence of protein S deficiency is between 1% to 5% of persons who experience a venous thrombotic event.

Warfarin:

Skin necrosis is a rare by potentially severe complication of warfarin therapy. The risk of this reaction is increased in patients with deficiency in protein C and/or S.

May Alter Pharmacodynamics of Warfarin

Laboratory Evaluation Future studies may support genotyping for the protein S polymorphisms in potential warfarin users with a family history of thrombosis.

Clinical Recommendations Warfarin should be avoided or started in low doses with concurrent heparin therapy and gradually dose increases over several weeks in patients with a genetic predisposition for protein S deficiency.

Prothrombin

Synonyms PT

Chromosome Location 11p11-12

Clinically-Important Polymorphisms G20210A

Discussion Prothrombin is the circulating precursor to thrombin, which catalyzes the conversion of fibrinogen into fibrin. The variant prothrombin gene results in higher circulating concentrations of thrombin, and results in a hypercoagulable state. Approximately 1% to 2% of the general population is heterozygous for the prothrombin gene mutation. It appears to be more common in Caucasians, and has been found to be relatively uncommon in the native populations of India, Korea, Africa, and North America. The highest rate of carriage has been in Spain, where rates as high as 6% have been reported. The *G20210A* mutation in the prothrombin gene is an established risk factor for venous thrombosis.

Oral contraceptives:

The risk of cerebral vein thrombosis is increased in patients with the prothrombin gene mutation. When coupled with oral contraceptive use, the risk of cerebral vein thrombosis in patients with the *G20210A* mutation was increased nearly 20-fold, resulting in an odds ratio of 149.3. Since cerebral vein thrombosis is a rare event, the authors concluded that screening for the prothrombin mutation would not be cost-effective (Martinelli et al 1998).

May Alter Pharmacokinetics of The prothrombin gene is not known to alter the pharmacokinetics of any drugs.

May Alter Pharmacodynamics of Oral contraceptives, estrogen

May Affect Disease Predisposition of Thrombosis

Laboratory Evaluation Screening for the *G20210A* polymorphism should be considered in potential oral contraceptive users with a positive family history of thrombosis.

Clinical Recommendations Individuals with the *20210A* allele who use oral contraceptives are at a markedly increased risk for thromboembolic events. Clinicians should consider alternative contraceptive methods in *20210A* allele carriers, especially if the factor V Leiden mutation is also present.

References

Martinelli I, Sacchi E, Landi G, et al, "High Risk of Cerebral-Vein Thrombosis in Carriers of a Prothrombin-Tene Mutation and in Users of Oral Contraceptives," *N Engl J Med*, 1998, 338(25):1793-7.

- ◆ **PT** *see* Prothrombin *on page 219*
- ◆ **Quinone Oxidoreductase** *see* NAD(P)H Quinone Oxidoreductase *on page 212*
- ◆ **SCN5A** *see* Cardiac Sodium Channel *on page 178*
- ◆ **SERT** *see* 5HT Transporter *on page 204*
- ◆ **SLC6A4** *see* 5HT Transporter *on page 204*

Stromelysin-1

Synonyms Matrix Metalloproteinase 3; MMP3

Chromosome Location 11q22.3

(Continued)

Stromelysin-1 *(Continued)*.

Clinically-Important Polymorphisms Presence of five (5A) or 6 (6A) adenines in the promoter region at nucleotide -1612 [-1612 (5A/6A)]

Discussion Stromelysin-1 is a member of the matrix metalloproteinase family and is believed to be involved in the remodeling of the extracellular matrix of atherosclerotic lesions. The *6A* allele has been associated with reduced stromelysin-1 activity and a faster progression of coronary atherosclerosis (as determined by angiography) (Ye et al 1996, de Maat et al 1999). The *5A* allele has been associated with an increased risk of acute myocardial infarction in patients with unstable angina.

HMG CoA reductase inhibitors:

Among men with coronary artery disease, pravastatin reduced the incidence of coronary artery restenosis and repeat angioplasty in those with the *5A6A* and *6A6A* genotypes, but not in those with the *5A5A* genotype (de Maat et al 1999).

May Alter Pharmacokinetics of Stromelysin-I is not known to alter the metabolism of any drugs.

May Alter Pharmacodynamics of HMG CoA reductase inhibitors

May Affect Disease Predisposition of Atherosclerosis

Clinical Recommendations Data suggest that the stromelysin-1 genotype may be useful in predicting regression of atherosclerotic lesions during HMG CoA reductase inhibitor therapy. However, the effect of this gene on clinical outcomes with HMG CoA reductase inhibitor therapy should be determined before genotyping for the stromelysin-1 polymorphism is considered clinically useful.

Counseling Points Carrier status for the *6A* allele has been associated with greater disease progression in individuals with coronary heart disease. Individuals with coronary heart disease who carry this allele should be encouraged to discuss the implications of their carrier status with their clinician or another healthcare professional.

References

de Maat MP, Jukema JW, Ye S, et al, "Effect of the Stromelysin-1 Promoter on Efficacy of Pravastatin in Coronary Atherosclerosis and Restenosis," *Am J Cardiol*, 1999, 83(6):852-6.

Ye S, Eriksson P, Hamsten A, et al, "Progression of Coronary Atherosclerosis Is Associated With a Common Genetic Variant of the Human Stromelysin-1 Promoter Which Results in Reduced Gene Expression," *J Biol Chem*, 1996, 271(22):13055-60.

Thiopurine Methyltransferase

Synonyms TPMT

Chromosome Location 6p22.3

Clinically-Important Polymorphisms Eight TPMT alleles have been described. However, three alleles account for the majority (80% to 95%) of cases with low or intermediate activity. These are *TPMT*2* (G238C), *TPMT*3A*, and *TPMT*3C*.

Discussion Thiopurine methyltransferase is responsible for the S-methylation of a number of compounds, including azathioprine, mercaptopurine, and thioguanine. A deficiency in this enzyme is inherited as an autosomal recessive trait. Approximately 10% of Caucasians exhibit diminished activity of this enzyme, while 0.3% of patients are estimated to carry a complete deficiency of the enzyme. Patients with diminished, but detectable activity, are heterozygous at the TPMT locus. Of note, aminosalicylates have been identified as inhibitors of this enzyme. Individuals with diminished activity are susceptible to severe, and potentially life-threatening, toxicities following exposure to these agents. The use of standard dosages in a patient with a complete deficiency of this enzyme may be fatal.

Azathiopurine:
A heart-transplant patient receiving azathioprine as part of routine immunosuppression developed severe neutropenia and sepsis. Ultimately, the episode proved to be fatal, and the patient was demonstrated to have very low TPMT activity (Schutz et al 1993).

Mercaptopurine:
The inactivation of mercaptopurine requires metabolism by the enzyme thiopurine methyl transferase (TPMT). TPMT polymorphisms were noted to be substantially over-represented in a population of patients with severe adverse reactions to mercaptopurine (Evans et al 2001).

Some centers have initiated screening programs for patients who are to receive chemotherapy of ALL (McLeod et al 1999, McLeod et al 2000). Dosage adjustments, including a 10-fold to 15-fold reduction in TPMT-deficient patients, and a twofold decrease in heterozygotes, have been reported to permit successful treatment without substantial toxicity.

May Alter Pharmacokinetics of Azathioprine, mercaptopurine (6-MP)

Laboratory Evaluation Commercial testing available

References
Black AJ, McLeod HL, Capell HA, et al, "Thiopurine Methyltransferase Genotype Predicts Therapy-Limiting Severe Toxicity From Azathioprine," *Ann Intern Med*, 1998, 129(9):716-8.

Evans WE, Hon YY, Bomgaars, et al, "Preponderance of Thiopurine S-Methyltransferase Deficiency and Heterozygosity Among Patients Intolerant to Mercaptopurine or Azathioprine," *J Clin Oncol*, 2001, 19(8):2293-301.

McLeod HL, Coulthard S, Thomas AE, et al, "Analysis of Thiopurine Methyltransferase Variant Alleles in Childhood Acute Lymphoblastic Leukaemia," *Br J Hem*, 1999, 105(3):696-700.

McLeod HL, Krynetski EY, Relling MV, et al, "Genetic Polymorphism of Thiopurine Methyltransferase and Its Clinical Relevance for Childhood Acute Lymphoblastic Leukemia," *Leukemia*, 2000, 14(4):567-72 (review).

Schutz E, Gummert J, Mohr F, et al, "Azathioprine-Induced Myelosuppression in Thiopurine Methyltransferase Deficient Heart Transplant Recipient," *Lancet*, 1993, 341(8842):436.

Thymydilate Synthetase
Synonyms TS; TSER; TYMS

Chromosome Location 18p11.32

Clinically-Important Polymorphisms TSER*2, TSER*3, TSER*4, TSER*9

(Continued)

Thymydilate Synthetase *(Continued)*

Discussion Thymydilate synthetase catalyzes the reductive methylation of 5,10-methylenetetrahydrofolate to dTMP. Thymydilate synthetase is an important synthetic enzyme, since this reaction is a critical step in the synthesis of DNA.

Fluorouracil:

Thymydilate synthetase is the intracellular target of 5FU. Several studies have demonstrated that induction of this enzyme is associated with fluorouracil resistance, while decreases in tumor expression of thymydilate synthetase are associated with improved sensitivity (Wang et al 2001). Endogenous expression is regulated by polymorphic variation in the enhancer region of the thymydilate synthetase gene. A tandem repeat sequence of 28 base pairs may be repeated for two, three, four, or nine copies (*TSER*2, TSER*3, TSER*4, TSER*9*). The presence of these repeated sequences alters enzyme activity. *In vitro* assays demonstrate that thymydilate synthetase expression of the *TSER*3* is 2.6 times that of the *TSER*2* allele.

In an analysis of patients with colon cancer, 29% of patients were homozygous for *TSER*3*, 16% were homozygous for the *TSER*2*, and 55% were heterozygous (Marsh 2001). From a total of 24 patients who received 5FU, 40% of responders were homozygous for the *TSER*2*, compared to 20% of nonresponders. Individuals with the *TSER*2* polymorphism had an improvement in median survival as compared to the *TSER*3* (16 months vs 12 months).

May Alter Pharmacokinetics of Fluorouracil

Clinical Recommendations Currently, routine clinical assessment of TS polymorphisms is not recommended.

References

Marsh S, McKay JA, Cassidy J, et al, "Polymorphism in the Thymidylate Synthase Promoter Enhancer Region in Colorectal Cancer," *Int J Oncol*, 2001, 19(2):383-6.

Wang W, Marsh S, Cassidy J, et al, "Pharmacogenomic Dissection of Resistance to Thymidylate Synthase Inhibitors," *Cancer Res*, 2001, 61(14):5505-10.

TNF-Alpha

Clinically-Important Polymorphisms The *-308G/A* polymorphism has been associated with schizophrenia and a recent report showed a trend of significance between the *A* allele and weight gain from antipsychotics (Basile et al 2001). Those genotyped as *A/A* homozygous had a twofold greater weight gain.

Discussion TNF-alpha is a cytokine that mediates local phagocytic-cell emigration and activation as well as release of lipid-derived mediators such as prostaglandin E2, thromboxane, and platelet-activating factor.

TNF-alpha has been shown to be expressed in adipose tissue and skeletal muscle and TNF-alpha receptors have been discovered in adipocytes (Hotamisligil et al 1995, Saghizadeh et al 1996). Increased levels of TNF-alpha are known to cause sedation, hyperinsulinemia, insulin resistance, and hypertriglyceridemia (Hotamisligil et al 1995, Argiles et al 1997).

Clozapine:
Clozapine increases serum levels of TNF-alpha (Hinze-Selch et al 2000, Haack et al 1999, Pollmacher et al 1996).

Olanzapine:
Olanzapine produced a rapid increase in soluble TNF-alpha receptor 1 and TNF-alpha receptor 2 following 1 week of treatment in patients with schizophrenia (Schuld et al 2000).

Tricyclic antidepressants:
Activate the TNF-alpha system by increasing TNF-alpha or its soluble receptors (Hinze-Selch et al 2000).

May Alter Pharmacodynamics of Clozapine, olanzapine, amitriptyline, paroxetine

References
Argiles JM, Lopez-Soriano J, Busquets S, et al, "Journey From Cachexia to Obesity by TNF," *FASEB J*, 1997 11(10):743-51 (review).

Basile VS, Masellis M, McIntyre RS, et al, "Genetic Dissection of Atypical Antipsychotic-Induced Weight Gain: Novel Preliminary Data on the Pharmacogenetic Puzzle," *J Clin Psychiatry*, 2001, 62(Suppl 23):45-66 (review).

Haack M, Hinze-Selch D, Fenzel T, et al, "Plasma Levels of Cytokines and Soluble Cytokine Receptors in Psychiatric Patients Upon Hospital Admission: Effects of Confounding Factors and Diagnosis," *J Psychiatr Res*, 1999, 33(5):407-18.

Hinze-Selch D, Schuld A, Kraus T, et al, "Effects of Antidepressants on Weight and on the Plasma Levels of Leptin, TNF-Alpha and Soluble TNF Receptors: A Longitudinal Study in Patients Treated With Amitriptyline or Paroxetine," *Neuropsychopharmacology*, 2000, 23(1):13-9.

Hotamisligil GS, Arner P, Caro JF, et al, "Increased Adipose Tissue Expression of Tumor Necrosis Factor-Alpha in Human Obesity and Insulin Resistance," *J Clin Invest*, 1995, 95(5):2409-15.

Pollmacher T, Hinze-Selch D, and Mullington J, "Effects of Clozapine on Plasma Cytokine and Soluble Cytokine Receptor Levels," *J Clin Psychopharmacol*, 1996, 16(5):403-9.

Saghizadeh M, Ong JM, Garvey WT, et al, "The Expression of TNF Alpha by Human Muscle. Relationship to Insulin Resistance," *J Clin Invest*, 1996, 97(4):1111-6.

Schuld A, Kraus T, Haack M, et al, "Plasma Levels of Cytokines and Soluble Cytokine Receptors During Treatment With Olanzapine," *Schizophr Res*, 2000, 43(2-3):164-6.

♦ **TPH** see Tryptophan Hydroxylase *on page 223*

♦ **TPMT** see Thiopurine Methyltransferase *on page 220*

Tryptophan Hydroxylase
Synonyms TPH

Chromosome Location 12q15 (neuronal); 11p15.3-p14

Clinically-Important Polymorphisms A218C in intron 7

Discussion Tryptophan hydroxylase is the enzyme responsible for the conversion of tryptophan to 5-hydroxytryptophan. It is the rate-limiting enzyme in the production of serotonin. It is not regulated by end product inhibition and brain tryptophan hydroxylase is not saturated with substrate. Therefore, the amount of substrate, tryptophan, controls the amount of serotonin produced.

Several studies have evaluated the role of tryptophan hydroxylase in affective disorders and suicidal behavior. The *A218C* polymorphism was evaluated in 927 patients (527 bipolar, 400 unipolar) in the European Collaborative Project on Affective Disorder study. This study failed to detect an association between the *A218C* polymorphism of
(Continued)

Tryptophan Hydroxylase *(Continued)*

the tryptophan hydroxylase gene and bipolar and unipolar disorders in the samples (Souery et al 2001).

Paroxetine:

Genetic variation in the tryptophan hydroxylase gene has been evaluated with respect to a difference in response to paroxetine therapy. The *A218C* variant was characterized in 121 patients with major depression. The *TPH*A/A* and *TPH*A/C* variants were associated with a decreased response to paroxetine as compared to patients with the *TPH*C/C* genotype (p=0.005). Other variables, including the presence of psychotic features, baseline severity of depressive symptoms and paroxetine plasma level, were not associated with the outcome. *TPH* gene variants may be a marker and/or modulator of paroxetine antidepressant activity (Serretti et al 2001).

May Alter Pharmacodynamics of Paroxetine

May Affect Disease Predisposition of Affective disorder

References
Serretti A, Zanardi R, Cusin C, et al, "Tryptophan Hydroxylase Gene Associated With Paroxetine Antidepressant Activity," *Eur Neuropsychopharmacol*, 2001, 11(5):375-80.

Souery D, Van Gestel S, Massat I, et al, "Tryptophan Hydroxylase Polymorphism and Suicidality in Unipolar and Bipolar Affective Disorders: A Multicenter Association Study," *Biol Psychiatry*, 2001, 49(5):405-9.

- **TS** *see* Thymydilate Synthetase *on page 221*
- **TSER** *see* Thymydilate Synthetase *on page 221*
- **TYMS** *see* Thymydilate Synthetase *on page 221*

UDP-Glucuronosyltransferase

Synonyms UGT 1A1

Chromosome Location 2q37

Clinically-Important Polymorphisms UGT 1A1*28

Discussion Irinotecan's active metabolite, SN-38 is glucuronidated by the 1A1 isoform of UDP-glucuronyl transferase. A clinically-important variant, UGT *1A1*28*, occurs in 3% to 10% of the population, is a risk factor for both severe neutropenia and diarrhea. This appears to be related to a decrease in the glucuronidation of SN-38, resulting in a prolongation of its half-life and an increase in the AUC (Innocenti et al 2002, Iyer et al 1999). It should be noted that severe toxicity may develop in individuals who do not carry this allele, indicating other factors are involved in the development of severe irinotecan toxicity.

May Alter Pharmacokinetics of Irinotecan

Clinical Recommendations Currently, routine clinical assessment of UGT polymorphisms is not recommended.

References
Innocenti F and Ratain MJ, "Update on Pharmacogenetics in Cancer Chemotherapy," *Eur J Cancer*, 2002, 38(5):639-44 (review).

Iyer L, Hall D, Das S, et al, "Phenotype-Genotype Correlation of *in vitro* SN-38 (Active Metabolite of Irinotecan) and Bilirubin Glucuronidation in Human Liver Tissue With UGT1A1 Promoter Polymorphism," *Clin Pharmacol Ther*, 1999, 65(5):576-82.

- **UGT 1A1** *see* UDP-Glucuronosyltransferase *on page 224*
- **val-COMT** *see* COMT *on page 180*

INDEX OF POLYMORPHISMS AND DRUGS POTENTIALLY AFFECTED

INDEX OF POLYMORPHISMS AND DRUGS POTENTIALLY AFFECTED

Aldosterone Synthase
Amlodipine and Benazepril 49
Benazepril 55
Candesartan 59
Captopril 60
Cilazapril 64
Enalapril 78
Eprosartan 78
Fosinopril 90
Irbesartan 99
Lisinopril 104
Lisinopril and Hydrochlorothiazide 104
Losartan 105
Losartan and Hydrochlorothiazide 105
Moexipril 114
Olmesartan 122
Perindopril Erbumine 126
Quinapril 133
Ramipril 135
Spirapril 141
Telmisartan 145
Trandolapril 150
Valsartan 153

Alpha-1 Adrenergic Receptor
Acetophenazine 45
Amitriptyline 48
Amitriptyline and Chlordiazepoxide 48
Amitriptyline and Perphenazine 49
Amoxapine 49
Aripiprazole 51
ChlorproMAZINE 63
Chlorprothixene 63
ClomiPRAMINE 66
Clozapine 67
Desipramine 71
Doxepin 76
Droperidol 76
Flupenthixol 88
Fluphenazine 88
Haloperidol 93
Imipramine 97
Loxapine 106
Mesoridazine 109
Mirtazapine 113
Molindone 114
Nefazodone 117
Nortriptyline 120
Olanzapine 121
Perphenazine 126
Pimozide 127
Prochlorperazine 130
Protriptyline 133
Quetiapine 133

INDEX OF POLYMORPHISMS AND DRUGS POTENTIALLY AFFECTED

Risperidone 137
Thioridazine 147
Thiothixene 148
Trazodone 151
Trifluoperazine 151
Trimipramine 152
Ziprasidone 157

Alpha-Adducin

Bendroflumethiazide 55
Chlorothiazide 63
Chlorthalidone 63
Furosemide 91
Hydrochlorothiazide 94
Hydroflumethiazide 95
Indapamide 98
Lisinopril and Hydrochlorothiazide 104
Losartan and Hydrochlorothiazide 105
Methyclothiazide 110
Metolazone 111
Polythiazide 128
Torsemide 150
Trichlormethiazide 151

Angiotensin-Converting Enzyme

Amlodipine and Benazepril 49
Atorvastatin 53
Benazepril 55
Bezafibrate 56
Bisoprolol 56
Candesartan 59
Captopril 60
Carvedilol 61
Cilazapril 64
Clofibrate 66
Enalapril 78
Eprosartan 78
Fenofibrate 86
Fluvastatin 89
Fosinopril 90
Gemfibrozil 91
Irbesartan 99
Lisinopril 104
Lisinopril and Hydrochlorothiazide 104
Losartan 105
Losartan and Hydrochlorothiazide 105
Lovastatin 106
Metoprolol 112
Moexipril 114
Olmesartan 122
Perindopril Erbumine 126
Pravastatin 129
Quinapril 133
(Continued)

227

INDEX OF POLYMORPHISMS AND DRUGS POTENTIALLY AFFECTED

Angiotensin-Converting Enzyme *(Continued)*
    Ramipril 135
    Rosuvastatin 138
    Simvastatin 140
    Spirapril 141
    Telmisartan 145
    Trandolapril 150
    Valsartan 153

Angiotensin II Type 1 Receptor
    Amlodipine and Benazepril 49
    Benazepril 55
    Candesartan 59
    Captopril 60
    Cilazapril 64
    Enalapril 78
    Eprosartan 78
    Fosinopril 90
    Irbesartan 99
    Lisinopril 104
    Lisinopril and Hydrochlorothiazide 104
    Losartan 105
    Losartan and Hydrochlorothiazide 105
    Moexipril 114
    Olmesartan 122
    Perindopril Erbumine 126
    Quinapril 133
    Ramipril 135
    Spirapril 141
    Telmisartan 145
    Trandolapril 150
    Valsartan 153

Angiotensinogen
    Amlodipine and Benazepril 49
    Benazepril 55
    Candesartan 59
    Captopril 60
    Cilazapril 64
    Enalapril 78
    Eprosartan 78
    Fosinopril 90
    Irbesartan 99
    Lisinopril 104
    Lisinopril and Hydrochlorothiazide 104
    Losartan 105
    Losartan and Hydrochlorothiazide 105
    Moexipril 114
    Olmesartan 122
    Perindopril Erbumine 126
    Quinapril 133
    Ramipril 135
    Spirapril 141
    Telmisartan 145

INDEX OF POLYMORPHISMS AND DRUGS POTENTIALLY AFFECTED

    Trandolapril 150
    Valsartan 153

Apolipoprotein E
    Atorvastatin 53
    Donepezil 75
    Fluvastatin 89
    Galantamine 91
    Lovastatin 106
    Pravastatin 129
    Rivastigmine 137
    Rosuvastatin 138
    Simvastatin 140
    Tacrine 144

Beta-1 Adrenergic Receptor
    Acebutolol 44
    Atenolol 53
    Betaxolol 56
    Bisoprolol 56
    Carvedilol 61
    Esmolol 80
    Metoprolol 112
    Nadolol 116
    Propranolol 132
    Sotalol 141
    Timolol 148

Beta-2 Adrenergic Receptor
    Albuterol 46
    Bitolterol 56
    Fenoterol 86
    Fluticasone and Salmeterol 89
    Formoterol 90
    Ipratropium and Albuterol 98
    Isoproterenol 99
    Levalbuterol 102
    Metaproterenol 109
    Pirbuterol 128
    Salmeterol 138
    Terbutaline 146

Beta-3 Adrenergic Receptor
    Clozapine 67
    Sibutramine 140

Beta-Fibrinogen
    Atorvastatin 53
    Fluvastatin 89
    Lovastatin 106
    Pravastatin 129
    Rosuvastatin 138
    Simvastatin 140

Bradykinin B2 Receptor
    Amlodipine and Benazepril 49
    Benazepril 55
    Captopril 60
    (Continued)

INDEX OF POLYMORPHISMS AND DRUGS POTENTIALLY AFFECTED

Bradykinin B2 Receptor *(Continued)*
    Cilazapril 64
    Enalapril 78
    Fosinopril 90
    Lisinopril 104
    Lisinopril and Hydrochlorothiazide 104
    Moexipril 114
    Perindopril Erbumine 126
    Quinapril 133
    Ramipril 135
    Spirapril 141
    Trandolapril 150

BRCA Genes
    Estradiol and Medroxyprogesterone 81
    Ethinyl Estradiol and Desogestrel 82
    Ethinyl Estradiol and Drospirenone 82
    Ethinyl Estradiol and Ethynodiol Diacetate 83
    Ethinyl Estradiol and Etonogestrel 83
    Ethinyl Estradiol and Levonorgestrel 83
    Ethinyl Estradiol and Norelgestromin 83
    Ethinyl Estradiol and Norethindrone 84
    Ethinyl Estradiol and Norgestimate 84
    Ethinyl Estradiol and Norgestrel 84
    Levonorgestrel 103
    MedroxyPROGESTERone 107
    Mestranol and Norethindrone 109
    Norethindrone 119
    Norgestrel 119

Cardiac Potassium Ion Channel
    Amiodarone 48
    Amitriptyline 48
    Amitriptyline and Chlordiazepoxide 48
    Amitriptyline and Perphenazine 49
    Arsenic Trioxide 51
    Bepridil 55
    Bretylium 57
    ChlorproMAZINE 63
    Chlorprothixene 63
    Cisapride 64
    Clarithromycin 65
    Disopyramide 74
    Dofetilide 75
    Domperidone 75
    Droperidol 76
    Erythromycin 79
    Erythromycin and Sulfisoxazole 80
    Flecainide 87
    Fluoxetine 88
    Flupenthixol 88
    Foscarnet 90
    Gatifloxacin 91
    Halofantrine 93

INDEX OF POLYMORPHISMS AND DRUGS POTENTIALLY AFFECTED

Haloperidol 93
Ibutilide 97
Imipramine 97
Indapamide 98
Isradipine 100
Levofloxacin 102
Levomethadyl Acetate Hydrochloride 102
Loxapine 106
Mesoridazine 109
Moxifloxacin 115
Octreotide 121
Pentamidine 125
Pimozide 127
Procainamide 130
Quetiapine 133
Quinidine 134
Risperidone 137
Sotalol 141
Sparfloxacin 141
Thioridazine 147
Thiothixene 148
Tizanidine 149
Ziprasidone 157
Zuclopenthixol 158

Cardiac Sodium Channel
Amiodarone 48
Amitriptyline 48
Amitriptyline and Chlordiazepoxide 48
Amitriptyline and Perphenazine 49
Arsenic Trioxide 51
Bepridil 55
Bretylium 57
ChlorproMAZINE 63
Chlorprothixene 63
Cisapride 64
Clarithromycin 65
Disopyramide 74
Dofetilide 75
Domperidone 75
Droperidol 76
Erythromycin 79
Erythromycin and Sulfisoxazole 80
Flecainide 87
Fluoxetine 88
Flupenthixol 88
Foscarnet 90
Gatifloxacin 91
Halofantrine 93
Haloperidol 93
Ibutilide 97
Imipramine 97
Indapamide 98
Isradipine 100
Levofloxacin 102
(Continued)

INDEX OF POLYMORPHISMS AND DRUGS POTENTIALLY AFFECTED

Cardiac Sodium Channel *(Continued)*
Levomethadyl Acetate Hydrochloride 102
Loxapine 106
Mesoridazine 109
Moxifloxacin 115
Octreotide 121
Pentamidine 125
Pimozide 127
Procainamide 130
Quetiapine 133
Quinidine 134
Risperidone 137
Sotalol 141
Sparfloxacin 141
Thioridazine 147
Thiothixene 148
Tizanidine 149
Ziprasidone 157

Cholesteryl Ester Transfer Protein
Atorvastatin 53
Bezafibrate 56
Clofibrate 66
Fenofibrate 86
Fluvastatin 89
Gemfibrozil 91
Lovastatin 106
Pravastatin 129
Rosuvastatin 138
Simvastatin 140

COMT
Acetaminophen and Codeine 44
Acetaminophen and Phenyltoloxamine 45
Acetaminophen and Tramadol 45
Alfentanil 47
Aspirin and Codeine 52
Belladonna and Opium 55
Buprenorphine 57
Buprenorphine and Naloxone 58
Butalbital, Acetaminophen, Caffeine, and Codeine 58
Butalbital, Aspirin, Caffeine, and Codeine 59
Butorphanol 59
Codeine 67
Dihydrocodeine, Aspirin, and Caffeine 73
Fentanyl 86
Hydrocodone and Acetaminophen 94
Hydrocodone and Aspirin 94
Hydrocodone and Ibuprofen 95
Hydromorphone 96
Levomethadyl Acetate Hydrochloride 102
Levorphanol 103
Meperidine 108
Meperidine and Promethazine 108
Methadone 110

232

INDEX OF POLYMORPHISMS AND DRUGS POTENTIALLY AFFECTED

Methotrimeprazine 110
Morphine Sulfate 115
Nalbuphine 116
Opium Tincture 122
Oxycodone 123
Oxycodone and Acetaminophen 123
Oxycodone and Aspirin 123
Oxymorphone 124
Paregoric 124
Pentazocine 125
Pentazocine Combinations 125
Promethazine and Codeine 131
Propoxyphene 132
Propoxyphene and Acetaminophen 132
Propoxyphene and Aspirin 132
Remifentanil 135
Sufentanil 142
Tramadol 150

CYP1A2

Aminophylline 48
Betaxolol 56
ClomiPRAMINE 66
Clozapine 67
Cyclobenzaprine 69
Dacarbazine 69
Doxepin 76
Estradiol 80
Estradiol and Medroxyprogesterone 81
Estrogens (Conjugated A/Synthetic) 81
Estrogens (Conjugated/Equine) 81
Estrogens (Esterified) 82
Estropipate 82
Flutamide 89
Fluvoxamine 90
Guanabenz 93
Mexiletine 112
Mirtazapine 113
Pimozide 127
Propranolol 132
Rifabutin 136
Riluzole 136
Ropinirole 138
Tacrine 144
Theophylline 147
Thiothixene 148
Trifluoperazine 151

CYP2C9

Amiodarone 48
Bosentan 56
Carvedilol 61
Dicumarol 72
Erythromycin and Sulfisoxazole 80
Fluoxetine 88
(Continued)

233

INDEX OF POLYMORPHISMS AND DRUGS POTENTIALLY AFFECTED

CYP2C9 *(Continued)*

- Fosphenytoin ... 90
- Glimepiride ... 92
- GlipiZIDE ... 92
- Ifosfamide ... 97
- Ketamine ... 101
- Losartan ... 105
- Losartan and Hydrochlorothiazide ... 105
- Montelukast ... 115
- Nateglinide ... 117
- Paclitaxel ... 124
- Phenytoin ... 127
- Pioglitazone ... 128
- Propofol ... 131
- Rifampin ... 136
- Rosiglitazone ... 138
- Selegiline ... 139
- Sertraline ... 139
- SulfaDIAZINE ... 143
- Sulfamethoxazole and Trimethoprim ... 143
- Sulfinpyrazone ... 143
- SulfiSOXAZOLE ... 144
- Tamoxifen ... 145
- TOLBUTamide ... 149
- Torsemide ... 150
- Trimethoprim ... 152
- Voriconazole ... 155
- Warfarin ... 155
- Zafirlukast ... 156
- Zopiclone ... 157

CYP2C19

- Carisoprodol ... 61
- Citalopram ... 64
- ClomiPRAMINE ... 66
- Cyclophosphamide ... 69
- Diazepam ... 72
- Escitalopram ... 80
- Fosphenytoin ... 90
- Ifosfamide ... 97
- Imipramine ... 97
- Lansoprazole ... 102
- Mephobarbital ... 108
- Methsuximide ... 110
- Moclobemide ... 114
- Nilutamide ... 118
- Omeprazole ... 122
- Pentamidine ... 125
- Phenobarbital ... 127
- Phenytoin ... 127
- Propranolol ... 132
- Rabeprazole ... 134
- Sertraline ... 139
- Trimipramine ... 152

INDEX OF POLYMORPHISMS AND DRUGS POTENTIALLY AFFECTED

CYP2D6

- Acetaminophen and Codeine ... 44
- Acetaminophen and Tramadol ... 45
- Amiodarone ... 48
- Amitriptyline and Perphenazine ... 49
- Aspirin and Codeine ... 52
- Atomoxetine ... 53
- Azelastine ... 54
- Betaxolol ... 56
- BuPROPion ... 58
- Butalbital, Acetaminophen, Caffeine, and Codeine ... 58
- Butalbital, Aspirin, Caffeine, and Codeine ... 59
- Carvedilol ... 61
- Chlorpheniramine ... 63
- Cimetidine ... 64
- Clemastine ... 65
- ClomiPRAMINE ... 66
- Cocaine ... 67
- Codeine ... 67
- Dexmedetomidine ... 71
- Dihydrocodeine, Aspirin, and Caffeine ... 73
- Flecainide ... 87
- Fluoxetine ... 88
- Haloperidol ... 93
- Methadone ... 110
- Metoprolol ... 112
- Mexiletine ... 112
- Oxycodone ... 123
- Oxycodone and Acetaminophen ... 123
- Oxycodone and Aspirin ... 123
- Paroxetine ... 124
- Pergolide ... 126
- Perphenazine ... 126
- Pimozide ... 127
- Promethazine and Codeine ... 131
- Propafenone ... 131
- Quinidine ... 134
- Quinine ... 134
- Ritonavir ... 137
- Ropinirole ... 138
- Thioridazine ... 147
- Timolol ... 148
- Tramadol ... 150

CYP3A4

- Alfentanil ... 47
- Alprazolam ... 47
- Amitriptyline and Chlordiazepoxide ... 48
- Amlodipine ... 49
- Amlodipine and Benazepril ... 49
- Aprepitant ... 50
- Aripiprazole ... 51
- Atorvastatin ... 53
- Benzphetamine ... 55
- Bisoprolol ... 56

(Continued)

INDEX OF POLYMORPHISMS AND DRUGS POTENTIALLY AFFECTED

CYP3A4 *(Continued)*

- Bosentan 56
- Bromazepam 57
- Bromocriptine 57
- Buprenorphine 57
- Buprenorphine and Naloxone 58
- BusPIRone 58
- Busulfan 58
- Carbamazepine 60
- Chlordiazepoxide 62
- Chlorpheniramine 63
- Cisapride 64
- Citalopram 64
- Clarithromycin 65
- Clobazam 65
- Clonazepam 66
- Clorazepate 67
- Cocaine 67
- Colchicine 68
- CycloSPORINE 69
- Dantrolene 70
- Dapsone 70
- Diazepam 72
- Digitoxin 73
- Dihydroergotamine 73
- Diltiazem 74
- Disopyramide 74
- Docetaxel 75
- Doxepin 76
- DOXOrubicin 76
- Eletriptan 77
- Eplerenone 78
- Ergoloid Mesylates 79
- Ergonovine 79
- Ergotamine 79
- Erythromycin 79
- Erythromycin and Sulfisoxazole 80
- Escitalopram 80
- Ethosuximide 85
- Etoposide 85
- Felbamate 85
- Felodipine 86
- Fentanyl 86
- Flurazepam 88
- Flutamide 89
- Halofantrine 93
- Haloperidol 93
- Ifosfamide 97
- Imatinib 97
- Irinotecan 99
- Isosorbide Dinitrate 100
- Isradipine 100
- Ketamine 101
- Levomethadyl Acetate Hydrochloride 102

INDEX OF POLYMORPHISMS AND DRUGS POTENTIALLY AFFECTED

Lidocaine 103
Lidocaine and Prilocaine 104
Lovastatin 106
Mefloquine 108
Methadone 110
Methylergonovine 111
Methysergide 111
Midazolam 112
Mirtazapine 113
Modafinil 114
Moricizine 115
Nateglinide 117
Nefazodone 117
NiCARdipine 118
NIFEdipine 118
Nimodipine 118
Nisoldipine 119
Nitrendipine 119
Paclitaxel 124
Pergolide 126
Phencyclidine 127
Pimozide 127
Pioglitazone 128
Quetiapine 133
Quinidine 134
Repaglinide 136
Sertraline 139
Sibutramine 140
Sildenafil 140
Simvastatin 140
Sirolimus 141
Spiramycin 141
Sufentanil 142
Tacrolimus 144
Tamsulosin 145
Teniposide 146
Theophylline 147
Tiagabine 148
Tolterodine 149
Trazodone 151
Triazolam 151
Trimipramine 152
Venlafaxine 154
Verapamil 154
VinBLAStine 154
VinCRIStine 155
Vinorelbine 155
Zolpidem 157
Zonisamide 157
Zopiclone 157

D2 Receptor

Acetophenazine 45
Amitriptyline and Perphenazine 49
Aripiprazole 51
(Continued)

INDEX OF POLYMORPHISMS AND DRUGS POTENTIALLY AFFECTED

D2 Receptor *(Continued)*
- ChlorproMAZINE 63
- Chlorprothixene 63
- Clozapine 67
- Droperidol 76
- Flupenthixol 88
- Fluphenazine 88
- Haloperidol 93
- Loxapine 106
- Mesoridazine 109
- Metoclopramide 111
- Molindone 114
- Olanzapine 121
- Perphenazine 126
- Pimozide 127
- Prochlorperazine 130
- Quetiapine 133
- Risperidone 137
- Thioridazine 147
- Thiothixene 148
- Trifluoperazine 151
- Ziprasidone 157

D3 Receptor
- Aripiprazole 51
- Clozapine 67
- Haloperidol 93
- Olanzapine 121
- Risperidone 137
- Ziprasidone 157

D4 Receptor
- Clozapine 67
- Haloperidol 93
- Risperidone 137

Dihydropyrimidine Dehydrogenase
- Capecitabine 60
- Fluorouracil 87

Epithelial Sodium Channel Beta-Subunit
- Amiloride 47

Factor V
- Estradiol 80
- Estradiol and Medroxyprogesterone 81
- Estrogens (Conjugated A/Synthetic) 81
- Estrogens (Conjugated/Equine) 81
- Estrogens (Conjugated/Equine) and Medroxyprogesterone 81
- Estrogens (Esterified) 82
- Estropipate 82
- Ethinyl Estradiol and Desogestrel 82
- Ethinyl Estradiol and Drospirenone 82
- Ethinyl Estradiol and Ethynodiol Diacetate 83
- Ethinyl Estradiol and Etonogestrel 83
- Ethinyl Estradiol and Levonorgestrel 83
- Ethinyl Estradiol and Norelgestromin 83

INDEX OF POLYMORPHISMS AND DRUGS POTENTIALLY AFFECTED

    Ethinyl Estradiol and Norethindrone 84
    Ethinyl Estradiol and Norgestimate 84
    Ethinyl Estradiol and Norgestrel 84

Glucose-6-Phosphate Dehydrogenase
    Chloramphenicol 62
    Chloroquine 62
    Dapsone 70
    Dimercaprol 74
    Erythromycin and Sulfisoxazole 80
    Furazolidone 91
    Hydroxychloroquine 96
    Lidocaine and Prilocaine 104
    Mafenide 107
    Methylene Blue 110
    Nalidixic Acid 116
    Nitrofurantoin 119
    Primaquine 130
    Probenecid 130
    Quinidine 134
    Quinine 134
    Rasburicase 135
    Silver Sulfadiazine 140
    Sulfacetamide 142
    SulfaDIAZINE 143
    Sulfadoxine and Pyrimethamine 143
    Sulfamethoxazole and Trimethoprim 143
    Sulfasalazine 143
    SulfiSOXAZOLE 144

Glycoprotein IIIa Receptor
    Abciximab 44
    Aspirin 51
    Aspirin and Codeine 52
    Aspirin and Dipyridamole 52
    Atorvastatin 53
    Cilostazol 64
    Clopidogrel 66
    Dipyridamole 74
    Eptifibatide 78
    Fluvastatin 89
    Hydrocodone and Aspirin 94
    Ipratropium and Albuterol 98
    Lovastatin 106
    Oxycodone and Aspirin 123
    Pravastatin 129
    Rosuvastatin 138
    Simvastatin 140
    Ticlopidine 148
    Tirofiban 149

G-Protein Beta-3 Subunit
    Amitriptyline 48
    Amitriptyline and Chlordiazepoxide 48
    Amitriptyline and Perphenazine 49
    Amoxapine 49
    (Continued)

INDEX OF POLYMORPHISMS AND DRUGS POTENTIALLY AFFECTED

G-Protein Beta-3 Subunit *(Continued)*

- Bendroflumethiazide 55
- Chlorothiazide 63
- Chlorthalidone 63
- Citalopram 64
- ClomiPRAMINE 66
- Clozapine 67
- Desipramine 71
- Doxepin 76
- Escitalopram 80
- Fluoxetine 88
- Fluvoxamine 90
- Hydrochlorothiazide 94
- Hydroflumethiazide 95
- Imipramine 97
- Indapamide 98
- Lisinopril and Hydrochlorothiazide 104
- Losartan and Hydrochlorothiazide 105
- Methyclothiazide 110
- Metolazone 111
- Mirtazapine 113
- Nefazodone 117
- Nortriptyline 120
- Paroxetine 124
- Polythiazide 128
- Protriptyline 133
- Sertraline 139
- Trazodone 151
- Trichlormethiazide 151
- Trimipramine 152

Gs Protein Alpha-Subunit

- Acebutolol 44
- Amitriptyline 48
- Amitriptyline and Chlordiazepoxide 48
- Amitriptyline and Perphenazine 49
- Amoxapine 49
- Atenolol 53
- Betaxolol 56
- Bisoprolol 56
- Carvedilol 61
- Citalopram 64
- ClomiPRAMINE 66
- Clozapine 67
- Desipramine 71
- Doxepin 76
- Escitalopram 80
- Esmolol 80
- Fluoxetine 88
- Fluvoxamine 90
- Imipramine 97
- Metoprolol 112
- Mirtazapine 113
- Nadolol 116

INDEX OF POLYMORPHISMS AND DRUGS POTENTIALLY AFFECTED

    Nefazodone 117
    Nortriptyline 120
    Paroxetine 124
    Propranolol 132
    Protriptyline 133
    Sertraline 139
    Sotalol 141
    Timolol 148
    Trazodone 151
    Trimipramine 152

Histamine 1 and 2 Receptors
    Clozapine 67
    Olanzapine 121

HLA-A1
    Clozapine 67

5HT1A Receptor
    Aripiprazole 51
    Clozapine 67
    Ziprasidone 157

5HT2A Receptor
    Aripiprazole 51
    Clozapine 67
    Olanzapine 121
    Risperidone 137
    Ziprasidone 157

5HT2C Receptor
    Aripiprazole 51
    Clozapine 67
    Olanzapine 121
    Risperidone 137
    Ziprasidone 157

5HT6 Receptor
    Clozapine 67
    Olanzapine 121

5HT Transporter
    Citalopram 64
    Clozapine 67
    Escitalopram 80
    Fluoxetine 88
    Fluvoxamine 90
    Paroxetine 124
    Sertraline 139

Human Leukocyte Antigen
    Abacavir 44

Leukotriene C4 Synthase
    Aspirin 51
    Aspirin and Codeine 52
    Aspirin and Dipyridamole 52
    Celecoxib 61
    Diclofenac 72
    (Continued)

INDEX OF POLYMORPHISMS AND DRUGS POTENTIALLY AFFECTED

Leukotriene C4 Synthase *(Continued)*
    Diclofenac and Misoprostol 72
    Diflunisal 73
    Etodolac 85
    Fenoprofen 86
    Flurbiprofen 89
    Hydrocodone and Aspirin 94
    Hydrocodone and Ibuprofen 95
    Ibuprofen 96
    Indomethacin 98
    Ipratropium and Albuterol 98
    Ketoprofen 101
    Ketorolac 101
    Meclofenamate 107
    Mefenamic Acid 108
    Meloxicam 108
    Montelukast 115
    Nabumetone 116
    Naproxen 117
    Oxaprozin 123
    Oxycodone and Aspirin 123
    Piroxicam 128
    Rofecoxib 137
    Sulindac 144
    Tiaprofenic Acid 148
    Tolmetin 149
    Valdecoxib 153
    Zafirlukast 156

5-Lipoxygenase
    Montelukast 115
    Zafirlukast 156

Low-Density Lipoprotein Receptor
    Atorvastatin 53
    Fluvastatin 89
    Lovastatin 106
    Pravastatin 129
    Rosuvastatin 138
    Simvastatin 140

Methylenetetrahydrofolate Reductase
    Fluorouracil 87
    Raltitrexed 135

N-Acetyltransferase 2 Enzyme
    Erythromycin and Sulfisoxazole 80
    HydrALAZINE 94
    Isoniazid 99
    Procainamide 130
    Sulfacetamide 142
    SulfaDIAZINE 143
    Sulfamethoxazole and Trimethoprim 143
    SulfiSOXAZOLE 144

NAD(P)H Quinone Oxidoreductase
    Mitomycin 113

INDEX OF POLYMORPHISMS AND DRUGS POTENTIALLY AFFECTED

None known

Acyclovir	45
Alendronate	46
Allopurinol	47
Amoxicillin	49
Amoxicillin and Clavulanate Potassium	50
Azithromycin	54
Benzonatate	55
Budesonide	57
Cefdinir	61
Cefprozil	61
Cephalexin	62
Cetirizine	62
Ciprofloxacin	64
Clindamycin	65
Clonidine	66
Desloratadine	71
Dextroamphetamine and Amphetamine	72
Doxazosin	76
Doxycycline	76
Esomeprazole	80
Famotidine	85
Ferrous Sulfate	87
Fluconazole	87
Fluticasone	89
Gabapentin	91
GlyBURIDE	92
Glyburide and Metformin	92
Insulin Preparations	98
Latanoprost	102
Levothyroxine	103
Loratadine	105
Lorazepam	105
Meclizine	107
Metaxalone	109
Metformin	109
Methylphenidate	111
MethylPREDNISolone	111
Metronidazole	112
Minocycline	113
Mometasone Furoate	114
Mupirocin	116
Olopatadine	122
Pantoprazole	124
Penicillin V Potassium	125
Potassium Chloride	128
PredniSONE	129
Promethazine	131
Raloxifene	134
Risedronate	137
Spironolactone	142
Sumatriptan	144
Temazepam	145
Terazosin	146

(Continued)

INDEX OF POLYMORPHISMS AND DRUGS POTENTIALLY AFFECTED

None known *(Continued)*

Tetracycline 146
Topiramate 150
Triamcinolone 151
Valacyclovir 153
Valproic Acid and Derivatives 153

P-Glycoprotein

Amiodarone 48
Amitriptyline 48
Amitriptyline and Chlordiazepoxide 48
Amitriptyline and Perphenazine 49
Aspirin and Dipyridamole 52
Atorvastatin 53
Azelastine 54
Carvedilol 61
ChlorproMAZINE 63
Cimetidine 64
Clarithromycin 65
CycloSPORINE 69
Desipramine 71
Dexrazoxane 71
Digoxin 73
Diltiazem 74
Dipyridamole 74
Disulfiram 75
Doxepin 76
Erythromycin 79
Erythromycin and Sulfisoxazole 80
Felodipine 86
Fexofenadine 87
Fluphenazine 88
Haloperidol 93
Hydrocortisone 95
HydrOXYzine 96
Imipramine 97
Itraconazole 100
Ivermectin 100
Ketoconazole 101
Lidocaine 103
Lidocaine and Prilocaine 104
Lovastatin 106
Maprotiline 107
Mefloquine 108
Midazolam 112
Mifepristone 113
Mitomycin 113
Nefazodone 117
Nelfinavir 118
NiCARdipine 118
NIFEdipine 118
Nitrendipine 119
Nortriptyline 120
Ofloxacin 121

INDEX OF POLYMORPHISMS AND DRUGS POTENTIALLY AFFECTED

Paclitaxel	124
Phenytoin	127
Probenecid	130
Prochlorperazine	130
Progesterone	131
Propafenone	131
Propranolol	132
Quinidine	134
Quinine	134
Ranitidine	135
Reserpine	136
Rifampin	136
Ritonavir	137
Saquinavir	139
Simvastatin	140
Tacrolimus	144
Tamoxifen	145
Testosterone	146
Trimipramine	152
Verapamil	154
VinBLAStine	154

Platelet Fc Gamma Receptor
Heparin	93

Protein C
Warfarin	155

Protein S
Warfarin	155

Prothrombin
Estradiol	80
Estradiol and Medroxyprogesterone	81
Estrogens (Conjugated A/Synthetic)	81
Estrogens (Conjugated/Equine)	81
Estrogens (Conjugated/Equine) and Medroxyprogesterone	81
Estrogens (Esterified)	82
Estropipate	82
Ethinyl Estradiol and Desogestrel	82
Ethinyl Estradiol and Drospirenone	82
Ethinyl Estradiol and Ethynodiol Diacetate	83
Ethinyl Estradiol and Etonogestrel	83
Ethinyl Estradiol and Levonorgestrel	83
Ethinyl Estradiol and Norelgestromin	83
Ethinyl Estradiol and Norethindrone	84
Ethinyl Estradiol and Norgestimate	84
Ethinyl Estradiol and Norgestrel	84
Levonorgestrel	103
MedroxyPROGESTERone	107
Mestranol and Norethindrone	109
Norethindrone	119
Norgestrel	119

Stromelysin-1
Atorvastatin	53
Fluvastatin	89
(Continued)	

INDEX OF POLYMORPHISMS AND DRUGS POTENTIALLY AFFECTED

Stromelysin-1 *(Continued)*
- Lovastatin 106
- Pravastatin 129
- Rosuvastatin 138
- Simvastatin 140

Thiopurine Methyltransferase
- Azathioprine 54
- Mercaptopurine 109
- Thioguanine 147

Thymydilate Synthetase
- Fluorouracil 87

TNF-Alpha
- Amitriptyline 48
- Amitriptyline and Chlordiazepoxide 48
- Amitriptyline and Perphenazine 49
- Clozapine 67
- Olanzapine 121
- Paroxetine 124

Tryptophan Hydroxylase
- Paroxetine 124

UDP-Glucuronosyltransferase
- Irinotecan 99

ALPHABETICAL INDEX

ALPHABETICAL INDEX

Abacavir	44
ABC20 see P-Glycoprotein	213
ABCB1 see P-Glycoprotein	213
Abciximab	44
Abilify™ see Aripiprazole	51
Accolate® see Zafirlukast	156
AccuNeb™ see Albuterol	46
Accupril® see Quinapril	133
ACE see Angiotensin-Converting Enzyme	163
ACE see Captopril	60
Acebutolol	44
Aceon® see Perindopril Erbumine	126
Acetaminophen and Codeine	44
Acetaminophen and Hydrocodone see Hydrocodone and Acetaminophen	94
Acetaminophen and Oxycodone see Oxycodone and Acetaminophen	123
Acetaminophen and Phenyltoloxamine	45
Acetaminophen and Propoxyphene see Propoxyphene and Acetaminophen	132
Acetaminophen and Tramadol	45
Acetaminophen, Caffeine, Codeine, and Butalbital see Butalbital, Acetaminophen, Caffeine, and Codeine	58
Acetophenazine	45
Acetoxymethylprogesterone see MedroxyPROGESTERone	107
Acetylsalicylic Acid see Aspirin	51
Achromycin see Tetracycline	146
Aciclovir see Acyclovir	45
Aciphex® see Rabeprazole	134
Actiq® see Fentanyl	86
Actonel® see Risedronate	137
Actos® see Pioglitazone	128
Acular® see Ketorolac	101
Acular® PF see Ketorolac	101
ACV see Acyclovir	45
Acycloguanosine see Acyclovir	45
Acyclovir	45
Adalat® CC see NIFEdipine	118
Adalat® XL® (Can) see NIFEdipine	118
ADDA see Alpha-Adducin	162
Adderall® see Dextroamphetamine and Amphetamine	72
Adderall XR™ see Dextroamphetamine and Amphetamine	72
Adoxa™ see Doxycycline	76
ADR see DOXOrubicin	76
ADRB1 see Beta-1 Adrenergic Receptor	171
ADRB2 see Beta-2 Adrenergic Receptor	171
ADRB3 see Beta-3 Adrenergic Receptor	174
Adria see DOXOrubicin	76
Adriamycin® (Can) see DOXOrubicin	76
Adriamycin PFS® see DOXOrubicin	76
Adriamycin RDF® see DOXOrubicin	76
Adrucil® see Fluorouracil	87
Advair™ Diskus® see Fluticasone and Salmeterol	89
Advil® [OTC] see Ibuprofen	96

ALPHABETICAL INDEX

Advil® Children's [OTC] see Ibuprofen 96
Advil® Infants' Concentrated Drops [OTC] see Ibuprofen 96
Advil® Junior [OTC] see Ibuprofen 96
Advil® Migraine [OTC] see Ibuprofen 96
Aerius® (Can) see Desloratadine 71
Aggrastat® see Tirofiban 149
Aggrenox™ see Aspirin and Dipyridamole 52
AGT see Angiotensinogen 167
AG TR1 see Angiotensin II Type 1 Receptor 166
A-hydroCort® see Hydrocortisone 95
Airomir (Can) see Albuterol 46
Akne-Mycin® see Erythromycin 79
AK-Sulf® see Sulfacetamide 142
Alavert™ [OTC] see Loratadine 105
Albert® Glyburide (Can) see GlyBURIDE 92
Albert® Tiafen (Can) see Tiaprofenic Acid 148
Albuterol 46
Albuterol and Ipratropium see Ipratropium and Albuterol 98
Aldactone® see Spironolactone 142
Aldosterone Synthase 160
Alendronate 46
Alertec® (Can) see Modafinil 114
Alesse® see Ethinyl Estradiol and Levonorgestrel 83
Aleve® [OTC] see Naproxen 117
Alfenta® see Alfentanil 47
Alfentanil 47
Allegra® see Fexofenadine 87
Aller-Chlor® [OTC] see Chlorpheniramine 63
Allopurinol 47
Allopurinol Sodium Injection see Allopurinol 47
Aloprim™ see Allopurinol 47
Alora® see Estradiol 80
ALOX5 see 5-Lipoxygenase 208
Alpha-1 Adrenergic Receptor 161
Alpha-Adducin 162
Alprazolam 47
Alprazolam Intensol® see Alprazolam 47
Altace® see Ramipril 135
Alti-Acyclovir (Can) see Acyclovir 45
Alti-Alprazolam (Can) see Alprazolam 47
Alti-Amiodarone (Can) see Amiodarone 48
Alti-Amoxi-Clav® (Can) see Amoxicillin and Clavulanate Potassium ... 50
Alti-Azathioprine (Can) see Azathioprine 54
Alti-Captopril (Can) see Captopril 60
Alti-Clindamycin (Can) see Clindamycin 65
Alti-Clobazam (Can) see Clobazam 65
Alti-Clonazepam (Can) see Clonazepam 66
Alti-Desipramine (Can) see Desipramine 71
Alti-Diltiazem CD (Can) see Diltiazem 74
Alti-Divalproex (Can) see Valproic Acid and Derivatives 153
Alti-Domperidone (Can) see Domperidone 75
Alti-Doxazosin (Can) see Doxazosin 76
Alti-Fluoxetine (Can) see Fluoxetine 88
Alti-Flurbiprofen (Can) see Flurbiprofen 89

ALPHABETICAL INDEX

Alti-Fluvoxamine (Can) *see* Fluvoxamine	90
Alti-Metformin (Can) *see* Metformin	109
Alti-Minocycline (Can) *see* Minocycline	113
Alti-Moclobemide (Can) *see* Moclobemide	114
Alti-MPA (Can) *see* MedroxyPROGESTERone	107
Alti-Nadolol (Can) *see* Nadolol	116
Alti-Nortriptyline (Can) *see* Nortriptyline	120
Alti-Ranitidine (Can) *see* Ranitidine	135
Alti-Salbutamol (Can) *see* Albuterol	46
Alti-Sotalol (Can) *see* Sotalol	141
Alti-Sulfasalazine (Can) *see* Sulfasalazine	143
Alti-Terazosin (Can) *see* Terazosin	146
Alti-Ticlopidine (Can) *see* Ticlopidine	148
Alti-Timolol (Can) *see* Timolol	148
Alti-Trazodone (Can) *see* Trazodone	151
Alti-Verapamil (Can) *see* Verapamil	154
Alti-Zopiclone (Can) *see* Zopiclone	157
Altocor™ *see* Lovastatin	106
Alupent® *see* Metaproterenol	109
Amaryl® *see* Glimepiride	92
Ambien® *see* Zolpidem	157
A-Methapred® *see* MethylPREDNISolone	111
Amiloride	47
2-Amino-6-Mercaptopurine *see* Thioguanine	147
2-Amino-6-Trifluoromethoxy-Benzothiazole *see* Riluzole	136
Aminophylline	48
Amiodarone	48
Amitriptyline	48
Amitriptyline and Chlordiazepoxide	48
Amitriptyline and Perphenazine	49
Amlodipine	49
Amlodipine and Benazepril	49
Amlodipine Besylate *see* Amlodipine	49
Amoxapine	49
Amoxicillin	49
Amoxicillin and Clavulanate Potassium	50
Amoxicillin and Clavulanic Acid *see* Amoxicillin and Clavulanate Potassium	50
Amoxil® *see* Amoxicillin	49
Amoxycillin *see* Amoxicillin	49
Amphetamine and Dextroamphetamine *see* Dextroamphetamine and Amphetamine	72
Anafranil® *see* ClomiPRAMINE	66
Anandron® (Can) *see* Nilutamide	118
Anaprox® *see* Naproxen	117
Anaprox® DS *see* Naproxen	117
Andriol® (Can) *see* Testosterone	146
Androderm® *see* Testosterone	146
AndroGel® *see* Testosterone	146
Andropository (Can) *see* Testosterone	146
Anestacon® *see* Lidocaine	103
Anexsia® *see* Hydrocodone and Acetaminophen	94
Angiotensin-Converting Enzyme	163
Angiotensin II Type 1 Receptor	166

ALPHABETICAL INDEX

Angiotensinogen 167
Ansaid® see Flurbiprofen 89
Ansamycin see Rifabutin 136
Antabuse® see Disulfiram 75
Antihist-1® [OTC] see Clemastine 65
Antivert® see Meclizine 107
Anturane see Sulfinpyrazone 143
Anucort-HC® see Hydrocortisone 95
Anusol-HC® see Hydrocortisone 95
Anusol® HC-1 [OTC] see Hydrocortisone 95
APAP and Tramadol see Acetaminophen and Tramadol 45
Apo®-Acebutolol (Can) see Acebutolol 44
Apo®-Acyclovir (Can) see Acyclovir 45
Apo®-Allopurinol (Can) see Allopurinol 47
Apo®-Alpraz (Can) see Alprazolam 47
Apo®-Amitriptyline (Can) see Amitriptyline 48
Apo®-Amoxi (Can) see Amoxicillin 49
Apo®-Amoxi-Clav (Can) see Amoxicillin and Clavulanate Potassium
. . . . 50
Apo®-Atenol (Can) see Atenolol 53
Apo®-Azathioprine (Can) see Azathioprine 54
Apo®-Bromazepam (Can) see Bromazepam 57
Apo® Bromocriptine (Can) see Bromocriptine 57
Apo®-Buspirone (Can) see BusPIRone 58
Apo®-Butorphanol (Can) see Butorphanol 59
Apo®-Capto (Can) see Captopril 60
Apo®-Carbamazepine (Can) see Carbamazepine 60
Apo®-Carbamazepine CR (Can) see Carbamazepine 60
Apo®-Cephalex (Can) see Cephalexin 62
Apo®-Cetirizine (Can) see Cetirizine 62
Apo®-Chlordiazepoxide (Can) see Chlordiazepoxide 62
Apo®-Chlorpromazine (Can) see ChlorproMAZINE 63
Apo®-Chlorthalidone (Can) see Chlorthalidone 63
Apo®-Cimetidine (Can) see Cimetidine 64
Apo®-Clomipramine (Can) see ClomiPRAMINE 66
Apo®-Clonazepam (Can) see Clonazepam 66
Apo®-Clonidine (Can) see Clonidine 66
Apo®-Clorazepate (Can) see Clorazepate 67
Apo®-Cyclobenzaprine (Can) see Cyclobenzaprine 69
Apo®-Desipramine (Can) see Desipramine 71
Apo®-Diazepam (Can) see Diazepam 72
Apo®-Diclo (Can) see Diclofenac 72
Apo®-Diclo Rapide (Can) see Diclofenac 72
Apo®-Diclo SR (Can) see Diclofenac 72
Apo®-Diflunisal (Can) see Diflunisal 73
Apo®-Diltiaz (Can) see Diltiazem 74
Apo®-Diltiaz CD (Can) see Diltiazem 74
Apo®-Diltiaz SR (Can) see Diltiazem 74
Apo®-Dipyridamole FC (Can) see Dipyridamole 74
Apo®-Divalproex (Can) see Valproic Acid and Derivatives 153
Apo®-Domperidone (Can) see Domperidone 75
Apo®-Doxazosin (Can) see Doxazosin 76
Apo®-Doxepin (Can) see Doxepin 76
Apo®-Doxy (Can) see Doxycycline 76

ALPHABETICAL INDEX

Apo®-Doxy Tabs (Can) *see* Doxycycline 76
APOE *see* Apolipoprotein E.. 168
Apo®-Erythro Base (Can) *see* Erythromycin 79
Apo®-Erythro E-C (Can) *see* Erythromycin 79
Apo®-Erythro-ES (Can) *see* Erythromycin 79
Apo®-Erythro-S (Can) *see* Erythromycin 79
Apo®-Etodolac (Can) *see* Etodolac 85
Apo®-Famotidine (Can) *see* Famotidine 85
Apo®-Fenofibrate (Can) *see* Fenofibrate 86
Apo®-Feno-Micro (Can) *see* Fenofibrate 86
Apo®-Ferrous Sulfate (Can) *see* Ferrous Sulfate 87
Apo®-Fluconazole (Can) *see* Fluconazole 87
Apo®-Fluoxetine (Can) *see* Fluoxetine 88
Apo®-Fluphenazine (Can) *see* Fluphenazine 88
Apo®-Fluphenazine Decanoate (Can) *see* Fluphenazine 88
Apo®-Flurazepam (Can) *see* Flurazepam 88
Apo®-Flurbiprofen (Can) *see* Flurbiprofen 89
Apo®-Flutamide (Can) *see* Flutamide 89
Apo®-Fluvoxamine (Can) *see* Fluvoxamine 90
Apo®-Furosemide (Can) *see* Furosemide 91
Apo®-Gabapentin (Can) *see* Gabapentin 91
Apo®-Gemfibrozil (Can) *see* Gemfibrozil 91
Apo®-Glyburide (Can) *see* GlyBURIDE 92
Apo®-Haloperidol (Can) *see* Haloperidol 93
Apo®-Haloperidol LA (Can) *see* Haloperidol 93
Apo®-Hydralazine (Can) *see* HydrALAZINE 94
Apo®-Hydro (Can) *see* Hydrochlorothiazide 94
Apo®-Hydroxyzine (Can) *see* HydrOXYzine 96
Apo®-Ibuprofen (Can) *see* Ibuprofen 96
Apo®-Imipramine (Can) *see* Imipramine 97
Apo®-Indapamide (Can) *see* Indapamide 98
Apo®-Indomethacin (Can) *see* Indomethacin 98
Apo®-ISDN (Can) *see* Isosorbide Dinitrate 100
Apo®-K (Can) *see* Potassium Chloride 128
Apo®-Keto (Can) *see* Ketoprofen 101
Apo®-Ketoconazole (Can) *see* Ketoconazole 101
Apo®-Keto-E (Can) *see* Ketoprofen 101
Apo®-Ketorolac (Can) *see* Ketorolac 101
Apo®-Ketorolac Injectable (Can) *see* Ketorolac 101
Apo®-Keto SR (Can) *see* Ketoprofen 101
Apolipoprotein E.. 168
Apo®-Lisinopril (Can) *see* Lisinopril 104
Apo®-Loratadine (Can) *see* Loratadine 105
Apo®-Lorazepam (Can) *see* Lorazepam 105
Apo®-Lovastatin (Can) *see* Lovastatin 106
Apo®-Loxapine (Can) *see* Loxapine 106
Apo®-Mefenamic (Can) *see* Mefenamic Acid 108
Apo®-Metformin (Can) *see* Metformin 109
Apo®-Methoprazine (Can) *see* Methotrimeprazine 110
Apo®-Metoclop (Can) *see* Metoclopramide 111
Apo®-Metoprolol (Can) *see* Metoprolol 112
Apo®-Metronidazole (Can) *see* Metronidazole 112
Apo®-Midazolam (Can) *see* Midazolam 112
Apo®-Minocycline (Can) *see* Minocycline 113

ALPHABETICAL INDEX

Apo®-Moclobemide (Can) *see* Moclobemide 114
Apo®-Nabumetone (Can) *see* Nabumetone 116
Apo®-Nadol (Can) *see* Nadolol 116
Apo®-Napro-Na (Can) *see* Naproxen 117
Apo®-Napro-Na DS (Can) *see* Naproxen 117
Apo®-Naproxen (Can) *see* Naproxen 117
Apo®-Naproxen SR (Can) *see* Naproxen 117
Apo®-Nefazodone (Can) *see* Nefazodone 117
Apo®-Nifed (Can) *see* NIFEdipine 118
Apo®-Nifed PA (Can) *see* NIFEdipine 118
Apo®-Nitrofurantoin (Can) *see* Nitrofurantoin 119
Apo®-Nortriptyline (Can) *see* Nortriptyline 120
Apo®-Oflox (Can) *see* Ofloxacin 121
Apo®-Oxaprozin (Can) *see* Oxaprozin 123
Apo®-Pen VK (Can) *see* Penicillin V Potassium 125
Apo®-Perphenazine (Can) *see* Perphenazine 126
Apo®-Piroxicam (Can) *see* Piroxicam 128
Apo®-Pravastatin (Can) *see* Pravastatin 129
Apo®-Prednisone (Can) *see* PredniSONE 129
Apo®-Procainamide (Can) *see* Procainamide 130
Apo®-Prochlorperazine (Can) *see* Prochlorperazine 130
Apo®-Propafenone (Can) *see* Propafenone 131
Apo®-Propranolol (Can) *see* Propranolol 132
Apo®-Quin-G (Can) *see* Quinidine 134
Apo®-Quinidine (Can) *see* Quinidine 134
Apo®-Ranitidine (Can) *see* Ranitidine 135
Apo®-Salvent (Can) *see* Albuterol 46
Apo®-Selegiline (Can) *see* Selegiline 139
Apo®-Sertraline (Can) *see* Sertraline 139
Apo®-Simvastatin (Can) *see* Simvastatin 140
Apo®-Sotalol (Can) *see* Sotalol 141
Apo®-Sulfatrim (Can) *see* Sulfamethoxazole and Trimethoprim . 143
Apo®-Sulfinpyrazone (Can) *see* Sulfinpyrazone 143
Apo®-Sulin (Can) *see* Sulindac 144
Apo®-Tamox (Can) *see* Tamoxifen 145
Apo®-Temazepam (Can) *see* Temazepam 145
Apo®-Terazosin (Can) *see* Terazosin 146
Apo®-Tetra (Can) *see* Tetracycline 146
Apo®-Theo LA (Can) *see* Theophylline 147
Apo®-Thioridazine (Can) *see* Thioridazine 147
Apo®-Tiaprofenic (Can) *see* Tiaprofenic Acid 148
Apo®-Ticlopidine (Can) *see* Ticlopidine 148
Apo®-Timol (Can) *see* Timolol 148
Apo®-Timop (Can) *see* Timolol 148
Apo®-Tolbutamide (Can) *see* TOLBUTamide 149
Apo®-Trazodone (Can) *see* Trazodone 151
Apo®-Trazodone D (Can) *see* Trazodone 151
Apo®-Triazo (Can) *see* Triazolam 151
Apo®-Trifluoperazine (Can) *see* Trifluoperazine 151
Apo®-Trimethoprim (Can) *see* Trimethoprim 152
Apo®-Trimip (Can) *see* Trimipramine 152
Apo®-Verap (Can) *see* Verapamil 154
Apo®-Warfarin (Can) *see* Warfarin 155
Apo®-Zopiclone (Can) *see* Zopiclone 157

ALPHABETICAL INDEX

Aprepitant	50
Apresoline [DSC] *see* HydrALAZINE	94
Apri® *see* Ethinyl Estradiol and Desogestrel	82
Aquacort® (Can) *see* Hydrocortisone	95
Aquanil™ HC [OTC] *see* Hydrocortisone	95
Aquatensen® *see* Methyclothiazide	110
Aquazide® H *see* Hydrochlorothiazide	94
Aralen® Phosphate *see* Chloroquine	62
Aricept® *see* Donepezil	75
Aripiprazole	51
Aristocort® *see* Triamcinolone	151
Aristocort® A *see* Triamcinolone	151
Aristocort® Forte *see* Triamcinolone	151
Aristospan® *see* Triamcinolone	151
Arsenic Trioxide	51
Arthrotec® *see* Diclofenac and Misoprostol	72
ASA *see* Aspirin	51
Asaphen (Can) *see* Aspirin	51
Asaphen E.C. (Can) *see* Aspirin	51
Ascriptin® [OTC] *see* Aspirin	51
Ascriptin® Arthritis Pain [OTC] *see* Aspirin	51
Ascriptin® Enteric [OTC] *see* Aspirin	51
Ascriptin® Extra Strength [OTC] *see* Aspirin	51
Asendin [DSC] *see* Amoxapine	49
Aspercin [OTC] *see* Aspirin	51
Aspercin Extra [OTC] *see* Aspirin	51
Aspergum® [OTC] *see* Aspirin	51
Aspirin	51
Aspirin and Codeine	52
Aspirin and Dipyridamole	52
Aspirin and Extended-Release Dipyridamole *see* Aspirin and Dipyridamole	52
Aspirin and Hydrocodone *see* Hydrocodone and Aspirin	94
Aspirin and Oxycodone *see* Oxycodone and Aspirin	123
Aspirin and Propoxyphene *see* Propoxyphene and Aspirin	132
Aspirin, Caffeine, and Dihydrocodeine *see* Dihydrocodeine, Aspirin, and Caffeine	73
Aspirin, Caffeine, Codeine, and Butalbital *see* Butalbital, Aspirin, Caffeine, and Codeine	59
Astelin® *see* Azelastine	54
Astramorph/PF™ *see* Morphine Sulfate	115
AT$_1$R *see* Angiotensin II Type 1 Receptor	166
Atacand® *see* Candesartan	59
Atarax® *see* HydrOXYzine	96
Atenolol	53
Ativan® *see* Lorazepam	105
Atomoxetine	53
Atorvastatin	53
Atromid-S® *see* Clofibrate	66
A/T/S® *see* Erythromycin	79
Augmentin® *see* Amoxicillin and Clavulanate Potassium	50
Augmentin ES-600® *see* Amoxicillin and Clavulanate Potassium	50
Augmentin XR™ *see* Amoxicillin and Clavulanate Potassium	50
Avandia® *see* Rosiglitazone	138

ALPHABETICAL INDEX

Avapro® *see* Irbesartan 99
Avelox® *see* Moxifloxacin 115
Avelox® I.V. *see* Moxifloxacin 115
Aventyl® (Can) *see* Nortriptyline 120
Aventyl® HCl *see* Nortriptyline 120
Aviane™ *see* Ethinyl Estradiol and Levonorgestrel 83
Avinza™ *see* Morphine Sulfate 115
Avlosulfon [DSC] *see* Dapsone 70
Aygestin® *see* Norethindrone 119
Azathioprine 54
Azelastine 54
Azithromycin 54
Azmacort® *see* Triamcinolone 151
Azulfidine® *see* Sulfasalazine 143
Azulfidine® EN-tabs® *see* Sulfasalazine 143
B1AR *see* Beta-1 Adrenergic Receptor 171
B2AR *see* Beta-2 Adrenergic Receptor 171
B3AR *see* Beta-3 Adrenergic Receptor 174
Bactrim™ *see* Sulfamethoxazole and Trimethoprim 143
Bactrim™ DS *see* Sulfamethoxazole and Trimethoprim 143
Bactroban® *see* Mupirocin 116
Bactroban® Nasal *see* Mupirocin 116
BAL *see* Dimercaprol 74
BAL in Oil® *see* Dimercaprol 74
Bancap HC® *see* Hydrocodone and Acetaminophen 94
Band-Aid® Hurt-Free™ Antiseptic Wash [OTC] *see* Lidocaine .. 103
Bayer® Aspirin [OTC] *see* Aspirin 51
Bayer® Aspirin Extra Strength [OTC] *see* Aspirin 51
Bayer® Aspirin Regimen Adult Low Strength [OTC] *see* Aspirin . 51
Bayer® Aspirin Regimen Adult Low Strength with Calcium [OTC]
  see Aspirin 51
Bayer® Aspirin Regimen Children's [OTC] *see* Aspirin 51
Bayer® Aspirin Regimen Regular Strength [OTC] *see* Aspirin .. 51
Bayer® Plus Extra Strength [OTC] *see* Aspirin 51
BDKRB2 *see* Bradykinin B2 Receptor 175
Belladonna and Opium 55
Benazepril 55
Benazepril and Amlodipine *see* Amlodipine and Benazepril 49
Bendroflumethiazide 55
Benemid [DSC] *see* Probenecid 130
Benicar™ *see* Olmesartan 122
Benuryl™ (Can) *see* Probenecid 130
Benzonatate 55
Benzphetamine 55
Bepridil 55
Berotec® (Can) *see* Fenoterol 86
Beta-1 Adrenergic Receptor 171
Beta-2 Adrenergic Receptor 171
Beta-3 Adrenergic Receptor 174
Beta-Fibrinogen 174
Betaloc® (Can) *see* Metoprolol 112
Betaloc® Durules® (Can) *see* Metoprolol 112
Betapace® *see* Sotalol 141
Betapace AF® *see* Sotalol 141

ALPHABETICAL INDEX

Betaxolol	56
Betimol® see Timolol	148
Betoptic® S see Betaxolol	56
Bextra® see Valdecoxib	153
Bezafibrate	56
Bezalip® (Can) see Bezafibrate	56
Biaxin® see Clarithromycin	65
Biaxin® XL see Clarithromycin	65
Biocef see Cephalexin	62
BioQuin® Durules™ (Can) see Quinidine	134
Bishydroxycoumarin see Dicumarol	72
Bisoprolol	56
Bitolterol	56
BKB2R see Bradykinin B2 Receptor	175
Bleph®-10 see Sulfacetamide	142
Blocadren® see Timolol	148
BMS 337039 see Aripiprazole	51
Bonamine™ (Can) see Meclizine	107
Bonine® [OTC] see Meclizine	107
Bosentan	56
B&O Supprettes® see Belladonna and Opium	55
Bradykinin B2 Receptor	175
BRCA-1 see BRCA Genes	176
BRCA-2 see BRCA Genes	176
BRCA Genes	176
Brethine® see Terbutaline	146
Bretylium	57
Brevibloc® see Esmolol	80
Brevicon® see Ethinyl Estradiol and Norethindrone	84
Brevicon® 0.5/35 (Can) see Ethinyl Estradiol and Norethindrone	84
Brevicon® 1/35 (Can) see Ethinyl Estradiol and Norethindrone	84
Bricanyl® [DSC] (Can) see Terbutaline	146
British Anti-Lewisite see Dimercaprol	74
Bromazepam	57
Bromocriptine	57
Budesonide	57
Bufferin® [OTC] see Aspirin	51
Bufferin® Arthritis Strength [OTC] see Aspirin	51
Bufferin® Extra Strength [OTC] see Aspirin	51
Buprenex® see Buprenorphine	57
Buprenorphine	57
Buprenorphine and Naloxone	58
Buprenorphine Hydrochloride and Naloxone Hydrochloride Dihydrate see Buprenorphine and Naloxone	58
BuPROPion	58
Burnamycin [OTC] see Lidocaine	103
Burn Jel [OTC] see Lidocaine	103
Burn-O-Jel [OTC] see Lidocaine	103
BuSpar® see BusPIRone	58
Buspirex (Can) see BusPIRone	58
BusPIRone	58
Busulfan	58
Busulfex® see Busulfan	58
Butalbital, Acetaminophen, Caffeine, and Codeine	58

ALPHABETICAL INDEX

Butalbital, Aspirin, Caffeine, and Codeine 59
Butalbital Compound and Codeine *see* Butalbital, Aspirin, Caffeine,
   and Codeine 59
Butorphanol 59
C7E3 *see* Abciximab 44
Cafergor® (Can) *see* Ergotamine 79
Cafergot® *see* Ergotamine 79
Caffeine, Acetaminophen, Butalbital, and Codeine *see* Butalbital,
   Acetaminophen, Caffeine, and Codeine 58
Caffeine, Aspirin, and Dihydrocodeine *see* Dihydrocodeine, Aspirin,
   and Caffeine 73
Caffeine, Codeine, Butalbital Compound, and Aspirin *see* Butalbital,
   Aspirin, Caffeine, and Codeine 59
Calan® *see* Verapamil 154
Calan® SR *see* Verapamil 154
CaldeCORT® [OTC] *see* Hydrocortisone 95
Camila™ *see* Norethindrone 119
Camphorated Tincture of Opium *see* Paregoric 124
Camptosar® *see* Irinotecan 99
Camptothecin-11 *see* Irinotecan 99
Candesartan 59
Capecitabine 60
Capital® and Codeine *see* Acetaminophen and Codeine 44
Capoten® *see* Captopril 60
Captopril 60
Carac™ *see* Fluorouracil 87
Carapres® (Can) *see* Clonidine 66
Carbamazepine 60
Carbatrol® *see* Carbamazepine 60
Cardene® *see* NiCARdipine 118
Cardene® I.V. *see* NiCARdipine 118
Cardene® SR *see* NiCARdipine 118
Cardiac Potassium Ion Channel 177
Cardiac Sodium Channel 178
Cardizem® *see* Diltiazem 74
Cardizem® CD *see* Diltiazem 74
Cardizem® LA *see* Diltiazem 74
Cardizem® SR *see* Diltiazem 74
Cardura® *see* Doxazosin 76
Cardura-1™ (Can) *see* Doxazosin 76
Cardura-2™ (Can) *see* Doxazosin 76
Cardura-4™ (Can) *see* Doxazosin 76
Carisoprodate *see* Carisoprodol 61
Carisoprodol 61
Carmol® Scalp *see* Sulfacetamide 142
Cartia XT™ *see* Diltiazem 74
Carvedilol 61
Cataflam® *see* Diclofenac 72
Catapres® *see* Clonidine 66
Catapres-TTS®-1 *see* Clonidine 66
Catapres-TTS®-2 *see* Clonidine 66
Catapres-TTS®-3 *see* Clonidine 66
CBZ *see* Carbamazepine 60
Cedocard®-SR (Can) *see* Isosorbide Dinitrate 100

ALPHABETICAL INDEX

Cefdinir	61
Cefprozil	61
Cefzil® see Cefprozil	61
Celebrex® see Celecoxib	61
Celecoxib	61
Celexa™ see Citalopram	64
Celontin® see Methsuximide	110
Cenestin® see Estrogens (Conjugated A/Synthetic)	81
Cenestin (Can) see Estrogens (Conjugated/Equine)	81
Cephalexin	62
Cerebyx® see Fosphenytoin	90
C.E.S.® (Can) see Estrogens (Conjugated/Equine)	81
Cetacort® see Hydrocortisone	95
Cetamide™ (Can) see Sulfacetamide	142
Ceta-Plus® see Hydrocodone and Acetaminophen	94
Cetirizine	62
CETP see Cholesteryl Ester Transfer Protein	179
CFDN see Cefdinir	61
CGP 57148B see Imatinib	97
Chlo-Amine® [OTC] see Chlorpheniramine	63
Chloramphenicol	62
Chlordiazepoxide	62
Chlordiazepoxide and Amitriptyline see Amitriptyline and Chlordiazepoxide	48
Chlormeprazine see Prochlorperazine	130
Chloromycetin® see Chloramphenicol	62
Chloroptic® see Chloramphenicol	62
Chloroquine	62
Chlorothiazide	63
Chlorpheniramine	63
ChlorproMAZINE	63
Chlorprothixene	63
Chlorthalidone	63
Chlor-Trimeton® [OTC] see Chlorpheniramine	63
Chlor-Tripolon® (Can) see Chlorpheniramine	63
Cholesteryl Ester Transfer Protein	179
Chronovera® (Can) see Verapamil	154
Cilazapril	64
Cilostazol	64
Ciloxan® see Ciprofloxacin	64
Cimetidine	64
Cipro® see Ciprofloxacin	64
Ciprofloxacin	64
Cipro® XR see Ciprofloxacin	64
Cisapride	64
Citalopram	64
CI-719 see Gemfibrozil	91
Cla see Clarithromycin	65
Clarinex® see Desloratadine	71
Clarithromycin	65
Claritin® [OTC] see Loratadine	105
Claritin® Kids (Can) see Loratadine	105
Clavulin® (Can) see Amoxicillin and Clavulanate Potassium	50
Clemastine	65

ALPHABETICAL INDEX

Cleocin® see Clindamycin 65
Cleocin HCl® see Clindamycin 65
Cleocin Pediatric® see Clindamycin 65
Cleocin Phosphate® see Clindamycin 65
Cleocin T® see Clindamycin 65
Climara® see Estradiol 80
Clindagel™ see Clindamycin 65
Clindamycin... 65
Clindets® see Clindamycin................................. 65
Clinoril® see Sulindac.................................... 144
Clobazam 65
Clofibrate 66
ClomiPRAMINE 66
Clonapam (Can) see Clonazepam 66
Clonazepam 66
Clonidine 66
Clopidogrel 66
Clopixol® (Can) see Zuclopenthixol......................... 158
Clopixol-Acuphase® (Can) see Zuclopenthixol 158
Clopixol® Depot (Can) see Zuclopenthixol 158
Clorazepate... 67
Clozapine 67
Clozaril® see Clozapine 67
Cocaine.. 67
Codeine.. 67
Codeine, Acetaminophen, Butalbital, and Caffeine see Butalbital,
  Acetaminophen, Caffeine, and Codeine 58
Codeine and Acetaminophen see Acetaminophen and Codeine 44
Codeine and Aspirin see Aspirin and Codeine 52
Codeine and Butalbital Compound see Butalbital, Aspirin, Caffeine,
  and Codeine 59
Codeine and Promethazine see Promethazine and Codeine 131
Codeine, Butalbital, Aspirin, and Caffeine see Butalbital, Aspirin,
  Caffeine, and Codeine 59
CO Fluoxetine (Can) see Fluoxetine.......................... 88
Co-Gesic® see Hydrocodone and Acetaminophen................ 94
Cognex® see Tacrine 144
Colchicine 68
Colocort™ see Hydrocortisone 95
Combivent® see Ipratropium and Albuterol 98
Compazine® see Prochlorperazine 130
Compound F see Hydrocortisone 95
Compro™ see Prochlorperazine 130
COMT 180
COMT-L see COMT...................................... 180
Concerta® see Methylphenidate 111
Congest (Can) see Estrogens (Conjugated/Equine) 81
Cordarone® see Amiodarone 48
Coreg® see Carvedilol 61
Corgard® see Nadolol 116
Coronex® (Can) see Isosorbide Dinitrate 100
CortaGel® Maximum Strength [OTC] see Hydrocortisone 95
Cortaid® Intensive Therapy [OTC] see Hydrocortisone 95
Cortaid® Maximum Strength [OTC] see Hydrocortisone 95

ALPHABETICAL INDEX

Cortaid® Sensitive Skin With Aloe [OTC] see Hydrocortisone 95
Cortamed® (Can) see Hydrocortisone 95
Cortate® (Can) see Hydrocortisone 95
Cortef® see Hydrocortisone 95
Cortenema® (Can) see Hydrocortisone 95
Corticool® [OTC] see Hydrocortisone 95
Cortifoam® see Hydrocortisone 95
Cortisol see Hydrocortisone 95
Cortizone®-5 [OTC] see Hydrocortisone 95
Cortizone®-10 Maximum Strength [OTC] see Hydrocortisone 95
Cortizone®-10 Plus Maximum Strength [OTC] see Hydrocortisone 95
Cortizone® 10 Quick Shot [OTC] see Hydrocortisone 95
Cortizone® for Kids [OTC] see Hydrocortisone 95
Cortoderm (Can) see Hydrocortisone 95
Corvert® see Ibutilide 97
Coryphen® Codeine (Can) see Aspirin and Codeine 52
Co-Trimoxazole see Sulfamethoxazole and Trimethoprim 143
Coumadin® see Warfarin 155
Covera® (Can) see Verapamil 154
Covera-HS® see Verapamil 154
Coversyl® (Can) see Perindopril Erbumine 126
Cozaar® see Losartan 105
CPM see Cyclophosphamide 69
CPT-11 see Irinotecan 99
CPZ see ChlorproMAZINE 63
Crestor® (Can) see Rosuvastatin 138
Crinone® see Progesterone 131
Cryselle™ see Ethinyl Estradiol and Norgestrel 84
Crystodigin see Digitoxin 73
CSA see CycloSPORINE 69
CTM see Chlorpheniramine 63
CTX see Cyclophosphamide 69
Cutivate® see Fluticasone 89
CyA see CycloSPORINE 69
Cyclen® (Can) see Ethinyl Estradiol and Norgestimate 84
Cyclessa® see Ethinyl Estradiol and Desogestrel 82
Cyclobenzaprine 69
Cyclophosphamide 69
Cyclosporin A see CycloSPORINE 69
CycloSPORINE 69
CYP1A2 181
CYP2C9 183
CYP2C19 185
CYP2D6 186
CYP3A4 189
CYP11B2 see Aldosterone Synthase 160
CYT see Cyclophosphamide 69
Cytochrome P450 Enzymes: Substrates, Inhibitors, and Inducers ... 23
Cytochrome P450 Isoenzyme 1A2 see CYP1A2 181
Cytochrome P450 Isoenzyme 2C9 see CYP2C9 183
Cytochrome P450 Isoenzyme 2C19 see CYP2C19 185
Cytochrome P450 Isoenzyme 2D6 see CYP2D6 186
Cytoxan® see Cyclophosphamide 69
D_2 see D2 Receptor 190

ALPHABETICAL INDEX

D$_{2L}$ see D2 Receptor 190
D2 Receptor 190
D$_{2S}$ see D2 Receptor 190
D$_3$ see D3 Receptor 191
D3 Receptor 191
D$_4$ see D4 Receptor 192
D4 Receptor 192
Dacarbazine 69
Dalacin® C (Can) see Clindamycin 65
Dalacin® T (Can) see Clindamycin 65
Dalacin® Vagiral (Can) see Clindamycin 65
Dalmane® see Flurazepam 88
Damason-P® see Hydrocodone and Aspirin 94
Dantrium® see Dantrolene 70
Dantrolene 70
Dapsone 70
Darvocet-N® 50 see Propoxyphene and Acetaminophen 132
Darvocet-N® 100 see Propoxyphene and Acetaminophen 132
Darvon® see Propoxyphene 132
Darvon® Compound-65 Pulvules® see Propoxyphene and Aspirin ... 132
Darvon-N® see Propoxyphene 132
Daypro® see Oxaprozin 123
Dehydrobenzperidol see Droperidol 76
Delatestryl® see Testosterone 146
Delestrogen® see Estradiol 80
Deltacortisone see PredniSONE 129
Deltadehydrocortisone see PredniSONE 129
Deltasone® see PredniSONE 129
Demadex® see Torsemide 150
Demerol® see Meperidine 108
Demulen® see Ethinyl Estradiol and Ethynodiol Diacetate 83
Demulen® 30 (Can) see Ethinyl Estradiol and Ethynodiol Diacetate
 83
Depacon® see Valproic Acid and Derivatives 153
Depakene® see Valproic Acid and Derivatives 153
Depakote® Delayed Release see Valproic Acid and Derivatives ... 153
Depakote® ER see Valproic Acid and Derivatives 153
Depakote® Sprinkle® see Valproic Acid and Derivatives 153
Depo®-Estradiol see Estradiol 80
Depo-Medrol® see MethylPREDNISolone 111
Depo-Provera® see MedroxyPROGESTERone 107
Depo-Provera® Contraceptive see MedroxyPROGESTERone 107
Depotest® 100 (Can) see Testosterone 146
Depo®-Testosterone see Testosterone 146
Deprenyl see Selegiline 139
Dermarest Dricort® [OTC] see Hydrocortisone 95
Dermazin™ (Can) see Silver Sulfadiazine 140
Dermtex® HC [OTC] see Hydrocortisone 95
Desipramine 71
Desloratadine 71
Desmethylimipramine Hydrochloride see Desipramine 71
Desogen® see Ethinyl Estradiol and Desogestrel 82
Desogestrel and Ethinyl Estradiol see Ethinyl Estradiol and
 Desogestrel 82

ALPHABETICAL INDEX

Desyrel® *see* Trazodone	151
Detrol® *see* Tolterodine	149
Detrol® LA *see* Tolterodine	149
Dexmedetomidine	71
Dexrazoxane	71
Dextroamphetamine and Amphetamine	72
Dextropropoxyphene *see* Propoxyphene	132
DHE *see* Dihydroergotamine	73
D.H.E. 45® *see* Dihydroergotamine	73
Diaβeta® *see* GlyBURIDE	92
Diaminodiphenylsulfone *see* Dapsone	70
Diaphorase-4 *see* NAD(P)H Quinone Oxidoreductase	212
Diastat® (Can) *see* Diazepam	72
Diastat® Rectal Delivery System *see* Diazepam	72
Diazemuls® (Can) *see* Diazepam	72
Diazepam	72
Diazepam Intensol® *see* Diazepam	72
DIC *see* Dacarbazine	69
Diclofenac	72
Diclofenac and Misoprostol	72
Diclotec (Can) *see* Diclofenac	72
Dicumarol	72
Didrex® *see* Benzphetamine	55
Diflucan® *see* Fluconazole	87
Diflunisal	73
Digitek® *see* Digoxin	73
Digitoxin	73
Digoxin	73
Digoxin CSD (Can) *see* Digoxin	73
Dihydrocodeine, Aspirin, and Caffeine	73
Dihydrocodeine Compound *see* Dihydrocodeine, Aspirin, and Caffeine	73
Dihydroergotamine	73
Dihydroergotoxine *see* Ergoloid Mesylates	79
Dihydrogenated Ergot Alkaloids *see* Ergoloid Mesylates	79
Dihydrohydroxycodeinone *see* Oxycodone	123
Dihydromorphinone *see* Hydromorphone	96
Dihydropyrimidine Dehydrogenase	193
Dihydroxydeoxynorvinkaleukoblastine *see* Vinorelbine	155
Dilacor® XR *see* Diltiazem	74
Dilantin® *see* Phenytoin	127
Dilatrate®-SR *see* Isosorbide Dinitrate	100
Dilaudid® *see* Hydromorphone	96
Dilaudid-HP® *see* Hydromorphone	96
Dilaudid-HP-Plus® (Can) *see* Hydromorphone	96
Dilaudid® Sterile Powder (Can) *see* Hydromorphone	96
Dilaudid-XP® (Can) *see* Hydromorphone	96
Diltia XT® *see* Diltiazem	74
Diltiazem	74
Dimercaprol	74
Dimethyl Triazeno Imidazol Carboxamide *see* Dacarbazine	69
Diochloram® (Can) *see* Chloramphenicol	62
Diomycin® (Can) *see* Erythromycin	79
Diosulf™ (Can) *see* Sulfacetamide	142

ALPHABETICAL INDEX

Diovan® *see* Valsartan ... 153
Diphenylhydantoin *see* Phenytoin ... 127
Diprivan® *see* Propofol ... 131
Dipropylacetic Acid *see* Valproic Acid and Derivatives ... 153
Dipyridamole ... 74
Dipyridamole and Aspirin *see* Aspirin and Dipyridamole ... 52
Disopyramide ... 74
Disulfiram ... 75
Dithioglycerol *see* Dimercaprol ... 74
Diucardin® [DSC] *see* Hydroflumethiazide ... 95
Diuril® *see* Chlorothiazide ... 63
Divalproex Sodium *see* Valproic Acid and Derivatives ... 153
Dixarit® (Can) *see* Clonidine ... 66
Docetaxel ... 75
Dofetilide ... 75
Dolobid® *see* Diflunisal ... 73
Dolophine® *see* Methadone ... 110
Dom-Domperidone (Can) *see* Domperidone ... 75
Domperidone ... 75
Dom-Tiaprofenic® (Can) *see* Tiaprofenic Acid ... 148
Donepezil ... 75
Doryx® *see* Doxycycline ... 76
Doxazosin ... 76
Doxepin ... 76
DOXOrubicin ... 76
Doxy-100® *see* Doxycycline ... 76
Doxycin (Can) *see* Doxycycline ... 76
Doxycycline ... 76
Doxytec (Can) *see* Doxycycline ... 76
DPA *see* Valproic Acid and Derivatives ... 153
DPD *see* Dihydropyrimidine Dehydrogenase ... 193
DPH *see* Phenytoin ... 127
DPYD *see* Dihydropyrimidine Dehydrogenase ... 193
Dramamine® Less Drowsy Formula [OTC] *see* Meclizine ... 107
DRD2 *see* D2 Receptor ... 190
DRD3 *see* D3 Receptor ... 191
DRD4 *see* D4 Receptor ... 192
Droperidol ... 76
Drospirenone and Ethinyl Estradiol *see* Ethinyl Estradiol and
   Drospirenone ... 82
DT-Diaphorase *see* NAD(P)H Quinone Oxidoreductase ... 212
DTIC® (Can) *see* Dacarbazine ... 69
DTIC-Dome® *see* Dacarbazine ... 69
DTO *see* Opium Tincture ... 122
DuoNeb™ *see* Ipratropium and Albuterol ... 98
DuP 753 *see* Losartan ... 105
Duraclon™ *see* Clonidine ... 66
Duragesic® *see* Fentanyl ... 86
Duramorph® *see* Morphine Sulfate ... 115
Dynacin® *see* Minocycline ... 113
DynaCirc® *see* Isradipine ... 100
DynaCirc® CR *see* Isradipine ... 100
E_2C and MPA *see* Estradiol and Medroxyprogesterone ... 81
7E3 *see* Abciximab ... 44

ALPHABETICAL INDEX

E2020 see Donepezil	75
EarSol® HC see Hydrocortisone	95
Easprin® see Aspirin	51
EC 1.6.99.2 see NAD(P)H Quinone Oxidoreductase	212
EC-Naprosyn® see Naproxen	117
Ecotrin® [OTC] see Aspirin	51
Ecotrin® Low Adult Strength [OTC] see Aspirin	51
Ecotrin® Maximum Strength [OTC] see Aspirin	51
E.E.S.® see Erythromycin	79
Effexor® see Venlafaxine	154
Effexor® XR see Venlafaxine	154
Efudex® see Fluorouracil	87
ELA-Max® [OTC] see Lidocaine	103
ELA-Max® 5 [OTC] see Lidocaine	103
Elavil® see Amitriptyline	48
Eldepryl® see Selegiline	139
Eletriptan	77
Elitek™ see Rasburicase	135
Elixophyllin® see Theophylline	147
Elocon® see Mometasone Furoate	114
Eltroxin® (Can) see Levothyroxine	103
Emend® see Aprepitant	50
Emgel® see Erythromycin	79
EMLA® see Lidocaine and Prilocaine	104
Emo-Cort® (Can) see Hydrocortisone	95
Emtec-30 (Can) see Acetaminophen and Codeine	44
ENA 713 see Rivastigmine	137
ENaC-Beta see Epithelial Sodium Channel Beta-Subunit	194
Enalapril	78
Enalaprilat see Enalapril	78
Endocet® see Oxycodone and Acetaminophen	123
Endodan® see Oxycodone and Aspirin	123
Enduron® see Methyclothiazide	110
Enpresse™ see Ethinyl Estradiol and Levonorgestrel	83
Entocort™ EC see Budesonide	57
Entrophen® (Can) see Aspirin	51
Epipodophyllotoxin see Etoposide	85
Epithelial Sodium Channel Beta-Subunit	194
Epitol® see Carbamazepine	60
Epival® ER (Can) see Valproic Acid and Derivatives	153
Epival® I.V. (Can) see Valproic Acid and Derivatives	153
Eplerenone	78
Eprosartan	78
EPT see Teniposide	146
Eptifibatide	78
Ergoloid Mesylates	79
Ergomar® see Ergotamine	79
Ergometrine Maleate see Ergonovine	79
Ergonovine	79
Ergotamine	79
Ergotamine Tartrate and Caffeine see Ergotamine	79
Errin™ see Norethindrone	119
Erybid™ (Can) see Erythromycin	79
Eryc® see Erythromycin	79

ALPHABETICAL INDEX

Erycette® *see* Erythromycin 79
Eryderm® *see* Erythromycin 79
Erygel® *see* Erythromycin 79
EryPed® *see* Erythromycin 79
Ery-Tab® *see* Erythromycin 79
Erythra-Derm™ *see* Erythromycin 79
Erythrocin® *see* Erythromycin 79
Erythromid® (Can) *see* Erythromycin 79
Erythromycin 79
Erythromycin and Sulfisoxazole 80
Eryzole® *see* Erythromycin and Sulfisoxazole 80
Escitalopram 80
Escitalopram Oxalate *see* Escitalopram 80
Esclim® *see* Estradiol 80
Esmolol 80
Esomeprazole 80
Esterified Estrogens *see* Estrogens (Esterified) 82
Estrace® *see* Estradiol 80
Estraderm® *see* Estradiol 80
Estradiol 80
Estradiol and Medroxyprogesterone 81
Estradot® (Can) *see* Estradiol 80
Estratab® [DSC] *see* Estrogens (Esterified) 82
Estring® *see* Estradiol 80
Estrogel® (Can) *see* Estradiol 80
Estrogenic Substances, Conjugated *see* Estrogens (Conjugated/
    Equine) 81
Estrogens (Conjugated A/Synthetic) 81
Estrogens (Conjugated/Equine) 81
Estrogens (Conjugated/Equine) and Medroxyprogesterone 81
Estrogens (Esterified) 82
Estropipate 82
Estrostep® 21 [DSC] *see* Ethinyl Estradiol and Norethindrone ..84
Estrostep® Fe *see* Ethinyl Estradiol and Norethindrone 84
Ethinyl Estradiol and Desogestrel 82
Ethinyl Estradiol and Drospirenone 82
Ethinyl Estradiol and Ethynodiol Diacetate 83
Ethinyl Estradiol and Etonogestrel 83
Ethinyl Estradiol and Levonorgestrel 83
Ethinyl Estradiol and NGM *see* Ethinyl Estradiol and Norgestimate ...84
Ethinyl Estradiol and Norelgestromin 83
Ethinyl Estradiol and Norethindrone 84
Ethinyl Estradiol and Norgestimate 84
Ethinyl Estradiol and Norgestrel 84
Ethmozine® *see* Moricizine 115
Ethosuximide 85
Ethynodiol Diacetate and Ethinyl Estradiol *see* Ethinyl Estradiol and
    Ethynodiol Diacetate 83
Etodolac 85
Etonogestrel and Ethinyl Estradiol *see* Ethinyl Estradiol and
    Etonogestrel 83
Etoposide 85
Etrafon® *see* Amitriptyline and Perphenazine 49
Euflex® (Can) *see* Flutamide 89

ALPHABETICAL INDEX

Euglucon® (Can) see GlyBURIDE	92
Eulexin® see Flutamide	89
Everone® 200 (Can) see Testosterone	146
Evista® see Raloxifene	134
Evra™ (Can) see Ethinyl Estradiol and Norelgestromin	83
Exelon® see Rivastigmine	137
F5 see Factor V	194
Factor V	194
Famotidine	85
Fansidar® see Sulfadoxine and Pyrimethamine	143
Fc Gamma RIIa see Platelet Fc Gamma Receptor	216
FCG R2A see Platelet Fc Gamma Receptor	216
Felbamate	85
Felbatol® see Felbamate	85
Feldene® see Piroxicam	128
Felodipine	86
femhrt® see Ethinyl Estradiol and Norethindrone	84
Femring™ see Estradiol	80
Fenofibrate	86
Fenoprofen	86
Fenoterol	86
Fentanyl	86
Feratab® [OTC] see Ferrous Sulfate	87
Fer-Gen-Sol [OTC] see Ferrous Sulfate	87
Fer-In-Sol® [OTC] see Ferrous Sulfate	87
Fer-Iron® [OTC] see Ferrous Sulfate	87
Ferodan™ (Can) see Ferrous Sulfate	87
Ferrous Sulfate	87
FeSO$_4$ see Ferrous Sulfate	87
Fexofenadine	87
FGB see Beta-Fibrinogen	174
Fioricet® with Codeine see Butalbital, Acetaminophen, Caffeine, and Codeine	58
Fiorinal®-C 1/2 (Can) see Butalbital, Aspirin, Caffeine, and Codeine	59
Fiorinal®-C 1/4 (Can) see Butalbital, Aspirin, Caffeine, and Codeine	59
Fiorinal® With Codeine see Butalbital, Aspirin, Caffeine, and Codeine	59
FK506 see Tacrolimus	144
Flagyl® see Metronidazole	112
Flagyl ER® see Metronidazole	112
Flamazine® (Can) see Silver Sulfadiazine	140
Flecainide	87
Flexeril® see Cyclobenzaprine	69
Flexitec (Can) see Cyclobenzaprine	69
Flomax® see Tamsulosin	145
Flonase® see Fluticasone	89
Florazole® ER (Can) see Metronidazole	112
Flovent® see Fluticasone	89
Flovent® HFA (Can) see Fluticasone	89
Flovent® Rotadisk® see Fluticasone	89
Floxin® see Ofloxacin	121
Fluanxol® (Can) see Flupenthixol	88

ALPHABETICAL INDEX

Fluconazole	87
Fluoroplex® *see* Fluorouracil	87
Fluorouracil	87
5-Fluorouracil *see* Fluorouracil	87
Fluoxetine	88
Flupenthixol	88
Fluphenazine	88
Flurazepam	88
Flurbiprofen	89
Flutamide	89
Fluticasone	89
Fluticasone and Salmeterol	89
Fluvastatin	89
Fluvoxamine	90
Foradil® (Can) *see* Formoterol	90
Foradil® Aerolizer™ *see* Formoterol	90
Formoterol	90
Fortovase® *see* Saquinavir	139
Fosamax® *see* Alendronate	46
Foscarnet	90
Foscavir® *see* Foscarnet	90
Fosinopril	90
Fosphenytoin	90
Frisium® (Can) *see* Clobazam	65
Froben® (Can) *see* Flurbiprofen	89
Froben-SR® (Can) *see* Flurbiprofen	89
Frusemide *see* Furosemide	91
FTP-Domperidone Maleate (Can) *see* Domperidone	75
FU *see* Fluorouracil	87
5-FU *see* Fluorouracil	87
Furadantin® *see* Nitrofurantoin	119
Furazolidone	91
Furosemide	91
Furoxone® (Can) *see* Furazolidone	91
G6PD *see* Glucose-6-Phosphate Dehydrogenase	195
Gabapentin	91
Gabitril® *see* Tiagabine	148
Galantamine	91
Gantrisin® *see* SulfiSOXAZOLE	144
Gatifloxacin	91
GB3 *see* G-Protein Beta-3 Subunit	197
Gemfibrozil	91
Gen-Acebutolol (Can) *see* Acebutolol	44
Gen-Acyclovir (Can) *see* Acyclovir	45
Gen-Alprazolam (Can) *see* Alprazolam	47
Gen-Amiodarone (Can) *see* Amiodarone	48
Gen-Amoxicillin (Can) *see* Amoxicillin	49
Gen-Atenolol (Can) *see* Atenolol	53
Gen-Azathioprine (Can) *see* Azathioprine	54
Gen-Bromazepam (Can) *see* Bromazepam	57
Gen-Budesonide AQ (Can) *see* Budesonide	57
Gen-Buspirone (Can) *see* BusPIRone	58
Gen-Captopril (Can) *see* Captopril	60
Gen-Carbamazepine CR (Can) *see* Carbamazepine	60

ALPHABETICAL INDEX

Gen-Cimetidine (Can) *see* Cimetidine 64
Gen-Clomipramine (Can) *see* ClomiPRAMINE 66
Gen-Clonazepam (Can) *see* Clonazepam 66
Gen-Cyclobenzaprine (Can) *see* Cyclobenzaprine 69
Gen-Diltiazem (Can) *see* Diltiazem 74
Gen-Diltiazem SR (Can) *see* Diltiazem 74
Gen-Divalproex (Can) *see* Valproic Acid and Derivatives 153
Gen-Doxazosin (Can) *see* Doxazosin 76
Genesec® [OTC] *see* Acetaminophen and Phenyltoloxamine ... 45
Gen-Famotidine (Can) *see* Famotidine 85
Gen-Fenofibrate Micro (Can) *see* Fenofibrate 86
Gen-Fluoxetine (Can) *see* Fluoxetine 88
Gen-Gemfibrozil (Can) *see* Gemfibrozil 91
Gen-Glybe (Can) *see* GlyBURIDE 92
Gengraf™ *see* CycloSPORINE 69
Gen-Indapamide (Can) *see* Indapamide 98
Gen-Lovastatin (Can) *see* Lovastatin 106
Gen-Medroxy (Can) *see* MedroxyPROGESTERone 107
Gen-Metformin (Can) *see* Metformin 109
Gen-Minocycline (Can) *see* Minocycline 113
Gen-Nabumetone (Can) *see* Nabumetone 116
Gen-Naproxen EC (Can) *see* Naproxen 117
Gen-Nortriptyline (Can) *see* Nortriptyline 120
Gen-Piroxicam (Can) *see* Piroxicam 128
Genpril® [OTC] *see* Ibuprofen 96
Gen-Ranidine (Can) *see* Ranitidine 135
Gen-Salbutamol (Can) *see* Albuterol 46
Gen-Selegiline (Can) *see* Selegiline 139
Gen-Sertraline (Can) *see* Sertraline 139
Gen-Simvastatin (Can) *see* Simvastatin 140
Gen-Sotalol (Can) *see* Sotalol 141
Gen-Tamoxifen (Can) *see* Tamoxifen 145
Gen-Temazepam (Can) *see* Temazepam 145
Gen-Ticlopidine (Can) *see* Ticlopidine 148
Gen-Timolol (Can) *see* Timolol 148
Gen-Trazodone (Can) *see* Trazodone 151
Gen-Triazolam (Can) *see* Triazolam 151
Gen-Verapamil (Can) *see* Verapamil 154
Gen-Verapamil SR (Can) *see* Verapamil 154
Gen-Warfarin (Can) *see* Warfarin 155
Gen-Zopiclone (Can) *see* Zopiclone 157
Geodon® *see* Ziprasidone 157
GI87084B *see* Remifentanil 135
Gleevec™ *see* Imatinib 97
Glibenclamide *see* GlyBURIDE 92
Glimepiride 92
GlipiZIDE 92
Glivec *see* Imatinib 97
GlucoNorm® (Can) *see* Repaglinide 136
Glucophage® *see* Metformin 109
Glucophage® XR *see* Metformin 109
Glucose-6-Phosphate Dehydrogenase 195
Glucotrol® *see* GlipiZIDE 92
Glucotrol® XL *see* GlipiZIDE 92

ALPHABETICAL INDEX

Glucovance® *see* Glyburide and Metformin 92
Glybenclamide *see* GlyBURIDE 92
Glybenzcyclamide *see* GlyBURIDE 92
GlyBURIDE 92
Glyburide and Metformin 92
Glycon (Can) *see* Metformin 109
Glycoprotein IIIa Receptor 196
Glydiazinamide *see* GlipiZIDE 92
Glynase® PresTab® *see* GlyBURIDE 92
GNAS1 *see* Gs Protein Alpha-Subunit 198
GNB3 *see* G-Protein Beta-3 Subunit 197
GP170 *see* P-Glycoprotein 213
GPIIIa *see* Glycoprotein IIIa Receptor 196
G-Protein Beta-3 Subunit 197
Gs Protein Alpha-Subunit 198
Guanabenz 93
Gynodiol® *see* Estradiol 80
Halcion® *see* Triazolam 151
Haldol® *see* Haloperidol 93
Haldol® Decanoate *see* Haloperidol 93
Halfprin® [OTC] *see* Aspirin 51
Halofantrine 93
Haloperidol 93
Haloperidol-LA Omega (Can) *see* Haloperidol 93
Haloperidol Long Acting (Can) *see* Haloperidol 93
Haltran® [OTC] *see* Ibuprofen 96
HCTZ *see* Hydrochlorothiazide 94
Hemril-HC® *see* Hydrocortisone 95
Hepalean® (Can) *see* Heparin 93
Hepalean® Leo (Can) *see* Heparin 93
Hepalean®-LOK (Can) *see* Heparin 93
Heparin 93
Hep-Lock® *see* Heparin 93
Histamine 1 and 2 Receptors 199
HLA *see* Human Leukocyte Antigen 206
HLA-A1 200
HR1 *see* Histamine 1 and 2 Receptors 199
HR2 *see* Histamine 1 and 2 Receptors 199
5HT1A Receptor 200
5HT2A Receptor 201
5HT2C Receptor 202
5HT6 Receptor 203
HTR2 *see* 5HT2A Receptor 201
HTR2C *see* 5HT2C Receptor 202
HTR6 *see* 5HT6 Receptor 203
HTT *see* 5HT Transporter 204
5HTT *see* 5HT Transporter 204
5HTTLPR *see* 5HT Transporter 204
5HT Transporter 204
Humalog® *see* Insulin Preparations 98
Humalog® Mix 25™ (Can) *see* Insulin Preparations 98
Humalog® Mix 75/25™ *see* Insulin Preparations 98
Human Leukocyte Antigen 206
Humulin® (Can) *see* Insulin Preparations 98

ALPHABETICAL INDEX

Humulin® 50/50 *see* Insulin Preparations 98
Humulin® 70/30 *see* Insulin Preparations 98
Humulin® L *see* Insulin Preparations 98
Humulin® N *see* Insulin Preparations 98
Humulin® R *see* Insulin Preparations 98
Humulin® R (Concentrated) U-500 *see* Insulin Preparations 98
Humulin® U *see* Insulin Preparations 98
Hycort™ (Can) *see* Hydrocortisone 95
Hydergine [DSC] *see* Ergoloid Mesylates 79
Hyderm (Can) *see* Hydrocortisone 95
HydrALAZINE 94
Hydrocet® *see* Hydrocodone and Acetaminophen 94
Hydrochlorothiazide 94
Hydrochlorothiazide and Lisinopril *see* Lisinopril and
    Hydrochlorothiazide 104
Hydrochlorothiazide and Losartan *see* Losartan and
    Hydrochlorothiazide 105
Hydrocodone and Acetaminophen 94
Hydrocodone and Aspirin 94
Hydrocodone and Ibuprofen 95
Hydrocortisone 95
Hydrocortone® *see* Hydrocortisone 95
Hydrocortone® Phosphate *see* Hydrocortisone 95
Hydroflumethiazide 95
Hydrogesic® [DSC] *see* Hydrocodone and Acetaminophen 94
Hydromorph Contin® (Can) *see* Hydromorphone 96
Hydromorphone 96
Hydromorphone HP (Can) *see* Hydromorphone 96
HydroVal® (Can) *see* Hydrocortisone 95
Hydroxychloroquine 96
Hydroxydaunomycin Hydrochloride *see* DOXOrubicin 76
HydrOXYzine 96
Hygroton [DSC] *see* Chlorthalidone 63
Hytone® *see* Hydrocortisone 95
Hytrin® *see* Terazosin 146
Hyzaar® *see* Losartan and Hydrochlorothiazide 105
Hyzaar® DS (Can) *see* Losartan and Hydrochlorothiazide 105
Ibuprofen 96
Ibuprofen and Hydrocodone *see* Hydrocodone and Ibuprofen 95
Ibu-Tab® *see* Ibuprofen 96
Ibutilide 97
ICI 204, 219 *see* Zafirlukast 156
ICI-46474 *see* Tamoxifen 145
ICI-D1694 *see* Raltitrexed 135
ICRF-187 *see* Dexrazoxane 71
Ifex® *see* Ifosfamide 97
Ifosfamide 97
Iletin® II Pork (Can) *see* Insulin Preparations 98
Imatinib 97
Imidazol Carboxamide Dimethyltriazene *see* Dacarbazine 69
Imidazole Carboxamide *see* Dacarbazine 69
Imipramine 97
Imitrex® *see* Sumatriptan 144
Imovane® (Can) *see* Zopiclone 157

ALPHABETICAL INDEX

Imuran® *see* Azathioprine 54
Inapsine® *see* Droperidol 76
Indapamide 98
Inderal® *see* Propranolol 132
Inderal® LA *see* Propranolol 132
Indocid® (Can) *see* Indomethacin 98
Indocid® P.D.A. (Can) *see* Indomethacin 98
Indocin® *see* Indomethacin 98
Indocin® I.V. *see* Indomethacin 98
Indocin® SR *see* Indomethacin 98
Indo-Lemmon (Can) *see* Indomethacin 98
Indometacin *see* Indomethacin 98
Indomethacin 98
Indotec (Can) *see* Indomethacin 98
Infumorph® *see* Morphine Sulfate 115
INH *see* Isoniazid 99
Inhibace® (Can) *see* Cilazapril 64
Inspra™ *see* Eplerenone 78
Insulin Preparations 98
Integrilin® *see* Eptifibatide 78
Intrifiban *see* Eptifibatide 78
Invirase® *see* Saquinavir 139
Ipratropium and Albuterol 98
I-Prin [OTC] *see* Ibuprofen 96
Iproveratril Hydrochloride *see* Verapamil 154
Irbesartan 99
Irinotecan 99
Iron Sulfate *see* Ferrous Sulfate 87
ISD *see* Isosorbide Dinitrate 100
ISDN *see* Isosorbide Dinitrate 100
Isobamate *see* Carisoprodol 61
Isoniazid 99
Isonicotinic Acid Hydrazide *see* Isoniazid 99
Isonipecaine Hydrochloride *see* Meperidine 108
Isophosphamide *see* Ifosfamide 97
Isoproterenol 99
Isoptin® (Can) *see* Verapamil 154
Isoptin® I.V. (Can) *see* Verapamil 154
Isoptin® SR *see* Verapamil 154
Isordil® *see* Isosorbide Dinitrate 100
Isosorbide Dinitrate 100
Isotamine® (Can) *see* Isoniazid 99
Isradipine 100
Isuprel® *see* Isoproterenol 99
Itraconazole 100
Ivermectin 100
K+8 *see* Potassium Chloride 128
K+10 *see* Potassium Chloride 128
Kadian® (Can) *see* Morphine Sulfate 115
Kaon-Cl-10® *see* Potassium Chloride 128
Kaon-Cl® 20 *see* Potassium Chloride 128
Kariva™ *see* Ethinyl Estradiol and Desogestrel 82
Kay Ciel® *see* Potassium Chloride 128
K+ Care® *see* Potassium Chloride 128

ALPHABETICAL INDEX

k-channel *see* Cardiac Potassium Ion Channel 177
KCl *see* Potassium Chloride 128
K-Dur® 10 *see* Potassium Chloride 128
K-Dur® 20 *see* Potassium Chloride 128
Keflex® *see* Cephalexin 62
Keftab® *see* Cephalexin 62
Kenalog® *see* Triamcinolone 151
Kenalog-10® *see* Triamcinolone 151
Kenalog-40® *see* Triamcinolone 151
Kenalog® in Orabase® *see* Triamcinolone 151
Keoxifene Hydrochloride *see* Raloxifene 134
Kerlone® *see* Betaxolol 56
Ketalar® *see* Ketamine 101
Ketamine 101
Ketoconazole 101
Ketoderm® (Can) *see* Ketoconazole 101
Ketoprofen 101
Ketorolac 101
Klaron® *see* Sulfacetamide 142
Klonopin™ *see* Clonazepam 66
K-Lor™ *see* Potassium Chloride 128
Klor-Con® *see* Potassium Chloride 128
Klor-Con® 8 *see* Potassium Chloride 128
Klor-Con® 10 *see* Potassium Chloride 128
Klor-Con®/25 *see* Potassium Chloride 128
Klor-Con® M10 *see* Potassium Chloride 128
Klor-Con® M20 *see* Potassium Chloride 128
Klotrix® *see* Potassium Chloride 128
K-Lyte®/Cl (Can) *see* Potassium Chloride 128
K-Tab® *see* Potassium Chloride 128
L 754030 *see* Aprepitant 50
LactiCare-HC® *see* Hydrocortisone 95
Lanoxicaps® *see* Digoxin 73
Lanoxin® *see* Digoxin 73
Lansoprazole 102
Lantus® *see* Insulin Preparations 98
Lanvis® (Can) *see* Thioguanine 147
Largactil® (Can) *see* ChlorproMAZINE 63
Lariam® *see* Mefloquine 108
Lasix® *see* Furosemide 91
Lasix® Special (Can) *see* Furosemide 91
Latanoprost 102
LCR *see* VinCRIStine 155
L-Deprenyl *see* Selegiline 139
LDLR *see* Low-Density Lipoprotein Receptor 209
Lectopam® (Can) *see* Bromazepam 57
Lenoltec (Can) *see* Acetaminophen and Codeine 44
Lente® Iletin® II *see* Insulin Preparations 98
Lescol® *see* Fluvastatin 89
Lescol® XL *see* Fluvastatin 89
Lessina™ *see* Ethinyl Estradiol and Levonorgestrel 83
Leukotriene C4 Synthase 206
Leurocristine *see* VinCRIStine 155
Leurocristine Sulfate *see* VinCRIStine 155

ALPHABETICAL INDEX

Levalbuterol..102
Levaquin® *see* Levofloxacin..................................102
Levate® (Can) *see* Amitriptyline..............................48
Levlen® *see* Ethinyl Estradiol and Levonorgestrel..............83
Levlite™ *see* Ethinyl Estradiol and Levonorgestrel.............83
Levo-Dromoran® *see* Levorphanol.............................103
Levofloxacin...102
Levomepromazine *see* Methotrimeprazine......................110
Levomethadyl Acetate Hydrochloride..........................102
Levonorgestrel...103
Levonorgestrel and Ethinyl Estradiol *see* Ethinyl Estradiol and
 Levonorgestrel...83
Levora® *see* Ethinyl Estradiol and Levonorgestrel..............83
Levorphanol...103
Levothroid® *see* Levothyroxine..............................103
Levothyroxine...103
Levoxyl® *see* Levothyroxine.................................103
Lexapro™ *see* Escitalopram...................................80
Librium® *see* Chlordiazepoxide...............................62
LidaMantle® *see* Lidocaine..................................103
Lidocaine..103
Lidocaine and Prilocaine....................................104
Lidodan™ (Can) *see* Lidocaine...............................103
Lidoderm® *see* Lidocaine...................................103
Lignocaine Hydrochloride *see* Lidocaine......................103
Limbitrol® *see* Amitriptyline and Chlordiazepoxide.............48
Limbitrol® DS *see* Amitriptyline and Chlordiazepoxide..........48
Lin-Amox (Can) *see* Amoxicillin..............................49
Lin-Buspirone (Can) *see* BusPIRone...........................58
Lin-Nefazodone (Can) *see* Nefazodone.......................117
Lin-Pravastatin (Can) *see* Pravastatin.......................129
Lin-Sotalol (Can) *see* Sotalol...............................141
Lipidil Micro® (Can) *see* Fenofibrate..........................86
Lipidil Supra® (Can) *see* Fenofibrate.........................86
Lipitor® *see* Atorvastatin....................................53
5-Lipoxygenase..208
Lisinopril..104
Lisinopril and Hydrochlorothiazide............................104
LNg 20 *see* Levonorgestrel..................................103
5-LO *see* 5-Lipoxygenase...................................208
Locoid® (Can) *see* Hydrocortisone............................95
Locoid Lipocream® *see* Hydrocortisone........................95
Lodine® *see* Etodolac.......................................85
Lodine® XL *see* Etodolac....................................85
Loestrin® *see* Ethinyl Estradiol and Norethindrone.............84
Loestrin™ 1.5.30 (Can) *see* Ethinyl Estradiol and Norethindrone.....84
Loestrin® Fe *see* Ethinyl Estradiol and Norethindrone..........84
Lo/Ovral® *see* Ethinyl Estradiol and Norgestrel................84
Lopid® *see* Gemfibrozil......................................91
Lopressor® *see* Metoprolol.................................112
Loratadine..105
Lorazepam..105
Lorazepam Intensol® *see* Lorazepam........................105
Lorcet® 10/650 *see* Hydrocodone and Acetaminophen..........94

ALPHABETICAL INDEX

Lorcet®-HD *see* Hydrocodone and Acetaminophen	94
Lorcet® Plus *see* Hydrocodone and Acetaminophen	94
Lortab® *see* Hydrocodone and Acetaminophen	94
Losartan	105
Losartan and Hydrochlorothiazide	105
Losec® (Can) *see* Omeprazole	122
Lotensin® *see* Benazepril	55
Lotrel® *see* Amlodipine and Benazepril	49
Lovastatin	106
Low-Density Lipoprotein Receptor	209
Low-Ogestrel® *see* Ethinyl Estradiol and Norgestrel	84
5-LOX *see* 5-Lipoxygenase	208
Loxapine	106
Loxitane® *see* Loxapine	106
Loxitane® C *see* Loxapine	106
Lozide® (Can) *see* Indapamide	98
Lozol® *see* Indapamide	98
LTC(4) Synthase *see* Leukotriene C4 Synthase	206
L-Thyroxine Sodium *see* Levothyroxine	103
Lu-26-054 *see* Escitalopram	80
Ludiomil *see* Maprotiline	107
Luminal® Sodium *see* Phenobarbital	127
Lunelle™ *see* Estradiol and Medroxyprogesterone	81
Luvox® [DSC] *see* Fluvoxamine	90
LY139603 *see* Atomoxetine	53
LY170053 *see* Olanzapine	121
Macrobid® *see* Nitrofurantoin	119
Macrodantin® *see* Nitrofurantoin	119
Mafenide	107
Manerix® (Can) *see* Moclobemide	114
Maprotiline	107
Margesic® H *see* Hydrocodone and Acetaminophen	94
Marvelon® (Can) *see* Ethinyl Estradiol and Desogestrel	82
Matrix Metalloproteinase 3 *see* Stromelysin-1	219
Mavik® *see* Trandolapril	150
Maxair™ *see* Pirbuterol	128
Maxair™ Autohaler™ *see* Pirbuterol	128
Maxidone™ *see* Hydrocodone and Acetaminophen	94
MDR-1 *see* P-Glycoprotein	213
Mebaral® *see* Mephobarbital	108
Meclizine	107
Meclofenamate	107
Meclomen® (Can) *see* Meclofenamate	107
Med-Diltiazem (Can) *see* Diltiazem	74
Medrol® *see* MethylPREDNISolone	111
MedroxyPROGESTERone	107
Medroxyprogesterone Acetate *see* MedroxyPROGESTERone	107
Medroxyprogesterone Acetate and Estradiol Cypionate *see* Estradiol and Medroxyprogesterone	81
Medroxyprogesterone and Estradiol *see* Estradiol and Medroxyprogesterone	81
Medroxyprogesterone and Estrogens (Conjugated) *see* Estrogens (Conjugated/Equine) and Medroxyprogesterone	81
Mefenamic Acid	108

ALPHABETICAL INDEX

Mefloquine ... 108
Mellaril® [DSC] *see* Thioridazine ... 147
Meloxicam ... 108
Menadol® [OTC] *see* Ibuprofen ... 96
Menest® *see* Estrogens (Esterified) ... 82
Mepergan *see* Meperidine and Promethazine ... 108
Meperidine ... 108
Meperidine and Promethazine ... 108
Meperitab® *see* Meperidine ... 108
Mephobarbital ... 108
Mercaptopurine ... 109
6-Mercaptopurine *see* Mercaptopurine ... 109
Meridia® *see* Sibutramine ... 140
M-Eslon® (Can) *see* Morphine Sulfate ... 115
Mesoridazine ... 109
Mestranol and Norethindrone ... 109
Metadate® CD *see* Methylphenidate ... 111
Metadate™ ER *see* Methylphenidate ... 111
Metadol™ (Can) *see* Methadone ... 110
Metahydrin® (Can) *see* Trichlormethiazide ... 151
Metaproterenol ... 109
Metatensin® (Can) *see* Trichlormethiazide ... 151
Metaxalone ... 109
Metformin ... 109
Metformin and Glyburide *see* Glyburide and Metformin ... 92
Methadone ... 110
Methadone Intensol™ *see* Methadone ... 110
Methadose® *see* Methadone ... 110
Methaminodiazepoxide Hydrochloride *see* Chlordiazepoxide ... 62
Methergine® *see* Methylergonovine ... 111
Methotrimeprazine ... 110
Methsuximide ... 110
Methyclothiazide ... 110
Methylacetoxyprogesterone *see* MedroxyPROGESTERone ... 107
Methylene Blue ... 110
Methylenetetrahydrofolate Reductase ... 210
Methylergonovine ... 111
Methylin™ *see* Methylphenidate ... 111
Methylin™ ER *see* Methylphenidate ... 111
Methylmorphine *see* Codeine ... 67
Methylphenidate ... 111
Methylphenobarbital *see* Mephobarbital ... 108
MethylPREDNISolone ... 111
6-α-Methylprednisolone *see* MethylPREDNISolone ... 111
Methysergide ... 111
Metoclopramide ... 111
Metolazone ... 111
Metoprolol ... 112
MetroCream® *see* Metronidazole ... 112
MetroGel® *see* Metronidazole ... 112
MetroGel-Vaginal® *see* Metronidazole ... 112
MetroLotion® *see* Metronidazole ... 112
Metronidazole ... 112
Mevacor® *see* Lovastatin ... 106

ALPHABETICAL INDEX

Mevinolin *see* Lovastatin 106
Mexiletine 112
Mexitil® *see* Mexiletine 112
MHFR *see* Methylenetetrahydrofolate Reductase 210
Micardis® *see* Telmisartan 145
Microgestin™ Fe *see* Ethinyl Estradiol and Norethindrone 84
microK® *see* Potassium Chloride 128
microK® 10 *see* Potassium Chloride 128
Micro-K Extencaps® (Can) *see* Potassium Chloride 128
Micronase® *see* GlyBURIDE 92
Micronor® *see* Norethindrone 119
Microzide™ *see* Hydrochlorothiazide 94
Midamor® *see* Amiloride 47
Midazolam 112
Midol® Maximum Strength Cramp Formula [OTC] *see* Ibuprofen 96
Mifeprex® *see* Mifepristone 113
Mifepristone 113
Migranal® *see* Dihydroergotamine 73
Minestrin™ 1/20 (Can) *see* Ethinyl Estradiol and Norethindrone 84
Minocin® *see* Minocycline 113
Minocycline 113
Min-Ovral® (Can) *see* Ethinyl Estradiol and Levonorgestrel 83
Mircette® *see* Ethinyl Estradiol and Desogestrel 82
Mirena® *see* Levonorgestrel 103
Mirtazapine 113
Misoprostol and Diclofenac *see* Diclofenac and Misoprostol 72
Mitomycin 113
Mitomycin-C *see* Mitomycin 113
Mitomycin-X *see* Mitomycin 113
MK383 *see* Tirofiban 149
MK594 *see* Losartan 105
MK869 *see* Aprepitant 50
MMC-IA *see* HLA-A1 200
MMP3 *see* Stromelysin-1 219
Moban® *see* Molindone 114
MOBIC® *see* Meloxicam 108
Mobicox® (Can) *see* Meloxicam 108
Moclobemide 114
Modafinil 114
Modecate® (Can) *see* Fluphenazine 88
Modicon® *see* Ethinyl Estradiol and Norethindrone 84
Moditen® Enanthate (Can) *see* Fluphenazine 88
Moditen® HCl (Can) *see* Fluphenazine 88
Moexipril 114
Molindone 114
Mometasone Furoate 114
Monacolin K *see* Lovastatin 106
Monitan® (Can) *see* Acebutolol 44
Monocor® (Can) *see* Bisoprolol 56
Monodox® *see* Doxycycline 76
Monopril® *see* Fosinopril 90
Montelukast 115
Moricizine 115
Morning After Pill *see* Ethinyl Estradiol and Norgestrel 84

ALPHABETICAL INDEX

Morphine HP® (Can) *see* Morphine Sulfate 115
Morphine LP® Epidural (Can) *see* Morphine Sulfate 115
Morphine Sulfate 115
M.O.S.-Sulfate® (Can) *see* Morphine Sulfate 115
Motilium® (Can) *see* Domperidone 75
Motrin® *see* Ibuprofen 96
Motrin® Children's [OTC] *see* Ibuprofen 96
Motrin® IB [OTC] *see* Ibuprofen 96
Motrin® Infants' [OTC] *see* Ibuprofen 96
Motrin® Junior Strength [OTC] *see* Ibuprofen 96
Motrin® Migraine Pain [OTC] *see* Ibuprofen 96
Moxifloxacin 115
Moxilin® *see* Amoxicillin 49
6-MP *see* Mercaptopurine 109
MPA and Estrogens (Conjugated) *see* Estrogens (Conjugated/ Equine) and Medroxyprogesterone 81
MS *see* Morphine Sulfate 115
MS Contin® *see* Morphine Sulfate 115
MS-IR® (Can) *see* Morphine Sulfate 115
MTC *see* Mitomycin 113
MTHFR *see* Methylenetetrahydrofolate Reductase 210
Multidrug Resistance Gene *see* P-Glycoprotein 213
Mupirocin 116
Mutamycin® *see* Mitomycin 113
Mycobutin® *see* Rifabutin 136
Mykrox® *see* Metolazone 111
Myleran® *see* Busulfan 58
Nabumetone 116
N-Acetyltransferase 2 Enzyme 211
Nadolol 116
Nadopen-V® (Can) *see* Penicillin V Potassium 125
NAD(P)H Quinone Oxidoreductase 212
Nalbuphine 116
Nalfon® *see* Fenoprofen 86
Nalidixic Acid 116
Nalidixinic Acid *see* Nalidixic Acid 116
Naloxone and Buprenorphine *see* Buprenorphine and Naloxone 58
Naloxone Hydrochloride Dihydrate and Buprenorphine Hydrochloride *see* Buprenorphine and Naloxone 58
Naprelan® *see* Naproxen 117
Naprosyn® *see* Naproxen 117
Naproxen 117
Naqua® *see* Trichlormethiazide 151
Nasacort® *see* Triamcinolone 151
Nasacort® AQ *see* Triamcinolone 151
Nasonex® *see* Mometasone Furoate 114
NAT2 *see* N-Acetyltransferase 2 Enzyme 211
Nateglinide 117
Naturetin® *see* Bendroflumethiazide 55
Navane® *see* Thiothixene 148
Navelbine® *see* Vinorelbine 155
Naxen® (Can) *see* Naproxen 117
NebuPent® *see* Pentamidine 125
Necon® 0.5/35 *see* Ethinyl Estradiol and Norethindrone 84

ALPHABETICAL INDEX

Necon® 1/35 see Ethynyl Estradiol and Norethindrone 84
Necon® 1/50 see Mestranol and Norethindrone 109
Necon® 7/7/7 see Ethynyl Estradiol and Norethindrone 84
Necon® 10/11 see Ethynyl Estradiol and Norethindrone 84
Nefazodone 117
NegGram® see Nalidixic Acid 116
Nelfinavir 118
Neoral® see CycloSPORINE 69
Neosar® see Cyclophosphamide 69
Neurontin® see Gabapentin 91
Nexium® see Esomeprazole 80
NiCARdipine 118
Nidagel™ (Can) see Metronidazole 112
Nifedical™ XL see NIFEdipine 118
NIFEdipine 118
Niftolid see Flutamide 89
Nilandron® see Nilutamide 118
Nilutamide 118
Nimodipine 118
Nimotop® see Nimodipine 118
Nisoldipine 119
Nitalapram see Citalopram 64
Nitrendipine 119
4'-Nitro-3'-Trifluoromethylisobutyrantide see Flutamide 89
Nitrofurantoin 119
Nizoral® see Ketoconazole 101
Nizoral® A-D [OTC] see Ketoconazole 101
Nolvadex® see Tamoxifen 145
Nolvadex®-D (Can) see Tamoxifen 145
Norco® see Hydrocodone and Acetaminophen 94
Nordette® see Ethynyl Estradiol and Levonorgestrel 83
Norelgestromin and Ethynyl Estradiol see Ethynyl Estradiol and
    Norelgestromin 83
Norethindrone 119
Norethindrone Acetate and Ethynyl Estradiol see Ethynyl Estradiol
    and Norethindrone 84
Norethindrone and Mestranol see Mestranol and Norethindrone 109
Norethisterone see Norethindrone 119
Norgestimate and Ethynyl Estradiol see Ethynyl Estradiol and
    Norgestimate 84
Norgestrel 119
Norgestrel and Ethynyl Estradiol see Ethynyl Estradiol and
    Norgestrel 84
Norinyl® 1+35 see Ethynyl Estradiol and Norethindrone 84
Norinyl® 1+50 see Mestranol and Norethindrone 109
Noritate™ see Metronidazole 112
Norlutate® (Can) see Norethindrone 119
Norpace® see Disopyramide 74
Norpace® CR see Disopyramide 74
Norplant® Implant [DSC] see Levonorgestrel 103
Norpramin® see Desipramine 71
Nor-QD® see Norethindrone 119
Nortrel™ see Ethynyl Estradiol and Norethindrone 84
Nortrel™ 7/7/7 see Ethynyl Estradiol and Norethindrone 84

ALPHABETICAL INDEX

Nortriptyline 120
Norvasc® *see* Amlodipine 49
Norventyl (Can) *see* Nortriptyline 120
Norvir® *see* Ritonavir 137
Norvir® SEC (Can) *see* Ritonavir 137
Novamoxin® (Can) *see* Amoxicillin 49
Novasen (Can) *see* Aspirin 51
Novo-Acebutolol (Can) *see* Acebutolol 44
Novo-Alprazol (Can) *see* Alprazolam 47
Novo-Amiodarone (Can) *see* Amiodarone 48
Novo-Atenol (Can) *see* Atenolol 53
Novo-Bromazepam (Can) *see* Bromazepam 57
Novo-Buspirone (Can) *see* BusPIRone 58
Novo-Captopril (Can) *see* Captopril 60
Novo-Carbamaz (Can) *see* Carbamazepine 60
Novo-Chlorpromazine (Can) *see* ChlorproMAZINE 63
Novo-Cimetidine (Can) *see* Cimetidine 64
Novo-Clobazam (Can) *see* Clobazam 65
Novo-Clonazepam (Can) *see* Clonazepam 66
Novo-Clonidine® (Can) *see* Clonidine 66
Novo-Clopate® (Can) *see* Clorazepate 67
Novo-Clopramine (Can) *see* ClomiPRAMINE 66
Novo-Cycloprine® (Can) *see* Cyclobenzaprine 69
Novo-Desipramine (Can) *see* Desipramine 71
Novo-Difenac® (Can) *see* Diclofenac 72
Novo-Difenac K (Can) *see* Diclofenac 72
Novo-Difenac-SR® (Can) *see* Diclofenac 72
Novo-Diflunisal (Can) *see* Diflunisal 73
Novo-Digoxin (Can) *see* Digoxin 73
Novo-Diltazem (Can) *see* Diltiazem 74
Novo-Diltazem-CD (Can) *see* Diltiazem 74
Novo-Diltazem SR (Can) *see* Diltiazem 74
Novo-Dipiradol (Can) *see* Dipyridamole 74
Novo-Divalproex (Can) *see* Valproic Acid and Derivatives 153
Novo-Domperidone (Can) *see* Domperidone 75
Novo-Doxazosin (Can) *see* Doxazosin 76
Novo-Doxepin (Can) *see* Doxepin 76
Novo-Doxylin (Can) *see* Doxycycline 76
Novo-Famotidine (Can) *see* Famotidine 85
Novo-Fenofibrate (Can) *see* Fenofibrate 86
Novo-Fluoxetine (Can) *see* Fluoxetine 88
Novo-Flurprofen (Can) *see* Flurbiprofen 89
Novo-Flutamide (Can) *see* Flutamide 89
Novo-Fluvoxamine (Can) *see* Fluvoxamine 90
Novo-Furantoin (Can) *see* Nitrofurantoin 119
Novo-Gabapentin (Can) *see* Gabapentin 91
Novo-Gemfibrozil (Can) *see* Gemfibrozil 91
Novo-Glyburide (Can) *see* GlyBURIDE 92
Novo-Hydrazide (Can) *see* Hydrochlorothiazide 94
Novo-Hydroxyzin (Can) *see* HydrOXYzine 96
Novo-Hylazin (Can) *see* HydrALAZINE 94
Novo-Indapamide (Can) *see* Indapamide 98
Novo-Keto (Can) *see* Ketoprofen 101
Novo-Ketoconazole (Can) *see* Ketoconazole 101

ALPHABETICAL INDEX

Novo-Keto-EC (Can) *see* Ketoprofen 101
Novo-Ketorolac (Can) *see* Ketorolac 101
Novo-Lexin® (Can) *see* Cephalexin 62
Novolin® 70/30 *see* Insulin Preparations 98
Novolin® ge (Can) *see* Insulin Preparations 98
Novolin® L *see* Insulin Preparations 98
Novolin® N *see* Insulin Preparations 98
Novolin® R *see* Insulin Preparations 98
NovoLog® *see* Insulin Preparations 98
NovoLog® Mix 70/30 *see* Insulin Preparations 98
Novo-Lorazepam® (Can) *see* Lorazepam 105
Novo-Maprotiline (Can) *see* Maprotiline 107
Novo-Medrone (Can) *see* MedroxyPROGESTERone 107
Novo-Meprazine (Can) *see* Methotrimeprazine 110
Novo-Metformin (Can) *see* Metformin 109
Novo-Methacin (Can) *see* Indomethacin 98
Novo-Metoprolol (Can) *see* Metoprolol 112
Novo-Mexiletine (Can) *see* Mexiletine 112
Novo-Minocycline (Can) *see* Minocycline 113
Novo-Moclobemide (Can) *see* Moclobemide 114
Novo-Nadolol (Can) *see* Nadolol 116
Novo-Naproc EC (Can) *see* Naproxen 117
Novo-Naprox (Can) *see* Naproxen 117
Novo-Naprox Sodium (Can) *see* Naproxen 117
Novo-Naprox Sodium DS (Can) *see* Naproxen 117
Novo-Naprox SR (Can) *see* Naproxen 117
Novo-Nidazol (Can) *see* Metronidazole 112
Novo-Nifedin (Can) *see* NIFEdipine 118
Novo-Nortriptyline (Can) *see* Nortriptyline 120
Novo-Pen-VK® (Can) *see* Penicillin V Potassium 125
Novo-Peridol (Can) *see* Haloperidol 93
Novo-Pirocam (Can) *see* Piroxicam 128
Novo-Pravastatin (Can) *see* Pravastatin 129
Novo-Profen® (Can) *see* Ibuprofen 96
Novo-Quinidin (Can) *see* Quinidine 134
Novo-Ranitidine (Can) *see* Ranitidine 135
NovoRapid® (Can) *see* Insulin Preparations 98
Novo-Selegiline (Can) *see* Selegiline 139
Novo-Sertraline (Can) *see* Sertraline 139
Novo-Sorbide (Can) *see* Isosorbide Dinitrate 100
Novo-Sotalol (Can) *see* Sotalol 141
Novo-Soxazole® (Can) *see* SulfiSOXAZOLE 144
Novo-Spiroton (Can) *see* Spironolactone 142
Novo-Sundac (Can) *see* Sulindac 144
Novo-Tamoxifen (Can) *see* Tamoxifen 145
Novo-Temazepam (Can) *see* Temazepam 145
Novo-Terazosin (Can) *see* Terazosin 146
Novo-Tetra (Can) *see* Tetracycline 146
Novo-Theophyl SR (Can) *see* Theophylline 147
Novothyrox *see* Levothyroxine 103
Novo-Tiaprofenic (Can) *see* Tiaprofenic Acid 148
Novo-Trazodone (Can) *see* Trazodone 151
Novo-Trifluzine (Can) *see* Trifluoperazine 151
Novo-Trimel (Can) *see* Sulfamethoxazole and Trimethoprim 143

ALPHABETICAL INDEX

Novo-Trimel D.S. (Can) see Sulfamethoxazole and Trimethoprim ... 143
Novo-Tripramine (Can) see Trimipramine 152
Novo-Veramil (Can) see Verapamil 154
Novo-Veramil SR (Can) see Verapamil 154
Nozinan® (Can) see Methotrimeprazine 110
NPH Iletin® II see Insulin Preparations 98
NQO1 see NAD(P)H Quinone Oxidoreductase 212
NSC-752 see Thioguanine 147
NSC-755 see Mercaptopurine 109
NSC-26271 see Cyclophosphamide 69
NSC-26980 see Mitomycin 113
NSC-49842 see VinBLAStine 154
NSC-67574 see VinCRIStine 155
NSC-109724 see Ifosfamide 97
NSC-123127 see DOXOrubicin 76
NSC-125973 see Paclitaxel 124
NSC-147834 see Flutamide 89
NSC-180973 see Tamoxifen 145
NSC-628503 see Docetaxel 75
NSC-639186 see Raltitrexed 135
NSC-706363 see Arsenic Trioxide 51
Nu-Acebutolol (Can) see Acebutolol 44
Nu-Acyclovir (Can) see Acyclovir 45
Nu-Alprax (Can) see Alprazolam 47
Nu-Amoxi (Can) see Amoxicillin 49
Nu-Atenol (Can) see Atenolol 53
Nubain® see Nalbuphine 116
Nu-Bromazepam (Can) see Bromazepam 57
Nu-Buspirone (Can) see BusPIRone 58
Nu-Capto® (Can) see Captopril 60
Nu-Carbamazepine® (Can) see Carbamazepine 60
Nu-Cephalex® (Can) see Cephalexin 62
Nu-Cimet® (Can) see Cimetidine 64
Nu-Clonazepam (Can) see Clonazepam 66
Nu-Clonidine® (Can) see Clonidine 66
Nu-Cotrimox® (Can) see Sulfamethoxazole and Trimethoprim 143
Nu-Cyclobenzaprine (Can) see Cyclobenzaprine 69
Nu-Desipramine (Can) see Desipramine 71
Nu-Diclo (Can) see Diclofenac 72
Nu-Diclo-SR (Can) see Diclofenac 72
Nu-Diflunisal (Can) see Diflunisal 73
Nu-Diltiaz (Can) see Diltiazem 74
Nu-Diltiaz-CD (Can) see Diltiazem 74
Nu-Divalproex (Can) see Valproic Acid and Derivatives 153
Nu-Domperidone (Can) see Domperidone 75
Nu-Doxycycline (Can) see Doxycycline 76
Nu-Erythromycin-S (Can) see Erythromycin 79
Nu-Famotidine (Can) see Famotidine 85
Nu-Fenofibrate (Can) see Fenofibrate 86
Nu-Fluoxetine (Can) see Fluoxetine 88
Nu-Flurprofen (Can) see Flurbiprofen 89
Nu-Fluvoxamine (Can) see Fluvoxamine 90
Nu-Gemfibrozil (Can) see Gemfibrozil 91
Nu-Glyburide (Can) see GlyBURIDE 92

ALPHABETICAL INDEX

Nu-Hydral (Can) *see* HydrALAZINE	94
Nu-Ibuprofen (Can) *see* Ibuprofen	96
Nu-Indapamide (Can) *see* Indapamide	98
Nu-Indo (Can) *see* Indomethacin	98
Nu-Ketoprofen (Can) *see* Ketoprofen	101
Nu-Ketoprofen-E (Can) *see* Ketoprofen	101
Nu-Loraz (Can) *see* Lorazepam	105
Nu-Loxapine (Can) *see* Loxapine	106
Nu-Mefenamic (Can) *see* Mefenamic Acid	108
Nu-Metformin (Can) *see* Metformin	109
Nu-Metoclopramide (Can) *see* Metoclopramide	111
Nu-Metop (Can) *see* Metoprolol	112
Nu-Moclobemide (Can) *see* Moclobemide	114
Numorphan® *see* Oxymorphone	124
Nu-Naprox (Can) *see* Naproxen	117
Nu-Nifed (Can) *see* NIFEdipine	118
Nu-Nortriptyline (Can) *see* Nortriptyline	120
Nu-Pen-VK® (Can) *see* Penicillin V Potassium	125
Nupercainal® Hydrocortisone Cream [OTC] *see* Hydrocortisone	95
Nu-Pirox (Can) *see* Piroxicam	128
Nu-Prochlor (Can) *see* Prochlorperazine	130
Nu-Propranolol (Can) *see* Propranolol	132
Nu-Ranit (Can) *see* Ranitidine	135
Nu-Selegiline (Can) *see* Selegiline	139
Nu-Sotalol (Can) *see* Sotalol	141
Nu-Sulfinpyrazone (Can) *see* Sulfinpyrazone	143
Nu-Sundac (Can) *see* Sulindac	144
Nu-Temazepam (Can) *see* Temazepam	145
Nu-Terazosin (Can) *see* Terazosin	146
Nu-Tetra (Can) *see* Tetracycline	146
Nu-Tiaprofenic (Can) *see* Tiaprofenic Acid	148
Nu-Ticlopidine (Can) *see* Ticlopidine	148
Nu-Timolol (Can) *see* Timolol	148
Nutracort® *see* Hydrocortisone	95
Nu-Trazodone (Can) *see* Trazodone	151
Nu-Trimipramine (Can) *see* Trimipramine	152
NuvaRing® *see* Ethinyl Estradiol and Etonogestrel	83
Nu-Verap (Can) *see* Verapamil	154
Nu-Zopiclone (Can) *see* Zopiclone	157
NVB *see* Vinorelbine	155
Nydrazid® *see* Isoniazid	99
Octreotide	121
Ocu-Chlor® *see* Chloramphenicol	62
Ocufen® *see* Flurbiprofen	89
Ocuflox® *see* Ofloxacin	121
Ocusulf-10 *see* Sulfacetamide	142
Oesclim® (Can) *see* Estradiol	80
Ofloxacin	121
Ogen® *see* Estropipate	82
Ogestrel® *see* Ethinyl Estradiol and Norgestrel	84
Olanzapine	121
Olmesartan	122
Olopatadine	122
Omeprazole	122

ALPHABETICAL INDEX

Omnicef® see Cefdinir 61
Oncovin® [DSC] see VinCRIStine 155
Onxol™ see Paclitaxel 124
OPC13013 see Cilostazol 64
OPC14597 see Aripiprazole 51
Opium and Belladonna see Belladonna and Opium 55
Opium Tincture 122
Opium Tincture, Deodorized see Opium Tincture 122
Optivar™ see Azelastine 54
Oracort (Can) see Triamcinolone 151
Oramorph SR® see Morphine Sulfate 115
Orap® see Pimozide 127
Orciprenaline Sulfate see Metaproterenol 109
Oretic® see Hydrochlorothiazide 94
Orinase Diagnostic® [DSC] see TOLBUTamide 149
ORLAAM® see Levomethadyl Acetate Hydrochloride 102
Ortho® 0.5/35 (Can) see Ethinyl Estradiol and Norethindrone .. 84
Ortho® 1/35 (Can) see Ethinyl Estradiol and Norethindrone .. 84
Ortho® 7/7/7 (Can) see Ethinyl Estradiol and Norethindrone .. 84
Ortho-Cept® see Ethinyl Estradiol and Desogestrel 82
Ortho-Cyclen® see Ethinyl Estradiol and Norgestimate 84
Ortho-Est® see Estropipate 82
Ortho Evra™ see Ethinyl Estradiol and Norelgestromin ... 83
Ortho-Novum® see Ethinyl Estradiol and Norethindrone .. 84
Ortho-Novum® 1/50 see Mestranol and Norethindrone .. 109
Ortho Tri-Cyclen® see Ethinyl Estradiol and Norgestimate .. 84
Ortho Tri-Cyclen® Lo see Ethinyl Estradiol and Norgestimate .. 84
Orudis® [DSC] see Ketoprofen 101
Orudis® KT [OTC] see Ketoprofen 101
Orudis® SR (Can) see Ketoprofen 101
Oruvail® see Ketoprofen 101
Ovace™ see Sulfacetamide 142
Ovcon® see Ethinyl Estradiol and Norethindrone 84
Ovral® see Ethinyl Estradiol and Norgestrel 84
Ovrette® see Norgestrel 119
Oxaprozin 123
Oxeze® Turbuhaler® (Can) see Formoterol 90
Oxilapine Succinate see Loxapine 106
Oxycocet® (Can) see Oxycodone and Acetaminophen ... 123
Oxycodan® (Can) see Oxycodone and Aspirin 123
Oxycodone 123
Oxycodone and Acetaminophen 123
Oxycodone and Aspirin 123
OxyContin® see Oxycodone 123
Oxydose™ see Oxycodone 123
OxyFast® see Oxycodone 123
Oxy.IR® (Can) see Oxycodone 123
Oxymorphone 124
P-071 see Cetirizine 62
P-450 C18 11-Beta Hydroxylase see Aldosterone Synthase .. 160
Pacerone® see Amiodarone 48
Paclitaxel 124
Pamelor® see Nortriptyline 120
Pandel® see Hydrocortisone 95

ALPHABETICAL INDEX

Panto™ IV (Can) see Pantoprazole	124
Pantoloc™ (Can) see Pantoprazole	124
Pantoprazole	124
Paregoric	124
Pariet® (Can) see Rabeprazole	134
Pariprazole see Rabeprazole	134
Parlodel® see Bromocriptine	57
Paroxetine	124
Patanol® see Olopatadine	122
Paxil® see Paroxetine	124
Paxil® CR™ see Paroxetine	124
PCA see Procainamide	130
PCE® see Erythromycin	79
PCP see Phencyclidine	127
Pediazole® see Erythromycin and Sulfisoxazole	80
Penicillin V Potassium	125
Pentacarinat® (Can) see Pentamidine	125
Pentam-300® see Pentamidine	125
Pentamidine	125
Pentamycetin® (Can) see Chloramphenicol	62
Pentazocine	125
Pentazocine Combinations	125
Pen VK see Penicillin V Potassium	125
Pepcid® see Famotidine	85
Pepcid® AC [OTC] see Famotidine	85
Pepcid® I.V. (Can) see Famotidine	85
Percocet® (Can) see Oxycodone and Acetaminophen	123
Percocet® 2.5/325 see Oxycodone and Acetaminophen	123
Percocet® 5/325 see Oxycodone and Acetaminophen	123
Percocet® 7.5/325 see Oxycodone and Acetaminophen	123
Percocet® 7.5/500 see Oxycodone and Acetaminophen	123
Percocet® 10/325 see Oxycodone and Acetaminophen	123
Percocet® 10/650 see Oxycodone and Acetaminophen	123
Percocet®-Demi (Can) see Oxycodone and Acetaminophen	123
Percodan® see Oxycodone and Aspirin	123
Percodan®-Demi [DSC] see Oxycodone and Aspirin	123
Percogesic® [OTC] see Acetaminophen and Phenyltoloxamine	45
Percolone® [DSC] see Oxycodone	123
Pergolide	126
Peridol (Can) see Haloperidol	93
Perindopril Erbumine	126
Periostat® see Doxycycline	76
Permax® see Pergolide	126
Perphenazine	126
Perphenazine and Amitriptyline see Amitriptyline and Perphenazine	49
Persantine® see Dipyridamole	74
Pethidine Hydrochloride see Meperidine	108
Pexicam® (Can) see Piroxicam	128
PFA see Foscarnet	90
P-Glycoprotein	213
PGP see P-Glycoprotein	213
PGY1 see P-Glycoprotein	213
Phenaphen® With Codeine see Acetaminophen and Codeine	44

ALPHABETICAL INDEX

Phencyclidine 127
Phenergan® (Can) *see* Promethazine 131
Phenergan® With Codeine *see* Promethazine and Codeine 131
Phenobarbital 127
Phenobarbitone *see* Phenobarbital 127
Phenoxymethyl Penicillin *see* Penicillin V Potassium 125
Phenylethylmalonylurea *see* Phenobarbital 127
Phenylgesic® [OTC] *see* Acetaminophen and Phenyltoloxamine 45
Phenyltoloxamine and Acetaminophen *see* Acetaminophen and
   Phenyltoloxamine 45
Phenytek™ *see* Phenytoin 127
Phenytoin 127
Phosphonoformate *see* Foscarnet 90
Phosphonoformic Acid *see* Foscarnet 90
Phoxal-timolol (Can) *see* Timolol 148
p-Hydroxyampicillin *see* Amoxicillin 49
Phyllocontin® (Can) *see* Aminophylline 48
Phyllocontin®-350 (Can) *see* Aminophylline 48
Pimozide 127
Pioglitazone 128
Piperazine Estrone Sulfate *see* Estropipate 82
Pirbuterol 128
Piroxicam 128
p-Isobutylhydratropic Acid *see* Ibuprofen 96
Plan B® *see* Levonorgestrel 103
Plaquenil® *see* Hydroxychloroquine 96
Platelet Fc Gamma Receptor 216
Plavix® *see* Clopidogrel 66
Plendil® *see* Felodipine 86
Pletal® *see* Cilostazol 64
PMS-Amitriptyline (Can) *see* Amitriptyline 48
PMS-Atenolol (Can) *see* Atenolol 53
PMS-Bezafibrate (Can) *see* Bezafibrate 56
PMS-Bromocriptine (Can) *see* Bromocriptine 57
PMS-Buspirone (Can) *see* BusPIRone 58
PMS-Captopril® (Can) *see* Captopril 60
PMS-Carbamazepine (Can) *see* Carbamazepine 60
PMS-Cimetidine (Can) *see* Cimetidine 64
PMS-Clobazam (Can) *see* Clobazam 65
PMS-Clonazepam (Can) *see* Clonazepam 66
PMS-Desipramine (Can) *see* Desipramine 71
PMS-Diclofenac (Can) *see* Diclofenac 72
PMS-Diclofenac SR (Can) *see* Diclofenac 72
PMS-Erythromycin (Can) *see* Erythromycin 79
PMS-Fenofibrate Micro (Can) *see* Fenofibrate 86
PMS-Fluoxetine (Can) *see* Fluoxetine 88
PMS-Fluphenazine Decanoate (Can) *see* Fluphenazine 88
PMS-Flutamide (Can) *see* Flutamide 89
PMS-Fluvoxamine (Can) *see* Fluvoxamine 90
PMS-Gabapentin (Can) *see* Gabapentin 91
PMS-Gemfibrozil (Can) *see* Gemfibrozil 91
PMS-Glyburide (Can) *see* GlyBURIDE 92
PMS-Haloperidol LA (Can) *see* Haloperidol 93
PMS-Hydromorphone (Can) *see* Hydromorphone 96

ALPHABETICAL INDEX

PMS-Hydroxyzine (Can) *see* HydrOXYzine 96
PMS-Indapamide (Can) *see* Indapamide 98
PMS-Isoniazid (Can) *see* Isoniazid 99
PMS-Isosorbide (Can) *see* Isosorbide Dinitrate 100
PMS-Loxapine (Can) *see* Loxapine 106
PMS-Mefenamic Acid (Can) *see* Mefenamic Acid 108
PMS-Metformin (Can) *see* Metformin 109
PMS-Methylphenidate (Can) *see* Methylphenidate 111
PMS-Metoprolol (Can) *see* Metoprolol 112
PMS-Minocycline (Can) *see* Minocycline 113
PMS-Moclobemide (Can) *see* Moclobemide 114
PMS-Nortriptyline (Can) *see* Nortriptyline 120
PMS-Ranitidine (Can) *see* Ranitidine 135
PMS-Salbutamol (Can) *see* Albuterol 46
PMS-Sotalol (Can) *see* Sotalol 141
PMS-Tamoxifen (Can) *see* Tamoxifen 145
PMS-Temazepam (Can) *see* Temazepam 145
PMS-Terazosin (Can) *see* Terazosin 146
PMS-Theophylline (Can) *see* Theophylline 147
PMS-Tiaprofenic (Can) *see* Tiaprofenic Acid 148
PMS-Ticlopidine (Can) *see* Ticlopidine 148
PMS-Timolol (Can) *see* Timolol 148
PMS-Trazodone (Can) *see* Trazodone 151
PMS-Trifluoperazine (Can) *see* Trifluoperazine 151
PMS-Valproic Acid (Can) *see* Valproic Acid and Derivatives ... 153
PMS-Valproic Acid E.C. (Can) *see* Valproic Acid and Derivatives ... 153
Polythiazide 128
Ponstan® (Can) *see* Mefenamic Acid 108
Ponstel® *see* Mefenamic Acid 108
Portia™ *see* Ethinyl Estradiol and Levonorgestrel 83
Post Peel Healing Balm [OTC] *see* Hydrocortisone 95
Potassium Chloride 128
Prandin® *see* Repaglinide 136
Pravachol® *see* Pravastatin 129
Pravastatin 129
Precedex™ *see* Dexmedetomidine 71
PredniSONE 129
Prednisone Intensol™ *see* PredniSONE 129
Pregnenedione *see* Progesterone 131
Premarin® *see* Estrogens (Conjugated/Equine) 81
Premjact® [OTC] *see* Lidocaine 103
Premphase® *see* Estrogens (Conjugated/Equine) and
  Medroxyprogesterone 81
Premplus® (Can) *see* Estrogens (Conjugated/Equine) and
  Medroxyprogesterone 81
Prempro™ *see* Estrogens (Conjugated/Equine) and
  Medroxyprogesterone 81
Preparation H® Hydrocortisone [OTC] *see* Hydrocortisone 95
Prevacid® *see* Lansoprazole 102
PREVEN® *see* Ethinyl Estradiol and Levonorgestrel 83
Prevex® HC (Can) *see* Hydrocortisone 95
Prilocaine and Lidocaine *see* Lidocaine and Prilocaine 104
Prilosec® *see* Omeprazole 122
Primaquine 130

ALPHABETICAL INDEX

Primsol® see Trimethoprim	152
Prinivil® see Lisinopril	104
Prinzide® see Lisinopril and Hydrochlorothiazide	104
Probenecid	130
PROC see Protein C	217
Procainamide	130
Procaine Amide Hydrochloride see Procainamide	130
Procanbid® see Procainamide	130
Procan® SR (Can) see Procainamide	130
Procardia® see NIFEdipine	118
Procardia XL® see NIFEdipine	118
Procetofene see Fenofibrate	86
Prochieve™ see Progesterone	131
Prochlorperazine	130
Proctocort® see Hydrocortisone	95
ProctoCream® HC see Hydrocortisone	95
Proctofene see Fenofibrate	86
Proctosol-HC® see Hydrocortisone	95
Procytox® (Can) see Cyclophosphamide	69
Progestasert® see Progesterone	131
Progesterone	131
Progestin see Progesterone	131
Prograf® see Tacrolimus	144
Prolixin® see Fluphenazine	88
Prolixin Decanoate® see Fluphenazine	88
Prolixin Enanthate® [DSC] see Fluphenazine	88
Proloprim® see Trimethoprim	152
Promethazine	131
Promethazine and Codeine	131
Promethazine and Meperidine see Meperidine and Promethazine	108
Prometrium® see Progesterone	131
Pronap-100® see Propoxyphene and Acetaminophen	132
Pronestyl® see Procainamide	130
Pronestyl-SR® see Procainamide	130
Propafenone	131
Propofol	131
Propoxyphene	132
Propoxyphene and Acetaminophen	132
Propoxyphene and Aspirin	132
Propoxyphene Hydrochloride and Acetaminophen see Propoxyphene and Acetaminophen	132
Propoxyphene Hydrochloride and Aspirin see Propoxyphene and Aspirin	132
Propoxyphene Napsylate and Acetaminophen see Propoxyphene and Acetaminophen	132
Propoxyphene Napsylate and Aspirin see Propoxyphene and Aspirin	132
Propranolol	132
Propranolol Intensol™ see Propranolol	132
Propulsid® see Cisapride	64
2-Propylpentanoic Acid see Valproic Acid and Derivatives	153
2-Propylvaleric Acid see Valproic Acid and Derivatives	153
Protein C	217
Protein S	218

ALPHABETICAL INDEX

Prothrombin	219
Protonix® *see* Pantoprazole	124
Protopic® *see* Tacrolimus	144
Protriptyline	133
Proventil® *see* Albuterol	46
Proventil® HFA *see* Albuterol	46
Proventil® Repetabs® *see* Albuterol	46
Provera® *see* MedroxyPROGESTERone	107
Provigil® *see* Modafinil	114
Prozac® *see* Fluoxetine	88
Prozac® Weekly™ *see* Fluoxetine	88
Prudoxin™ *see* Doxepin	76
Prymaccone *see* Primaquine	130
Pseudomonic Acid A *see* Mupirocin	116
PT *see* Prothrombin	219
Pulmicort® (Can) *see* Budesonide	57
Pulmicort Respules® *see* Budesonide	57
Pulmicort Turbuhaler® *see* Budesonide	57
Pulmophylline (Can) *see* Theophylline	147
Purinethol® *see* Mercaptopurine	109
PVF® K (Can) *see* Penicillin V Potassium	125
Pyrimethamine and Sulfadoxine *see* Sulfadoxine and Pyrimethamine	143
Quetiapine	133
Quibron®-T *see* Theophylline	147
Quibron®-T/SR *see* Theophylline	147
Quinaglute® Dura-Tabs® *see* Quinidine	134
Quinapril	133
Quinate® (Can) *see* Quinidine	134
Quinidex® Extentabs® *see* Quinidine	134
Quinidine	134
Quinine	134
Quinine-Odan™ (Can) *see* Quinine	134
Quinone Oxidoreductase *see* NAD(P)H Quinone Oxidoreductase	212
Quixin™ *see* Levofloxacin	102
Rabeprazole	134
R-albuterol *see* Levalbuterol	102
Raloxifene	134
Raltitrexed	135
Ramipril	135
Ranitidine	135
Rapamune® *see* Sirolimus	141
Rasburicase	135
ratio-Acyclovir (Can) *see* Acyclovir	45
ratio-AmoxiClav (Can) *see* Amoxicillin and Clavulanate Potassium	50
ratio-Colchicine (Can) *see* Colchicine	68
ratio-Diltiazem CD (Can) *see* Diltiazem	74
Ratio-Domperidone (Can) *see* Domperidone	75
ratio-Famotidine (Can) *see* Famotidine	85
ratio-Glyburide (Can) *see* GlyBURIDE	92
ratio-Inspra-Sal (Can) *see* Albuterol	46
ratio-Lovastatin (Can) *see* Lovastatin	106
ratio-Morphine SR (Can) *see* Morphine Sulfate	115
ratio-Salbutamol (Can) *see* Albuterol	46

ALPHABETICAL INDEX

ratio-Sertraline (Can) *see* Sertraline 139
ratio-Theo-Bronc (Can) *see* Theophylline 147
Reactine™ (Can) *see* Cetirizine 62
Reglan® *see* Metoclopramide 111
Regular Iletin® II *see* Insulin Preparations 98
Relafen® *see* Nabumetone 116
Relpax® *see* Eletriptan 77
Remeron® *see* Mirtazapine 113
Remeron SolTab® *see* Mirtazapine 113
Remifentanil 135
Reminyl® *see* Galantamine 91
Renedil® (Can) *see* Felodipine 86
Renese® *see* Polythiazide 128
ReoPro® *see* Abciximab 44
Repaglinide 136
Requip® *see* Ropinirole 138
Reserpine 136
Restasis™ *see* CycloSPORINE 69
Restoril® *see* Temazepam 145
Rhinocort® [DSC] *see* Budesonide 57
Rhinocort® Aqua™ *see* Budesonide 57
Rhinocort® Turbuhaler® (Can) *see* Budesonide 57
Rho-Clonazepam (Can) *see* Clonazepam 66
Rhodacine® (Can) *see* Indomethacin 98
Rhodis™ (Can) *see* Ketoprofen 101
Rhodis-EC™ (Can) *see* Ketoprofen 101
Rhodis SR™ (Can) *see* Ketoprofen 101
Rho®-Metformin (Can) *see* Metformin 109
Rho®-Sotalol (Can) *see* Sotalol 141
Rhotral (Can) *see* Acebutolol 44
Rhotrimine® (Can) *see* Trimipramine 152
Rhovane® (Can) *see* Zopiclone 157
Rhoxal-amiodarone (Can) *see* Amiodarone 48
Rhoxal-atenolol (Can) *see* Atenolol 53
Rhoxal-clozapine (Can) *see* Clozapine 67
Rhoxal-cyclosporine (Can) *see* CycloSPORINE 69
Rhoxal-diltiazem CD (Can) *see* Diltiazem 74
Rhoxal-diltiazem SR (Can) *see* Diltiazem 74
Rhoxal-famotidine (Can) *see* Famotidine 85
Rhoxal-fluoxetine (Can) *see* Fluoxetine 88
Rhoxal-metformin FC (Can) *see* Metformin 109
Rhoxal-minocycline (Can) *see* Minocycline 113
Rhoxal-nabumetone (Can) *see* Nabumetone 116
Rhoxal-oxaprozin (Can) *see* Oxaprozin 123
Rhoxal-ranitidine (Can) *see* Ranitidine 135
Rhoxal-salbutamol (Can) *see* Albuterol 46
Rhoxal-sertraline (Can) *see* Sertraline 139
Rhoxal-ticlopidine (Can) *see* Ticlopidine 148
Rhoxal-valproic (Can) *see* Valproic Acid and Derivatives ... 153
Rifabutin 136
Rifadin® *see* Rifampin 136
Rifampicin *see* Rifampin 136
Rifampin 136
Rilutek® *see* Riluzole 136

ALPHABETICAL INDEX

Riluzole 136
Rimactane® see Rifampin 136
Riphenidate (Can) see Methylphenidate 111
Risedronate 137
Risperdal® see Risperidone 137
Risperdal Consta™ [Investigational] see Risperidone . 137
Risperdal M-Tab™ see Risperidone 137
Risperidone 137
Ritalin® see Methylphenidate 111
Ritalin® LA see Methylphenidate 111
Ritalin-SR® see Methylphenidate 111
Ritonavir 137
Riva-Diclofenac (Can) see Diclofenac 72
Riva-Diclofenac-K (Can) see Diclofenac 72
Riva-Famotidine (Can) see Famotidine 85
Riva-Lorazepam (Can) see Lorazepam 105
Riva-Naproxen (Can) see Naproxen 117
Riva-Simvastatin (Can) see Simvastatin 140
Rivastigmine 137
Rivotril® (Can) see Clonazepam 66
RMS® see Morphine Sulfate 115
Ro 11-1163 see Moclobemide 114
Rofact™ (Can) see Rifampin 136
Rofecoxib 137
Romycin® see Erythromycin 79
Ropinirole 138
Rosiglitazone 138
Rosuvastatin 138
Rovamycine® (Can) see Spiramycin 141
Roxanol® see Morphine Sulfate 115
Roxanol 100® see Morphine Sulfate 115
Roxanol®-T see Morphine Sulfate 115
Roxicet® see Oxycodone and Acetaminophen 123
Roxicet® 5/500 see Oxycodone and Acetaminophen 123
Roxicodone™ see Oxycodone 123
Roxicodone™ Intensol™ see Oxycodone 123
Roychlor® (Can) see Potassium Chloride 128
RP-6976 see Docetaxel 75
RP54274 see Riluzole 136
RU-486 see Mifepristone 113
RU-23908 see Nilutamide 118
RU-38486 see Mifepristone 113
Rubex® see DOXOrubicin 76
Rum-K® see Potassium Chloride 128
Rythmodan® (Can) see Disopyramide 74
Rythmodan®-LA (Can) see Disopyramide 74
Rythmol® see Propafenone 131
Salazopyrin® (Can) see Sulfasalazine 143
Salazopyrin En-Tabs® (Can) see Sulfasalazine 143
Salbu-2 (Can) see Albuterol 46
Salbu-4 (Can) see Albuterol 46
Salbutamol see Albuterol 46
Salicylazosulfapyridine see Sulfasalazine 143
Salmeterol 138

ALPHABETICAL INDEX

Salmeterol and Fluticasone *see* Fluticasone and Salmeterol 89
Saluron® [DSC] *see* Hydroflumethiazide 95
Sandimmune® *see* CycloSPORINE 69
Sandimmune® I.V. (Can) *see* CycloSPORINE 69
Sandostatin® *see* Octreotide 121
Sandostatin LAR® *see* Octreotide 121
Sansert® [DSC] *see* Methysergide 111
Saquinavir 139
Sarafem™ *see* Fluoxetine 88
Sarna® HC (Can) *see* Hydrocortisone 95
Sarnol®-HC [OTC] *see* Hydrocortisone 95
SCH 13521 *see* Flutamide 89
S-Citalopram *see* Escitalopram 80
SCN5A *see* Cardiac Sodium Channel 178
SDZ ENA 713 *see* Rivastigmine 137
Sectral® *see* Acebutolol 44
Select™ 1/35 (Can) *see* Ethinyl Estradiol and Norethindrone 84
Selegiline 139
Septra® *see* Sulfamethoxazole and Trimethoprim 143
Septra® DS *see* Sulfamethoxazole and Trimethoprim 143
Septra® Injection (Can) *see* Sulfamethoxazole and Trimethoprim ... 143
Serentil® *see* Mesoridazine 109
Serevent® *see* Salmeterol 138
Serevent® Diskus® *see* Salmeterol 138
Seroquel® *see* Quetiapine 133
SERT *see* 5HT Transporter 204
Sertraline 139
Serzone® *see* Nefazodone 117
Serzone-5HT$_2$® (Can) *see* Nefazodone 117
Sibutramine 140
Sildenafil 140
Silvadene® *see* Silver Sulfadiazine 140
Silver Sulfadiazine 140
Simvastatin 140
Sinequan® *see* Doxepin 76
Singulair® *see* Montelukast 115
Sirdalud® *see* Tizanidine 149
Sirolimus 141
Skelaxin® *see* Metaxalone 109
SLC6A4 *see* 5HT Transporter 204
Slow FE® [OTC] *see* Ferrous Sulfate 87
Slow-K® (Can) *see* Potassium Chloride 128
SMZ-TMP *see* Sulfamethoxazole and Trimethoprim 143
Sodium Sulamyd® (Can) *see* Sulfacetamide 142
Solaraze™ *see* Diclofenac 72
Solarcaine® Aloe Extra Burn Relief [OTC] *see* Lidocaine 103
Solu-Cortef® *see* Hydrocortisone 95
Solu-Medrol® *see* MethylPREDNISolone 111
Soma® *see* Carisoprodol 61
Sorine® *see* Sotalol 141
Sotacor® (Can) *see* Sotalol 141
Sotalol 141
Sparfloxacin 141
Spiramycin 141

ALPHABETICAL INDEX

Spirapril	141
Spironolactone	142
Sporanox® see Itraconazole	100
Sprintec™ see Ethinyl Estradiol and Norgestimate	84
SSD® see Silver Sulfadiazine	140
SSD® AF see Silver Sulfadiazine	140
Stadol® see Butorphanol	59
Stadol® NS see Butorphanol	59
Stagesic® see Hydrocodone and Acetaminophen	94
Starlix® see Nateglinide	117
Statex® (Can) see Morphine Sulfate	115
Staticin® see Erythromycin	79
Stelazine® see Trifluoperazine	151
Stemetil® (Can) see Prochlorperazine	130
Sterapred® see PredniSONE	129
Sterapred® DS see PredniSONE	129
STI571 see Imatinib	97
St. Joseph® Pain Reliever [OTC] see Aspirin	51
Strattera™ see Atomoxetine	53
Stromectol® see Ivermectin	100
Stromelysin-1	219
Sublimaze® see Fentanyl	86
Suboxone® see Buprenorphine and Naloxone	58
Subutex® see Buprenorphine	57
Sufenta® see Sufentanil	142
Sufentanil	142
Sular® see Nisoldipine	119
Sulf-10® see Sulfacetamide	142
Sulfacetamide	142
SulfaDIAZINE	143
Sulfadoxine and Pyrimethamine	143
Sulfamethoxazole and Trimethoprim	143
Sulfamylon® see Mafenide	107
Sulfasalazine	143
Sulfatrim see Sulfamethoxazole and Trimethoprim	143
Sulfinpyrazone	143
SulfiSOXAZOLE	144
Sulfisoxazole and Erythromycin see Erythromycin and Sulfisoxazole	80
Sulfizole® (Can) see SulfiSOXAZOLE	144
Sulindac	144
Sulphafurazole see SulfiSOXAZOLE	144
Sumatriptan	144
Summer's Eve® SpecialCare™ Medicated Anti-Itch Cream [OTC] see Hydrocortisone	95
Sumycin® see Tetracycline	146
Supeudol® (Can) see Oxycodone	123
Sureprin 81™ [OTC] see Aspirin	51
Surgam® (Can) see Tiaprofenic Acid	148
Surgam® SR (Can) see Tiaprofenic Acid	148
Surmontil® see Trimipramine	152
Synalgos®-DC see Dihydrocodeine, Aspirin, and Caffeine	73
Syn-Diltiazem® (Can) see Diltiazem	74
Synphasic® (Can) see Ethinyl Estradiol and Norethindrone	84

ALPHABETICAL INDEX

Synthroid® *see* Levothyroxine	103
T₄ *see* Levothyroxine	103
642® Tablet (Can) *see* Propoxyphene	132
Tac™-3 [DSC] *see* Triamcinolone	151
Tacrine	144
Tacrolimus	144
Tagamet® *see* Cimetidine	64
Tagamet® HB (Can) *see* Cimetidine	64
Tagamet® HB 200 [OTC] *see* Cimetidine	64
Talacen® *see* Pentazocine Combinations	125
Talwin® *see* Pentazocine	125
Talwin® NX *see* Pentazocine	125
TAM *see* Tamoxifen	145
Tambocor™ *see* Flecainide	87
Tamofen® (Can) *see* Tamoxifen	145
Tamoxifen	145
Tamsulosin	145
Tarka® (Can) *see* Verapamil	154
Taro-Carbamazepine Chewable (Can) *see* Carbamazepine	60
Taro-Warfarin (Can) *see* Warfarin	155
Tavist® *see* Clemastine	65
Tavist®-1 [OTC] *see* Clemastine	65
Taxol® *see* Paclitaxel	124
Taxotere® *see* Docetaxel	75
TCN *see* Tetracycline	146
Tecnal C 1/2 (Can) *see* Butalbital, Aspirin, Caffeine, and Codeine	59
Tecnal C 1/4 (Can) *see* Butalbital, Aspirin, Caffeine, and Codeine	59
Tegretol® *see* Carbamazepine	60
Tegretol®-XR *see* Carbamazepine	60
Telmisartan	145
Temazepam	145
Teniposide	146
Tenolin (Can) *see* Atenolol	53
Tenormin® *see* Atenolol	53
Tequin® *see* Gatifloxacin	91
Terazosin	146
Terbutaline	146
Terfluzine (Can) *see* Trifluoperazine	151
Tessalon® *see* Benzonatate	55
Testim™ *see* Testosterone	146
Testoderm® *see* Testosterone	146
Testoderm® TTS [DSC] *see* Testosterone	146
Testoderm® with Adhesive *see* Testosterone	146
Testopel® *see* Testosterone	146
Testosterone	146
Tetracycline	146
Tetrahydroaminoacrine *see* Tacrine	144
Teveten® *see* Eprosartan	78
Texacort® *see* Hydrocortisone	95
TG *see* Thioguanine	147
6-TG *see* Thioguanine	147
THA *see* Tacrine	144
Thalitone® *see* Chlorthalidone	63
Theo-24® *see* Theophylline	147

293

ALPHABETICAL INDEX

Theochron® see Theophylline 147
Theochron® SR (Can) see Theophylline 147
Theo-Dur® (Can) see Theophylline 147
Theolair™ see Theophylline 147
Theolair-SR® [DSC] see Theophylline 147
Theophylline 147
Theophylline Ethylenediamine see Aminophylline 48
Theracort® [OTC] see Hydrocortisone 95
Theramycin Z® see Erythromycin 79
Thermazene® see Silver Sulfadiazine 140
Thioguanine 147
6-Thioguanine see Thioguanine 147
Thiopurine Methyltransferase 220
Thioridazine 147
Thioridazine Intensol™ see Thioridazine 147
Thiothixene 148
Thorazine® see ChlorproMAZINE 63
Thymydilate Synthetase 221
Tiagabine 148
Tiaprofenic-200 (Can) see Tiaprofenic Acid 148
Tiaprofenic-300 (Can) see Tiaprofenic Acid 148
Tiaprofenic Acid 148
Tiazac® see Diltiazem 74
Ticlid® see Ticlopidine 148
Ticlopidine 148
Tikosyn™ see Dofetilide 75
Tim-AK (Can) see Timolol 148
Timolol 148
Timoptic® see Timolol 148
Timoptic® OcuDose® see Timolol 148
Timoptic-XE® see Timolol 148
Tioguanine see Thioguanine 147
Tiotixene see Thiothixene 148
Tirofiban 149
Tizanidine 149
TMP see Trimethoprim 152
TMP-SMZ see Sulfamethoxazole and Trimethoprim 143
TNF-Alpha 222
Tofranil® see Imipramine 97
Tofranil-PM® see Imipramine 97
TOLBUTamide 149
Tolectin® see Tolmetin 149
Tolectin® DS see Tolmetin 149
Tolmetin 149
Tol-Tab® see TOLBUTamide 149
Tolterodine 149
Tomoxetine see Atomoxetine 53
Tomudex® (Can) see Raltitrexed 135
Topamax® see Topiramate 150
Topicaine® [OTC] see Lidocaine 103
Topiramate 150
Toposar® see Etoposide 85
Toprol-XL® see Metoprolol 112
Toradol® see Ketorolac 101

ALPHABETICAL INDEX

Toradol® IM (Can) see Ketorolac 101
Tornalate [DSC] see Bitolterol 56
Torsemide 150
TPH see Tryptophan Hydroxylase 223
T-Phyl® see Theophylline 147
TPMT see Thiopurine Methyltransferase 220
Tracleer™ see Bosentan 56
Tramadol 150
Tramadol Hydrochloride and Acetaminophen see Acetaminophen
    and Tramadol 45
Trandolapril 150
Tranxene® see Clorazepate 67
Trazodone 151
Triaderm (Can) see Triamcinolone 151
Triamcinolone 151
Triatec-8 (Can) see Acetaminophen and Codeine 44
Triatec-8 Strong (Can) see Acetaminophen and Codeine 44
Triatec-30 (Can) see Acetaminophen and Codeine 44
Triavil® see Amitriptyline and Perphenazine 49
Triazolam 151
Trichlorex® (Can) see Trichlormethiazide 151
Trichlormethiazide 151
TriCor® see Fenofibrate 86
Tri-Cyclen® (Can) see Ethinyl Estradiol and Norgestimate ... 84
Triderm® see Triamcinolone 151
Trifluoperazine 151
Trilafon® [DSC] see Perphenazine 126
Tri-Levlen® see Ethinyl Estradiol and Levonorgestrel 83
Trimethoprim 152
Trimethoprim and Sulfamethoxazole see Sulfamethoxazole and
    Trimethoprim 143
Trimipramine 152
Trimox® see Amoxicillin 49
Trinasal® (Can) see Triamcinolone 151
Tri-Norinyl® see Ethinyl Estradiol and Norethindrone 84
Triphasil® see Ethinyl Estradiol and Levonorgestrel 83
Triquilar® (Can) see Ethinyl Estradiol and Levonorgestrel 83
Trisenox™ see Arsenic Trioxide 51
Trivora® see Ethinyl Estradiol and Levonorgestrel 83
Tryptophan Hydroxylase 223
TS see Thymydilate Synthetase 221
TSER see Thymydilate Synthetase 221
T-Stat® see Erythromycin 79
Tylenol® With Codeine see Acetaminophen and Codeine 44
Tylox® see Oxycodone and Acetaminophen 123
TYMS see Thymydilate Synthetase 221
UCB-P071 see Cetirizine 62
UDP-Glucuronosyltransferase 224
UGT 1A1 see UDP-Glucuronosyltransferase 224
UK-68-798 see Dofetilide 75
UK 92480UK-92480 see Sildenafil 140
UK-109496 see Voriconazole 155
Ultiva® see Remifentanil 135
Ultracet™ see Acetaminophen and Tramadol 45

295

ALPHABETICAL INDEX

Ultram® see Tramadol 150
Unidet® (Can) see Tolterodine 149
Uniphyl® see Theophylline 147
Uniphyl® SRT (Can) see Theophylline 147
Unithroid® see Levothyroxine 103
Univasc® see Moexipril 114
Urolene Blue® see Methylene Blue 110
Utradol™ (Can) see Etodolac 85
Vagifem® see Estradiol 80
Valacyclovir 153
val-COMT see COMT 180
Valdecoxib 153
Valium® see Diazepam 72
Valproate Semisodium see Valproic Acid and Derivatives 153
Valproate Sodium see Valproic Acid and Derivatives 153
Valproic Acid see Valproic Acid and Derivatives 153
Valproic Acid and Derivatives 153
Valsartan 153
Valtrex® see Valacyclovir 153
Vanatrip® see Amitriptyline 48
Vascor® see Bepridil 55
Vasotec® see Enalapril 78
Vasotec® I.V. see Enalapril 78
VCR see VinCRIStine 155
Veetids® see Penicillin V Potassium 125
Velban® [DSC] see VinBLAStine 154
Velosulin® BR (Buffered) see Insulin Preparations 98
Venlafaxine 154
Ventolin® see Albuterol 46
Ventolin® Diskus (Can) see Albuterol 46
Ventolin® HFA see Albuterol 46
Ventrodisk (Can) see Albuterol 46
VePesid® see Etoposide 85
Verapamil 154
Verelan® see Verapamil 154
Verelan® PM see Verapamil 154
Versed® [DSC] see Midazolam 112
VFEND® see Voriconazole 155
Viagra® see Sildenafil 140
Vibramycin® see Doxycycline 76
Vibra-Tabs® see Doxycycline 76
Vicodin® see Hydrocodone and Acetaminophen 94
Vicodin® ES see Hydrocodone and Acetaminophen 94
Vicodin® HP see Hydrocodone and Acetaminophen 94
Vicoprofen® see Hydrocodone and Ibuprofen 95
Vigamox™ see Moxifloxacin 115
VinBLAStine 154
Vincaleucoblastine see VinBLAStine 154
Vincaleukoblastine see VinBLAStine 154
Vincasar PFS® see VinCRIStine 155
VinCRIStine 155
Vinorelbine 155
Vioxx® see Rofecoxib 137
Viracept® see Nelfinavir 118

ALPHABETICAL INDEX

Virilon® IM (Can) see Testosterone 146
Vistaril® see HydrOXYzine 96
Vivactil® see Protriptyline 133
Vivelle® see Estradiol 80
Vivelle-Dot® see Estradiol 80
VLB see VinBLAStine 154
VM-26 see Teniposide 146
Volmax® see Albuterol 46
Voltaren® see Diclofenac 72
Voltaren Ophtha® (Can) see Diclofenac 72
Voltaren Ophthalmic® see Diclofenac 72
Voltaren Rapide® (Can) see Diclofenac 72
Voltaren®-XR see Diclofenac 72
Voriconazole 155
VoSpire ER™ see Albuterol 46
VP-16 see Etoposide 85
VP-16-213 see Etoposide 85
Vumon see Teniposide 146
Warfarin 155
Wellbutrin® see BuPROPion 58
Wellbutrin SR® see BuPROPion 58
Wesmycin® see Tetracycline 146
Westcort® see Hydrocortisone 95
Wigraine® see Ergotamine 79
Winpred™ (Can) see PredniSONE 129
WR-139007 see Dacarbazine 69
Wytensin® [DSC] see Guanabenz 93
Xalatan® see Latanoprost 102
Xanax® see Alprazolam 47
Xanax TS™ (Can) see Alprazolam 47
Xanax XR® see Alprazolam 47
Xeloda® see Capecitabine 60
Xopenex® see Levalbuterol 102
Xylocaine® see Lidocaine 103
Xylocaine® MPF see Lidocaine 103
Xylocaine® Viscous see Lidocaine 103
Xylocard® (Can) see Lidocaine 103
Yasmin® see Ethinyl Estradiol and Drospirenone 82
Z4942 see Ifosfamide 97
Zafirlukast 156
Zagam® see Sparfloxacin 141
Zanaflex® see Tizanidine 149
Zantac® see Ranitidine 135
Zantac® 75 [OTC] see Ranitidine 135
Zarontin® see Ethosuximide 85
Zaroxolyn® see Metolazone 111
Z-Chlopenthixol see Zuclopenthixol 158
ZD1694 see Raltitrexed 135
Zebeta® see Bisoprolol 56
Zeldox see Ziprasidone 157
Zestoretic® see Lisinopril and Hydrochlorothiazide 104
Zestril® see Lisinopril 104
Ziagen® see Abacavir 44
Zilactin® (Can) see Lidocaine 103

ALPHABETICAL INDEX

Zilactin-L® [OTC] see Lidocaine 103
Zinecard® see Dexrazoxane 71
Ziprasidone 157
Zithromax® see Azithromycin 54
Zithromax® TRI-PAK™ see Azithromycin 54
Zithromax® Z-PAK® see Azithromycin 54
Zocor® see Simvastatin 140
Zoloft® see Sertraline 139
Zolpidem 157
Zonalon® see Doxepin 76
Zonegran® see Zonisamide 157
Zonisamide 157
Zopiclone 157
ZORprin® see Aspirin 51
Zovia™ see Ethinyl Estradiol and Ethynodiol Diacetate 83
Zovirax® see Acyclovir 45
Zuclopenthixol 158
Zyban® see BuPROPion 58
Zydone® see Hydrocodone and Acetaminophen 94
Zyloprim® see Allopurinol 47
Zymar™ see Gatifloxacin 91
Zyprexa® see Olanzapine 121
Zyprexa® Zydis® see Olanzapine 121
Zyrtec® see Cetirizine 62

NOTES

NOTES

NOTES

NOTES

Other products offered by LEXI-COMP

DRUG INFORMATION HANDBOOK (International edition available)
by Charles Lacy, RPh, PharmD, FCSHP; Lora L. Armstrong, RPh, PharmD, BCPS;
Morton P. Goldman, PharmD, BCPS; and Leonard L. Lance, RPh, BSPharm

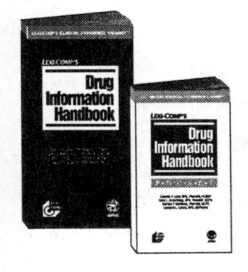

Specifically compiled and designed for the healthcare professional requiring quick access to concisely-stated comprehensive data concerning clinical use of medications.

The Drug Information Handbook is an ideal portable drug information resource, providing the reader with up to 34 key points of data concerning clinical use and dosing of the medication. Material provided in the Appendix section is recognized by many users to be, by itself, well worth the purchase of the handbook.

All medications found in the *Drug Information Handbook* are included in the abridged *Pocket* edition (select fields were extracted to maintain portability).

PEDIATRIC DOSAGE HANDBOOK (International edition available)
by Carol K. Taketomo, PharmD; Jane Hurlburt Hodding, PharmD; and Donna M. Kraus, PharmD

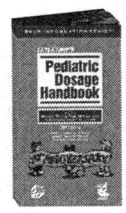

Special considerations must frequently be taken into account when dosing medications for the pediatric patient. This highly regarded quick reference handbook is a compilation of recommended pediatric doses based on current literature, as well as the practical experience of the authors and their many colleagues who work every day in the pediatric clinical setting.

Includes neonatal dosing, drug administration, and (in select monographs) extemporaneous preparations for medications used in pediatric medicine.

GERIATRIC DOSAGE HANDBOOK
by Todd P. Semla, PharmD, BCPS, FCCP; Judith L. Beizer, PharmD, FASCP; and
Martin D. Higbee, PharmD, CGP

2000 "Book of the Year" — *American Journal of Nursing*

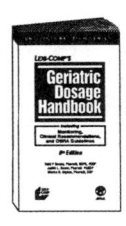

Many physiologic changes occur with aging, some of which affect the pharmacokinetics or pharmacodynamics of medications. Strong consideration should also be given to the effect of decreased renal or hepatic functions in the elderly, as well as the probability of the geriatric patient being on multiple drug regimens.

Healthcare professionals working with nursing homes and assisted living facilities will find the drug information contained in this handbook to be an invaluable source of helpful information.

An International Brand Name Index with names from 58 different countries is also included.

To order call toll free anywhere in the U.S.: 1-800-837-LEXI (5394)
Outside of the U.S. call: 330-650-6506 or online at www.lexi.com

Other products offered by LEXI-COMP

DRUG INFORMATION HANDBOOK FOR THE ALLIED HEALTH PROFESSIONAL
by Leonard L. Lance, RPh, BSPharm; Charles Lacy, RPh, PharmD, FCSHP; Lora L. Armstrong, RPh, PharmD, BCPS; and Morton P. Goldman, PharmD, BCPS

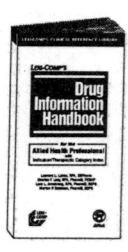

Working with clinical pharmacists, hospital pharmacy and therapeutics committees, and hospital drug information centers, the authors have assisted hundreds of hospitals in developing institution-specific formulary reference documentation.

The most current basic drug and medication data from those clinical settings have been reviewed, coalesced, and cross-referenced to create this unique handbook. The handbook offers quick access to abbreviated monographs for generic drugs.

This is a great tool for physician assistants, medical records personnel, medical transcriptionists and secretaries, pharmacy technicians, and other allied health professionals.

NATURAL THERAPEUTICS POCKET GUIDE
by Daniel L. Krinsky, RPh, MS; James B. LaValle, RPh, DHM, NMD, CCN; Ernest B. Hawkins, RPh, MS; Ross Pelton, RPh, PhD, CCN; Nancy Ashbrook Willis, BA, JD

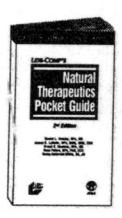

Provides condition-specific information on common uses of natural therapies. Each condition discussed includes the following: review of condition, decision tree, list of commonly recommended herbals, nutritional supplements, homeopathic remedies, lifestyle modifications, and special considerations.

Provides herbal/nutritional/nutraceutical monographs with over 10 fields including references, reported uses, dosage, pharmacology, toxicity, warnings & interactions, and cautions & contraindications.

The Appendix includes: drug-nutrient depletion, herb-drug interactions, drug-nutrient interaction, herbal medicine use in pediatrics, unsafe herbs, and reference of top herbals.

DRUG-INDUCED NUTRIENT DEPLETION HANDBOOK
by Ross Pelton, RPh, PhD, CCN; James B. LaValle, RPh, DHM, NMD, CCN; Ernest B. Hawkins, RPh, MS; Daniel L. Krinsky, RPh, MS

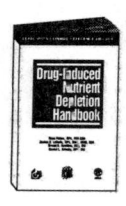

A complete and up-to-date listing of all drugs known to deplete the body of nutritional compounds.

This book is alphabetically organized and provides extensive cross-referencing to related information in the various sections of the book. Drug monographs identify the nutrients depleted and provide cross-references to the nutrient monographs for more detailed information on effects of depletion, biological function & effect, side effects & toxicity, RDA, dosage range, and dietary sources. this book also contains a studies & abstracts section, a valuable appendix, and alphabetical & pharmacological indexes.

To order call toll free anywhere in the U.S.: 1-800-837-LEXI (5394)
Outside of the U.S. call: 330-650-6506 or online at www.lexi.com

Other products offered by LEXI-COMP

DRUG INFORMATION HANDBOOK FOR ADVANCED PRACTICE NURSING
by Beatrice B. Turkoski, RN, PhD; Brenda R. Lance, RN, MSN; and Mark F. Bonfiglio, PharmD Foreword by: Margaret A. Fitzgerald, MS, RN, CS-FNP

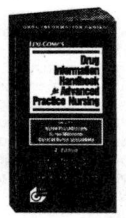

1999 "Book of the Year"
*American Journal of Nursing
Advanced Practice Nursing Category*

Designed specifically to meet the needs of nurse practitioners, clinical nurse specialists, nurse midwives, and graduate nursing students. The handbook is a unique resource for detailed, accurate information, which is vital to support the advanced practice nurse's role in patient drug therapy management. Over 4750 U.S., Canadian, and Mexican medications are covered in the 1000 monographs. Drug data is presented in an easy-to-use, alphabetically-organized format covering up to 46 key points of information (including dosing for pediatrics, adults, and geriatrics). Appendix contains over 230 pages of valuable comparison tables and additional information. Also included are two indexes, Pharmacologic Category and Controlled Substance, which facilitate comparison between agents.

DRUG INFORMATION HANDBOOK FOR NURSING
by Beatrice B. Turkoski, RN, PhD; Brenda R. Lance, RN, MSN; and Mark F. Bonfiglio, PharmD

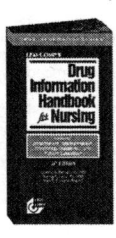

Registered professional nurses and upper-division nursing students involved with drug therapy will find this handbook provides quick access to drug data in a concise easy-to-use format.

Over 4000 U.S., Canadian, and Mexican medications are covered with up to 43 key points of information in each monograph. The handbook contains basic pharmacology concepts and nursing issues such as patient factors that influence drug therapy (ie, pregnancy, age, weight, etc) and general nursing issues (ie, assessment, administration, monitoring, and patient education). The Appendix contains over 230 pages of valuable information.

ANESTHESIOLOGY & CRITICAL CARE DRUG HANDBOOK
by Andrew J. Donnelly, PharmD; Francesca E. Cunningham, PharmD; Verna L. Baughman, MD

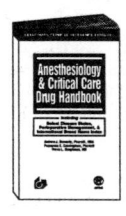

Contains the most common perioperative drugs in the critical care setting and also contains Special Issues and Topics including: Allergic Reaction, Cardiac Patients in Noncardiac Surgery, Obstetric Patients in Nonobstetric Surgery, Patients With Liver Disease, Chronic Pain Management, Chronic Renal Failure, Conscious Sedation, Perioperative Management of Patients on Antiseizure Medication, and more.

The Appendix includes Abbreviations & Measurements, Anesthesiology Information, Assessment of Liver & Renal Function, Comparative Drug Charts, Infectious Disease-Prophylaxis & Treatment, Laboratory Values, Therapy Recommendations, Toxicology information, *and much more.*
International Brand Name Index with names from over 58 different countries is also included.

To order call toll free anywhere in the U.S.: 1-800-837-LEXI (5394)
Outside of the U.S. call: 330-650-6506 or online at www.lexi.com

Other products offered by LEXI-COMP

INFECTIOUS DISEASES HANDBOOK
by Carlos M. Isada, MD; Bernard L. Kasten Jr., MD; Morton P. Goldman, PharmD; Larry D. Gray, PhD; and Judith A. Aberg, MD

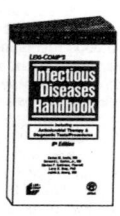

A four-in-one quick reference concerned with the identification and treatment of infectious diseases. Each of the four sections of the book contains related information and cross-referencing to one or more of the other three sections. The Disease Syndrome section provides the clinical presentation, differential diagnosis, diagnostic tests, and drug therapy recommended for treatment of more common infectious diseases. The Organism section presents the microbiology, epidemiology, diagnosis, and treatment of each organism. The Laboratory Diagnosis section describes performance of specific tests and procedures. The Antimicrobial Therapy section presents important facts and considerations regarding each drug recommended for specific diseases of organisms. Also contains an International Brand Name Index with names from 58 different countries.

DIAGNOSTIC PROCEDURES HANDBOOK by Frank Michota, MD

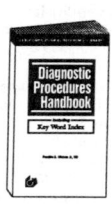

A comprehensive, yet concise, quick reference source for physicians, nurses, students, medical records personnel, or anyone needing quick access to diagnostic procedure information. This handbook is an excellent source of information in the following areas: allergy, rheumatology, and infectious disease; cardiology; computed tomography; diagnostic radiology; gastroenterology; invasive radiology; magnetic resonance imaging; nephrology, urology, and hematology; neurology; nuclear medicine; pulmonary function; pulmonary medicine and critical care; ultrasound; and women's health.

DRUG INFORMATION HANDBOOK FOR ONCOLOGY
by Dominic A. Solimando, Jr, MA, BCOP

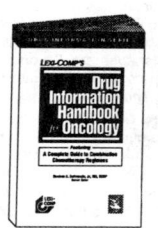

Presented in a concise and uniform format, this book contains the most comprehensive collection of oncology-related drug information available. Organized like a dictionary for ease of use, drugs can be found by looking up the *brand* or *generic name!*

This book contains individual monographs for both antineoplastic agents and ancillary medications.

The fields of information per monograph include: Use, U.S. Investigational, Bone Marrow/Blood Cell Transplantation, Vesicant, Emetic Potential. A Special Topics Section, Appendix, and Therapeutic Category & Key Word Index are valuable features of this book, as well.

To order call toll free anywhere in the U.S.: 1-800-837-LEXI (5394)
Outside of the U.S. call: 330-650-6506 or online at www.lexi.com

Other products offered by LEXI-COMP

CLINICIAN'S GUIDE TO LABORATORY MEDICINE—A Practical Approach by Samir P. Desai, MD and Sana Isa-Pratt, MD

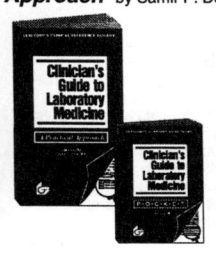

When faced with the patient presenting with abnormal laboratory tests, the clinician can now turn to the *Clinician's Guide to Laboratory Medicine: A Practical Approach*. This source is unique in its ability to lead the clinician from laboratory test abnormality to clinical diagnosis. Written for the busy clinician, this concise handbook will provide rapid answers to the questions that busy clinicians face in the care of their patients. No longer does the clinician have to struggle in an effort to find this information - *it's all here*.
Included is a **FREE** copy of *Clinician's Guide to Laboratory Medicine - Pocket*. Great to carry in your pocket! Perfect for use *"in the trenches."*

CLINICIAN'S GUIDE TO INTERNAL MEDICINE—A Practical Approach by Samir P. Desai, MD

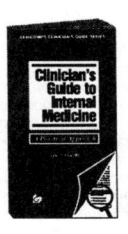

Provides quick access to essential information covering diagnosis, treatment, and management of commonly encountered patient problems in Internal Medicine. Contains up-to-date, clinically-relevant information in an easy-to-read format and is easily accessible. Contains practical approaches that are not readily available in standard textbooks. Contains algorithms to help you establish the diagnosis and select the appropriate therapy. There are numerous tables and boxes that summarize diagnostic and therapeutic strategies. It is an ideal reference for use at the point-of-care. This is a reference companion that will provide you with the tools necessary to tackle even the most challenging problems in Internal Medicine.

CLINICIAN'S GUIDE TO DIAGNOSIS—A Practical Approach
by Samir P. Desai, MD

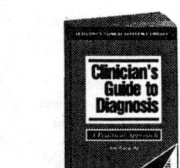

Symptoms are what prompt patients to seek medical care. In the evaluation of a patient's symptom, it is not unusual for healthcare professionals to ask "What do I do next?" This is precisely the question for which the *Clinician's Guide to Diagnosis: A Practical Approach* provides the answer. It will lead you from symptom to diagnosis through a series of steps designed to mimic the logical thought processes of seasoned clinicians. For the young clinician, this is an ideal book to help bridge the gap between the classroom and actual patient care. For the experienced clinician, this concise handbook offers rapid answers to the questions that are commonly encountered on a day-to-day basis. Let this guide become your companion, providing you with the tools necessary to tackle even the most challenging symptoms.

To order call toll free anywhere in the U.S.: 1-800-837-LEXI (5394)
Outside of the U.S. call: 330-650-6506 or online at www.lexi.com

Other products offered by LEXI-COMP

POISONING & TOXICOLOGY HANDBOOK
by Jerrold B. Leikin, MD and Frank P. Paloucek, PharmD

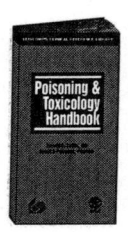

It's back by popular demand! The small size of our Poisoning & Toxicology Handbook is once again available. Better than ever, this comprehensive, portable reference contains 80 antidotes and drugs used in toxicology with 694 medicinal agents, 287 nonmedicinal agents, 291 biological agents, 57 herbal agents, and more than 200 laboratory tests. Monographs are extensively referenced and contain valuable information on overdose symptomatology and treatment considerations, as well as, admission criteria and impairment potential of select agents. Designed for quick reference with monographs arranged alphabetically, plus a cross-referencing index. The authors have expanded current information on drugs of abuse and use of antidotes, while providing concise tables, graphics, and other pertinent toxicology text.

LABORATORY TEST HANDBOOK & CONCISE version
by David S. Jacobs MD, FACP; Wayne R. DeMott, MD, FACP; and Dwight K. Oxley, MD, FACP

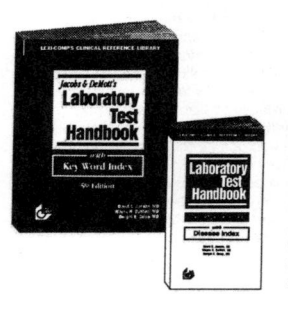

Contains over 900 clinical laboratory tests and is an excellent source of laboratory information for physicians of all specialties, nurses, laboratory professionals, students, medical personnel, or anyone who needs quick access to most routine and many of the more specialized testing procedures available in today's clinical laboratory. Each monograph contains test name, synonyms, patient care, specimen requirements, reference ranges, and interpretive information with footnotes, references, and selected websites. The *Laboratory Test Handbook Concise* is a portable, abridged (800 tests) version and is an ideal, quick reference for anyone requiring information concerning patient preparation, specimen collection and handling, and test result interpretation.

DENTAL OFFICE MEDICAL EMERGENCIES
by Timothy F. Meiller, DDS, PhD; Richard L. Wynn, BSPharm, PhD; Ann Marie McMullin, MD; Cynthia Biron, RDH, EMT, MA; and Harold L. Crossley, DDS, PhD

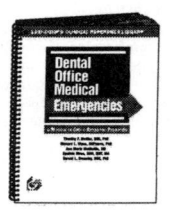

Designed specifically for general dentists during times of emergency. A tabbed paging system allows for quick access to specific crisis events. Created with urgency in mind, it is spiral bound and drilled with a hole for hanging purposes. Contains the following: Basic Action Plan for Stabilization; Allergic / Drug Reactions; Loss of Consciousness / Respiratory Distress / Chest Pain; Altered Sensation / Changes in Affect; Management of Acute Bleeding; Office Preparedness / Procedures and Protocols; Automated External Defibrillator (AED); Oxygen Delivery

To order call toll free anywhere in the U.S.: 1-800-837-LEXI (5394)
Outside of the U.S. call: 330-650-6506 or online at www.lexi.com

Other products offered by LEXI-COMP

DRUG INFORMATION HANDBOOK FOR PSYCHIATRY
by Matthew A. Fuller, PharmD and Martha Sajatovic, MD

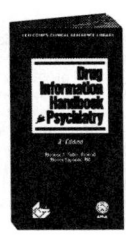

The source for comprehensive and clinically-relevant drug information for the mental health professional. Alphabetically arranged by generic and brand name for ease-of-use. There are up to 35 key fields of information including these unique fields: "Effect on Mental Status" and "Effect on Psychiatric Treatment."
A special topics/issues section includes psychiatric assessment, major psychiatric disorders, major classes of psychotropic medications, psychiatric emergencies, special populations, enhanced patient education information section, and DSM-IV classification. Also contains a valuable appendix section, Pharmacologic Index, and Alphabetical Index.

PSYCHOTROPIC DRUG INFORMATION HANDBOOK
by Matthew A. Fuller, PharmD and Martha Sajatovic, MD

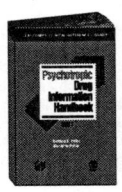

This portable, yet comprehensive guide to psychotropic drugs provides healthcare professionals with detailed information on use, drug interactions, pregnancy risk factors, warnings/precautions, adverse reactions, mechanism of action, and contraindications. Alphabetically organized by brand and generic name, this concise handbook provides quick access to the information you need and includes patient education sheets on the psychotropic medications. It is the perfect pocket companion to the *Drug Information for Psychiatry*.

RATING SCALES IN MENTAL HEALTH
by Martha Sajatovic, MD and Luis F. Ramirez, MD

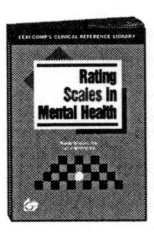

A basic guide to the rating scales in mental health, this is an ideal reference for psychiatrists, nurses, residents, psychologists, social workers, healthcare administrators, behavioral healthcare organizations, and outcome committees. It is designed to assist clinicians in determining the appropriate rating scale when assessing their client. A general concepts section provides text discussion on the use and history of rating scales, statistical evaluation, rating scale domains, and two clinical vignettes. Information on over 100 rating scales used in mental health is organized by condition. Appendix contains tables and charts in a quick reference format allowing clinicians to rapidly identify categories and characteristics of rating scales.

To order call toll free anywhere in the U.S.: 1-800-837-LEXI (5394)
Outside of the U.S. call: 330-650-6506 or online at www.lexi.com

Other products offered by LEXI-COMP

DRUG INFORMATION HANDBOOK FOR DENTISTRY
by Richard L. Wynn, BSPharm, PhD; Timothy F. Meiller, DDS, PhD; Harold L. Crossley, DDS, PhD

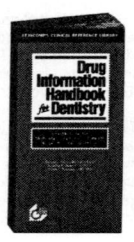

For all dental professionals requiring quick access to concisely-stated drug information pertaining to medications commonly prescribed by dentists and physicians. Designed and written by dentists for all dental professionals as a portable, chair-side resource. Includes drugs commonly prescribed by dentists or being taken by dental patients and written in an easy-to-understand format. There are 24 key points of information for each drug including **Local Anesthetic/Vasoconstrictor, Precautions, Effects on Dental Treatment**, and **Drug Interactions**. Includes information on dental treatment for medically-compromised patients and dental management of specific oral conditions.

Also contains Canadian & Mexican brand names.

CLINICIAN'S ENDODONTIC HANDBOOK
by Thom C. Dumsha, MS, DDS and James L. Gutmann, DDS, FACD, FICD

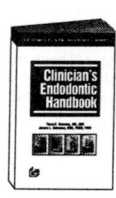

Designed for all general practice dentists. Highlights include quick referencing to address current endodontics; easy-to-use format and alphabetical index; latest techniques, procedures, and materials; root canal therapy: why's and why nots; guide to diagnosis and treatment of endodontic; emergencies; facts and rationale behind treating endodontically-involved teeth; straight-forward dental trauma management information; pulpal histology, access openings, bleaching, resorption, radiology, restoration, and periodontal / endodontic complications; frequently asked questions (faq) section and "clinical notes" sections.

MANUAL OF CLINICAL PERIODONTICS
by Francis G. Serio, DMD, MS and Charles E. Hawley, DDS, PhD

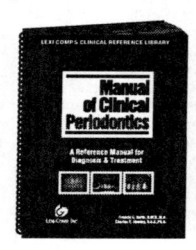

A reference manual for diagnosis and treatment including sample treatment plans. It is organized by basic principles and is visually-cued with over 220 high quality color photos. The presentation is in a "question & answer" format. There are 12 chapters tabbed for easy access: 1) Problem-based Periodontal Diagnosis; 2) Anatomy, Histology, and Physiology; 3) Etiology and Disease Classification; 4) Assessment, Diagnosis, and Treatment Planning; 5) Prevention and Maintenance; 6) Nonsurgical Treatment; 7) Surgical Treatment: Principles; 8) Repair, Resection, and Regeneration; 9) Periodontal Plastic Surgery; 10) Periodontal Emergencies; 11) Implant Considerations; 12) Appendix

To order call toll free anywhere in the U.S.: 1-800-837-LEXI (5394)
Outside of the U.S. call: 330-650-6506 or online at www.lexi.com

Other products offered by LEXI-COMP

ORAL SOFT TISSUE DISEASES
by J. Robert Newland, DDS, MS; Timothy F. Meiller, DDS, PhD; Richard L. Wynn, BSPharm, PhD; and Harold L.Crossley, DDS, PhD

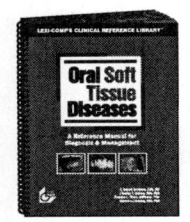

Designed for all dental professionals, a pictorial reference to assist in the diagnosis and management of oral soft tissue diseases (over 160 photos).

Easy-to-use, sections include:

Diagnosis process: obtaining a history, examining the patient, establishing a differential diagnosis, selecting appropriate diagnostic tests, interpreting the results, etc.; white lesions; red lesions; blistering-sloughing lesions; ulcerated lesions; pigmented lesions; papillary lesions; soft tissue swelling (each lesion is illustrated with a color representative photograph); specific medications to treat oral soft tissue diseases; sample prescriptions; and special topics.

ORAL HARD TISSUE DISEASES
by J. Robert Newland, DDS, MS

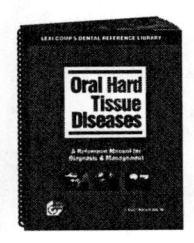

A reference manual for radiographic diagnosis, visually-cued with over 130 high quality radiographs is designed to require little more than visual recognition to make an accurate diagnosis. Each lesion is illustrated by one or more photographs depicting the typical radiographic features and common variations. There are 12 chapters tabbed for easy access: 1) Periapical Radiolucent Lesions; 2) Pericoronal Radiolucent Lesions; 3) Inter-Radicular Radiolucent Lesions; 4) Periodontal Radiolucent Lesions; 5) Radiolucent Lesions Not Associated With Teeth; 6) Radiolucent Lesions With Irregular Margins; 7) Periapical Radiopaque Lesions; 8) Periocoronal Radiopaque Lesions; 9) Inter-Radicular Radiopaque Lesions; 10) Radiopaque Lesions Not Associated With Teeth; 11) Radiopaque Lesions With Irregular Margins; 12) Selected Readings / Alphabetical Index

YOUR ROADMAP TO FINANCIAL INTEGRITY IN THE DENTAL OFFICE
by Donald P. Lewis, Jr., DDS, CFE

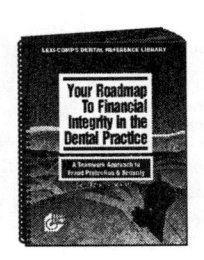

A Teamwork Approach to Fraud Protection & Security
Ideal practice management reference, designed and written by a dentist in private practice. Covers four basic areas of financial security. Utilizes tabbed paging system with 8 major tabs for quick reference.
Part I: Financial Transactions Incoming: Financial Arrangements, Billing, Accounts Receivable, Banking, Cash, Checks, and Credit Cards; **Part II: Financial Transactions Outgoing:** Accounts Payable, Supplies, Cash-on-hand, Payroll; **Part III: Internal Controls:** Banking, General Office Management, Human Resource (H/R) issues; **Part IV: Employees:** Employee Related Issues and Employees Manual Topics
Part V: Report Checklist: Daily, Weekly, Monthly, Quarterly, Semi-annually, Annually; **Additional Features:** Glossary terms for clarification, alphabetical index for quick reference, 1600 bulleted points of interest, over 180 checklist options, 12 real-life stories (names changed to protect the innocent!), 80-boxed topics of special interest for quick review.

To order call toll free anywhere in the U.S.: 1-800-837-LEXI (5394)
Outside of the U.S. call: 330-650-6506 or online at www.lexi.com

Other products offered by LEXI-COMP

A PATIENT GUIDE TO MENTAL HEALTH ISSUES FLIP CHART

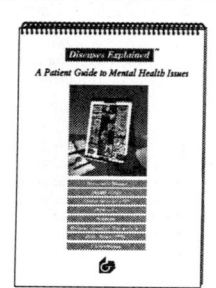

- ▶ Alzheimer's Disease
- ▶ Anxiety (GAD)
- ▶ Bipolar Disorder (BD)
- ▶ Depression
- ▶ Insomnia
- ▶ Obsessive-Compulsive Disorder (OCD)
- ▶ Panic Attacks (PD)
- ▶ Schizophrenia

A PATIENT GUIDE TO ROOT THERAPY FLIP CHART
Contributor Thom C. Dumsha, M.S., D.D.S., M.S.

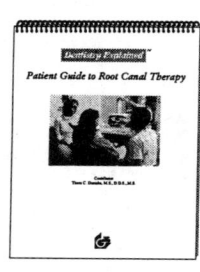

- An ideal tool used to educate and explain to your patients about root canals
- 8-1/2" x 11" colorful tabbed flip chart explaining each of the steps involved in a root canal
- Actual clinical photographs, radiographs, and diagrams

PATIENT GUIDE TO DENTAL IMPLANTS FLIP CHART
Contributor Marvin L. Baer, D.D.S., M.Sc.

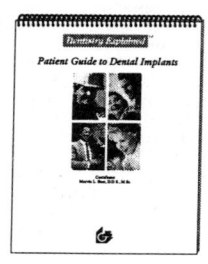

- An ideal tool used to educate and explain to your patients about dental implants
- 8-1/2" x 11" colorful tabbed flip chart explaining each of the steps involved in:
    1.) Single tooth restoration
    2.) Replacement of several teeth
    3.) Implants supported overdenture (4 implants/2 implants)
    4.) Screw-retained denture

To order call toll free anywhere in the U.S.: 1-800-837-LEXI (5394)
Outside of the U.S. call: 330-650-6506 or online at www.lexi.com

PATIENT EDUCATION
Wall Posters

Ideal for Waiting Rooms and Examination Rooms.

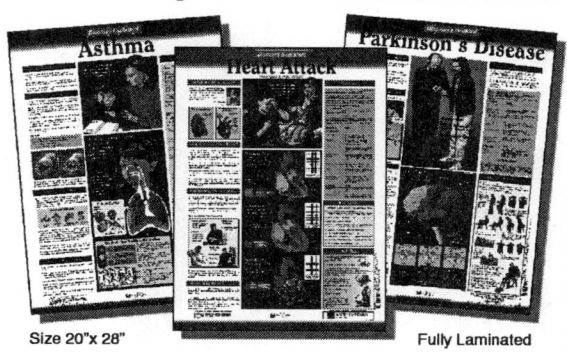

Size 20"x 28" Fully Laminated

Written in a layman's language and presented in an easy-to-follow, graphic style. Each condition is carefully described, along with the treatments available, and complex medical terms are explained.

Titles available

Acne	Heart Attack
Alzheimer's Disease	HIV and AIDS
Anemia	Hypertension
Angina	Irritable Bowel Syndrome
Anxiety	Incontinence
Asthma	Insomnia
Bipolar Disorder	Menopause
Breast Cancer	Migraine
Congestive Heart Failure	Multiple Sclerosis
Cholesterol	OCD
COPD	Osteoporosis
Depression	Otitis Media
Diabetes	Panic Attacks
Deep Vein Thrombosis	Parkinson's Disease
Enlarged Prostate (BPH)	Schizophrenia
Epilepsy	Spasticity
Essential Tremor	Stroke
Glaucoma	Thyroid Disease

To order a catalog, call Toll Free at: 1-877-837-5394
or visit us online at - **www.diseases-explained.com**

LEXI-COMP

Diseases Explained ™

DXLX04/1

Outside of the U.S. call: 330-650-6506

PATIENT EDUCATION Booklets

Promoting health education and self-help.

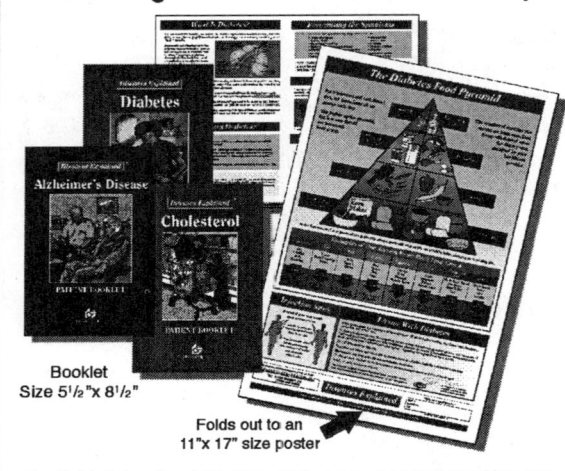

Booklet Size 5½"x 8½"

Folds out to an 11"x 17" size poster

Available in packs of 10, 50 or 100 pieces. Larger quantities are available custom printed with your own logo or clinic address.

Titles available

Acne	Depression	Menopause
Allergic Rhinitis	Diabetes	Migraine
Alzheimer's Disease	Epilepsy	Multiple Sclerosis
Angina	Hardening of	Obesity
Anxiety	The Arteries	OCD
Asthma	Heart Attack	Osteoporosis
Bipolar Disorder	Enlarged Prostate	Panic Attacks
Breast Cancer	GERD	Parkinson's Disease
Cholesterol	HIV & AIDS	Schizophrenia
COPD	Hypertension	Stroke
CHF	Incontinence	Thyroid Disorders
DVT	Insomnia	

To order a catalog, call Toll Free at: 1-877-837-5394
or visit us online at - www.diseases-explained.com

LEXI-COMP

Diseases Explained ™

DXLX05/1b

Outside of the U.S. call: 330-650-6506

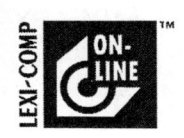

LEXI-COMP ONLINE™

Lexi-Comp Online™ integrates industry-leading reference databases and advanced searching technology to provide time-sensitive clinical information in a <u>single online resource</u>!

Lexi-Comp Online™ **includes:**

- Information from 4 distinct drug databases including *Lexi-Drugs Online*™ which integrates 7 different specialty databases into one comprehensive database and *Lexi-Drugs for Pediatrics*™
- Two nutritional supplement databases
- Four laboratory and diagnostic databases
- Two patient education databases - LEXI-PALS™ for adults and PEDI-PALS™ for pediatric patients
- Lexi-Interact™ - drug interaction analysis online for drug and herbal products
- Lexi-Drug ID™ - drug identification system
- Lexi-Drugs Online™ - updated daily

Visit our website www.lexi.com to sign up for a
FREE 30-day trial to *Lexi-Comp Online*™

Lexi-Comp Online™ licenses are available on an <u>individual</u>, <u>academic</u>, and <u>institutional</u> basis.

Also available on CD-ROM

To order call toll free anywhere in the U.S.: 1-800-837-LEXI (5394)
Outside of the U.S. call: 330-650-6506 or online at www.lexi.com

LEXI-COMP ON-HAND SOFTWARE LIBRARY
For Palm OS® and Windows™ Powered Pocket PC Devices

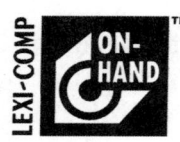

LEXI-COMP ON-HAND™ Lexi-Comp's handheld software solutions provide quick, portable access to clinical information needed at the point-of-care. Whether you need laboratory test or diagnostic procedure information, to validate a dose, or to check multiple medications and natural products for drug interactions, Lexi-Comp has the information you need in the palm of your hand. Lexi-Comp also provides advanced linking technology to allow you to hyperlink to related information topics within a title or to the same topic in another title for more extensive information. No longer will you have to exit 5MCC to look up a dose in Lexi-Drugs or lab test information in Lexi-Diagnostic Medicine — seamlessly link between all databases to **save valuable time**.

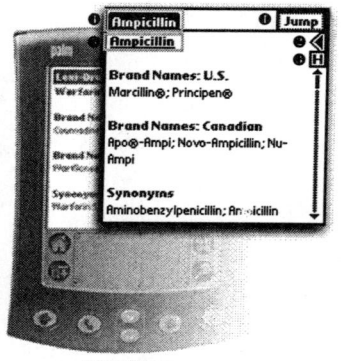

Palm OS® Device

New Navigational Tools:

❶ **"Jump"** provides a drop down list of available fields to easily navigate through information.

❷ **Back arrow** returns to the index from a monograph or to the "Installed Books" menu from the Index.

❸ **"H"** provides a linkable History to return to any of the last 12 Topics viewed during your session.

❹ **Title bar:** Tap the monograph or topic title bar to activate a menu to "Edit a Note" or return to the "Installed Books" menu.

❺ **Linking:** Link to another companion database by clicking the topic or monograph title link or within a database noted by various hyperlinked (colorized and underlined) text.

To order call toll free anywhere in the U.S.: 1-800-837-LEXI (5394)
Outside of the U.S. call: 330-650-6506 or online at www.lexi.com